The Gourmet's Companion™
German
Menu Guide
&
Translator

Other Titles by Bernard Rivkin

The Gourmet's Companion: French Menu Guide & Translator

The Gourmet's Companion: Italian Menu Guide & Translator

The Gourmet's Companion: Spanish Menu Guide & Translator

The Author wishes to express appreciation to the German government tourist office for their cooperation and assistance, and the supply of some of the information used in the preparation of this book.

The Gourmet's Companion™
German
Menu Guide
&
Translator

Bernard Rivkin

John Wiley & Sons, Inc.

New York • Chichester • Brisbane • Toronto • Singapore

Library of Congress Cataloging-in-Publication Data

Rivkin, Bernard.
    The gourmet's companion: German menu guide and
      translator / Bernard Rivkin.
      p. cm.
    Includes bibliographical references.
    ISBN 0-471-52516-2
    1. Food—Dictionaries. 2. Cookery, German—Dictionaries.
3. Cookery—Germany. I. Title.
TX349.R494   1991
641.5943'03—dc20   90-39307

Printed in the United States of America

91 92 10 9 8 7 6 5 4 3 2 1

This book is dedicated to my associate, Myrna Childs Rivkin, without whose patience, effort, and efficiency the project could not have been completed. Thank you! Dear wife.

Contents

1

Food and Drink in Germany: A Region by Region Guide

Germany's Surprising Variety of Dining Experiences

American visitors to Germany today expect to see magnificent cathedrals, castles overlooking the Rhine and Neckar Rivers, Hansel-and-Gretel villages nestled in enchanted forests, and towns and cities filled with the music of Bach, Beethoven, Handel, and other great German composers. They also may anticipate seeing Romanesque, Gothic, Baroque, and German Rococo architecture mixed with modern buildings. Other traditional strongholds of tourism include the Bavarian Alps, Romantic Road, Black Forest, the Rhine region, and lively cities such as Hamburg and Berlin.

If you are visiting Germany for the first time, you probably also have expectations about what you will be eating. You might think of Germany as a land of sausages, dumplings, and sauerkraut washed down with large steins of beer. But when you actually reach Germany, the great variety of the "German table" might surprise and even overwhelm you.

True, you will find the expected dishes, but in an incredible variety of forms, and flavor subtleties. You might also be overwhelmed by the incredible selection of eating establishments, ranging from lunch counters and tables in bakeries and department stores, to country inns, castles, revolving tower restaurants with panoramic views in larger cities, elegant meals served in Michelin Guide star-awarded restaurants, and inexpensive lunchtime eating places in Germany's finest museums. When you dine out in Germany you can expect to find every level of cuisine and many different levels of service and cost, and quite often with special menus for children and for the elderly.

In Germany, many specialties and dishes carry the names of the cities and districts where they originated. For example, *Regensburger,* a large, heavily spiced pork sausage, shares the name of its city of origin.

Germans are masters at sausage making, which explains why you can find at least 80 different kinds of sausage in this country. Most every one knows *Leberwurst*; it is a specialty of Hesse and is also served throughout the country. Among the *Bratwurst* family are the small pork sausages of Nuremberg, usually served fried or grilled.

Another renowned specialty, sauerbraten, begins with a basic recipe of beef that is marinated and cooked in vinegar or red wine with a bouquet of such spices as peppercorns, bay leaves, and cloves. Rhinelanders may distinguish their sauerbraten with seedless white raisins in a sweet-and-sour sauce, while Bavarian chefs will create regional favorites with a few dollops of sour cream or tomato puree.

Indeed, Germany is a composite of "culinary regions." A good many dishes reflect the influence of bordering countries and areas, including Scandinavia, Austria, and France. Northern German cuisine is characteristically sweet-and-sour; Eastern European flavors dominate with liberal lacings of sour cream, paprika, and caraway.

Pork is a perennial favorite on German menus, as is smoked or cured ham. (Has anyone *not* heard of Westphalian ham?)

Fish and seafood are featured throughout the year. The bounty of the northern coastline has inspired a wealth of delightful creations. Herring is especially popular for use in recipes. Smoked eel is a Northern German favorite, too, taken with rich, dark bread. And the regions of Southern Germany have spawned a rainbow of fresh-water selections, including trout and pike (baked in cream sauce, or shaped into delicate quenelles, or prepared as an elegant pâté with apples cooked in white wine).

Ducklings and chicken are popular, too, as is wild game. Venison, hare, wild boar, and pheasant are relished with gusto, especially in Bavaria and the southern provinces, where such fare is indigenous.

Vegetables? Germany serves up an astonishing array of them. Cabbage is a favorite, followed by potatoes that come deep fried, mashed, patted into crisp pancakes, shredded, and sliced and used in countless kinds of salads. During the growing season, from late April into June, asparagus becomes the aristocrat of vegetables for Germans and is prized by epicures throughout the world. Following the asparagus season, Germans turn to mushroom dishes in August and September. The Steinpilze mushrooms are especially favored.

As the meal comes to an end, a selection of desserts called *Süss-Speisen* (sweet dishes) is offered. Apple strudel or fruit pancakes, for example, alternate with rich puddings or exotic ice cream creations.

Try to visit at least one *Konditorei*, a cafe where Germans go in the afternoons to enjoy an incredible variety of cakes and pastries. There are seasonal delights, such as *Dresdener Christstollen* (a traditional Christmas cake), and year-round favorites like *Schwarzwälder Kirschtorte* (Black Forest cherry cake laced with kirsch).

Regional German Food and Drink

Food and drink in Germany are as varied and diverse as the regions of the country and the people who inhabit them. Of course, if you are a guest in large towns, you can find on the menus and wine-cards of the international hotels and restaurants just about everything you want, and you will have little difficulty finding a large number of foreign restaurants. But you will only notice the large variety of specialties in Germany's kitchens and cellars when you begin to visit different regions. The Bavarian eats and drinks differently from the Rhinelander, the Swabian differently from the North German. So, a trip through Germany is also a worthwhile culinary journey of discovery.

Bavaria

In this still very rural country, the most popular dish is roast pork with dumplings, made of potatoes or bread, preceded by a liver dumpling soup. So-called *Haxen*, a piece of veal or pork leg, is a genuine Bavarian meal that presupposes a hearty appetite. Very popular, too, is the famous Munich white sausage, which tastes best in the morning. All these dishes should be accompanied by beer, and since hops and barley thrive north and south of the Danube, innumerable large and small breweries produce a variety of beers according to the time of year. In the mountains, especially when the weather is rather raw, you will soon come to appreciate the strong, warming gentian schnapps. In the west of Bavaria, in the Allgäu, the cheese-lover will encounter an unrivaled selection.

Franconia

North of the Danube, living customs are quite different from those in the south. Here, the people are more fastidious and demanding in their food and drink. The creation of sausages, in particular—and first and foremost the Nuremberg fried sausages—has developed into a fine art. These sausages should be accompanied by the rather aromatic Franconian beer; brewers in the Bamberg area are particularly skilled at imparting a special smoky flavor to their beer. Northwest of Nuremberg, wine takes precedence over beer. In the district of Würzburg, wine is filled into small squat bottles, so-called bocksbeutel. A strange old custom is to sell the bottles in bakers' shops, together with bread and the small fried fish from the river Main. A signboard with a wine glass in the middle points the way.

Swabia

Lake Constance, also called the Swabian Sea, is home to the *felchen*, a delicious fish that belongs to the salmon family. Whether boiled or fried, felchen makes an excellent and inexpensive dish. This fish, of course, calls for wine, and the endless vineyards of the northern banks of the great lake contain all imaginable types of vines from the sylvaner and traminer to the riesling and burgundy. Swabia proper lies north of Lake Constance and is the land of *Spätzle* and *Maultaschen*, dishes made of dough and served with fried onions and grated cheese. These dishes should be eaten with red wine, which flourishes in the area of Stuttgart and Esslingen and further north on the rivers Rems, Jagst, and Kocher.

In the Black Forest

Here you will find some especially good dishes: nourishing ham or bacon, which is smoked over fragrant juniper, Black Forest onion soup, the best trout in Germany from the mountain streams (with which the excellent southern Baden wines are drunk) and dark fir honey, without which no breakfast in a forest is complete. But above all, apart from *Kirschwasser* (cherry schnapps) and *Himbeergeist* (raspberry schnapps), be sure to try the Black Forest cherry cake. It's true you can buy this cake in every German pastry shop, but only in Baden-Baden is it so dainty, so light and airy as the genuine article should be.

Left and Right of the Rhine

The best asparagus in Germany comes from Schwetzingen, south of Mannheim, where it grows in huge fields. Harvesting time is in May and June. Asparagus can be prepared in an incredible variety of ways, cold or hot, in over thirty different dishes.

In the Palatinate and on the Rhine, the wines dominate the menu: Here, it is not a question of what to drink with the meal, but of what to eat with the drink—rump steak, liver and crackling sausage, or white cheese of Mainz cheese. In Frankfurt, the apple wine, called *Appelwoi* locally, is accompanied by sausages or chops. In Hesse, wine is often accompanied by smoked ribs of pork, while in Cologne, the so-called *Reibekuchen*, a kind of pancake prepared from grated potatoes, is equally good with beer or wine.

Westphalia and Lower Saxony

In Westphalia and in the Münsterland, the north German way of life begins to become noticeable. The harsher climate calls for more substantial food. Rural dishes predominate, the most important of which is the famous Westphalian ham—a truly historical German specialty. During the reign of the Roman Emperors, Westphalian ham was delivered to Rome over the Alps. In Lower Saxony, Göttingen is famous for its university and its sausages, as Heinrich Heine wrote. With these you drink *Steinhäger*, a juniper schnapps, or corn brandy or aqua vitae. On the Lüneburg Heath—where a special kind of sheep is bred, the meat of which produces many excellent local dishes—*Ratzeputz* is taken before or after the meal; this is an exceptionally strong brandy produced from herbs. The local people call it "half devil, half Satan."

North Germany

In the north German coastal region, seafood dominates the menu; boiled or smoked eel, flounder, turbot, shrimp, crab, and lobster are here fresher and better than just about anywhere else. A favorite dish in this region is the so-called *Eintopf*, a mixture of different meats cut up with vegetables and potatoes and all boiled together. Many other dishes have been introduced by sailors. For example, the nourishing *Labskaus* is prepared from corned beef, potatoes, onions, and herring. From Kiel come the excellent Kiel sprats, packed in wooden boxes. Hamburg's specialty is an eel soup.

Although it is true that no wine grows on the North Sea and the Baltic, the three large Hanseatic towns and, in particular Lübeck, are famous for their wines, a fact that you can verify in the old town hall cellars. For centuries, Lübeck has been a center for importing, shipping, and storing French red wine from Bordeaux and Burgundy. The huge vaulted cellars under the quays of Lübeck are said to be especially suited—by their temperature and perhaps their mineralogical influences—to the storage of these noble red wines.

In the far north, in Flensburg, on the Danish border, the processing of rum imported from Central America has been made a specialty. This rum is the basis of the hot grog, one of the most popular and almost indispensable hot drinks on the whole of the North German coast.

Berlin also has its specialties. Old Berlin dishes like Eisbein (boiled or pickled knuckles of pork with sauerkraut), ribs of pork, boiled sausages, and meatballs are just as famous as the Berlin doughnuts and as good and cheap as ever. And the *Weisse mit Schuss*, pale ale with a clash of raspberry syrup, is an excellent summer drink that originated in Berlin but is now enjoyed throughout the whole of Germany.

Vines Grown in Germany and the Characteristic Tastes of Their Wines

White wine is derived from light grapes, while red is made from the darker varieties.

The German wine region stretches from the Lake of Constance along the Rhine and its tributaries to the Middle Rhine at Bonn—an area blessed with ideal growing conditions.

White Wine

Riesling is the finest and best known of the white vines grown in Germany. Its especially small grapes ripen late—in November or even December. Despite a lengthy ripening time, during which the grapes accumulate a great deal of glucose, Riesling does not taste too sweet, but remains richly piquant and vivacious with a fruity taste.

Silvaner vines, like Riesling, are cultivated over a quarter of the German wine area. Its fruit is bigger and ripens earlier. Also, yields are higher than Riesling. Typical Silvaner tastes mild and fruity.

Muller-Thurgau, the third most important German type of vine, is a cross between Riesling and Silvaner. The Muller-Thurgau Vine—developed by H. Muller from Switzerland—grows over a quarter of the German wine region. The berries ripen as early as September. Typical Muller-Thurgau tastes fruity and mild.

Rulander takes fourth place among German white wine vines. Its home is in the Rhenish Palatinate and Baden, although it originated in Burgundy. Today it can also be found in Rhenish Hesse. Typical Rulander, which was discovered in 1709 in the garden of a merchant called Ruland, is full bodied and pleasantly fruity.

Germany has many other strains of vine, but these are only of significance in single areas. Traminer and the Gewürztraminer have a richer boquet; while Scheurebe and Morio-Muskat are equally interesting. Not many of these grapes are cultivated, but they are distinguished by the piquancy of their boquet.

Red Wine

Spätburgunder, like Riesling among the white wines, is undisputed as the finest variety of German red wine. Originally from the old French province of Burgundy, it later became indigenous to Germany. Typical Spätburgunder is velvety and fruity.

Trollinger is light with an especially fresh taste. The vine was taken to Württemberg from its original home in the Tirol.

Portugieser, a red wine in no way associated with Portugal, comes from the Rhenish Palatinate and Hesse. More of it is drunk in Germany than any other German red wine. It is enjoyed as a good table wine.

The German Wine Regions

Germany has 11 designated wine-cultivation regions. Each region, despite all similarities, boasts a great variety of wines to attract the interest of wine tasters. Each specified region consists of two or more districts; each district contains several villages or parishes, which form a unit geologically and climatically. Within each village, there can be a variety of individual vineyards. The precise definitions of village, district, and specified region are strictly controlled and defined for labeling, so it is easy to identify each wine.

Baden

Baden is the southernmost wine region, on the right bank of the Rhine, lying between Lake Constance and Heidelberg. It includes the following districts: Lake Constance, Markgraflerland, Kaiserstuhl-Tuniberg, Breisgau, Ortenau, Badische Bergstrasse/Kraichgau, Badisches Frankenland.

Just about every resident of Baden takes at least a daily glass of wine, so that everybody in Baden is in fact a connoisseur of local wines.

About a dozen different varieties of wine come from Baden. For example, the full-bodied Rulander, the light aromatic Gutedel, and the spicy Kaiserstuhl wines of the heat-retaining volcanic soils, the potent wines of Lake Constance, and the popular Weissherbst all hail from Baden. Other favorites include the spicy boquet of Gewürztraminer and the Spätburgunder.

The Rheinpfalz (Rhenish Palatinate): Synonymous with Great Wines for Centuries

The most thickly forested of the German wine growing regions is the Palatinate. There is plenty to suit every taste, from the mild fresh wines produced from Silvaner and Muller-Thurgau vines, to the piquant varieties that flourish in the loamy soil of the Oberhaardt. Traminer, Muskateller, and the Rulander are also produced here.

The wines produced between Neustadt and Schweigen come from good stock. The flavor and aroma arise from gravelly, chalky sandstone; volcanic basalt; and mica. Protected by the Voges Mountains, the Pfälzer wood and Haardt are the great wine districts of the Rhenish Palatinate, which has been synonymous with quality wines for centuries.

Württemberg

Wines from this region are seldom encountered outside Württemberg, and red grapes are especially abundant. Typical of the region is the Trollinger vine. Early and late burgundies, black Riesling, and Lemberger are also grown here. But the strong-tasting white wines are the classic Württemberg specialty. Portugieser is considered best as an everyday drink, while Schiller wine—mixed red and white wine—is also popular.

Between Stuttgart and Heidelberg lie the districts of Remstal-Stuttgart, the Württemberg flat country, and Kocher-Jagst-Taubertal.

Wines from Franken (Franconia)

Franconian wine is the most robust of German wines. Along the Main, you will encounter rich strong Silvaner and piquant Muller-Thurgau. In Franconia, red wine lovers will find first-class, fiery wines. The benchmark of Franconian wine—which tastes deliciously fruity and juicy—is its typical flavor.

Cultivation in Franconia, which stretches from the Steigerwald to the other side of the Spessart, is confined to the warmest parts of the region: Steigerwald, Maindreieck, and Mainviereck.

Rheinhessen

These wines originate on the left bank of the Rhine, between Worms, Mainz, Bingen, and Alzey. With its variety of soils, Rhenish Hesse produces both wholesome table wines and top-quality vintages. It was in this ancient country that the Riesling vine was first given its name in 1404. Riesling, Silvaner, and Muller-Thurgau are found in Hesse. Scheurebe, Siegerrebe, Kanzlerrebe, and Morio-Muskat also are produced in Hesse, but are somewhat rarer because they come from a new breed of vine. Red wines also grow here: fine, spicy Spätburgunder—chiefly in the area of Ingelheim—and the tasty Portugieser, a light dinner wine. The provinces of Bingen, Nierstein, and Wonnegau are the districts of Rhenish Hesse.

Hessische Bergstrasse—A Small Wine Region

The local Riesling wines in Bergstrasse are strong and tangy. The districts of Hessische Bergstrasse are Starkenburg and Umstadt. During spring, the area around the magnificent medieval town of Heppenheim is alive with blossoming fruit trees, while in the first week of September, the famous Bergstrasse wine festival takes place in Bensheim.

The Rheingau

The slopes of the Rheingau lie between Rheinknie and Taunushöhen. The district is known as Johannisberg.

A wealth of monuments, monasteries and wine cellars—some from the time of Charles the Great—combined with the finest wine, contribute to the unique charm of the region.

In the Rheingau, chestnuts, almonds, figs, and lemons flourish in the open. So it is not surprising that the Riesling develops true perfection under the Rheingau's favorable climatic conditions. The Rheingau is also protected by the Taunus hills, while the river Rhine reflects the sun onto vineyards. Rheingau Riesling is distinguished by a spicy elegance, coupled with great fruit—a connoisseur's wine.

The Nahe Region

Kreuznach and Bockelheim, protected from the wind by the Soonwald heights, are the districts of the Nahe region. The most typical Nahe wines grow along the middle Nahe and Alsenz. Riesling, Silvaner, and Muller-Thurgau are the most common types of vine, which incorporate all quality grades from light table wines to the great grades.

The Mittelrhein (Middle Rhine)

The Middle Rhine, a beautiful region of terraced vineyards crowned with old castles, stretches on the right bank of the Rhine from the mouth of the Nahe to the Siebengebirge.

The local Riesling, so full of character, is lively and dry. And there is a red wine, too. The small district of Siebengebirge produces a Spätburgunder, called Dragon's Blood.

The Mosel-Saar-Ruwer

Wine lovers are well catered for in these impressive river valleys. A truly fine Riesling grows on the steep southern slopes below Trier, while the high-class and fruity wines of the Saar are equally renowned. The Mosel meanders between the protective slopes of the Hünsruck, with numerous bends on its way to the Rhine. With the tributaries Saar and Ruwer, the Mosel forms a climatic unit. The districts are Zell-Mosel, Bernkastel, Saar-Ruwer, and Upper Mosel.

The Ahr: For Red Wine Lovers

In this, the smallest of the German wine regions, the vines can ripen only because gravel and volcanic rock store up warmth and release it at night. This gives the red Spätburgunder its fine, fiery, velvety-soft character, to which the Ahr owes its reputation as Germany's favored red wine production area. Four pleasant, white table wines are also produced, and a refreshing, thirst-quenching Portugieser is available.

One of the biggest red wine areas in Germany lies in the Lower Ahr, on the slopes of the Eifel in the District of Walporzhein-Ahr.

How German Wine Law Helps

Guidance and consumer protection are paramount in German wine law, which lays down precise quality requirements for every German wine.

What the Wine Label Tells You: The Quality Grade

German wine is divided into three quality grades. Each grade must fulfill minimum legal requirements. The grade is shown on every wine label and gives a sure indication of quality.

The Four German Table Wine Growing Areas

The light, tasty wines from the table wine growing areas are produced from officially-approved vines that originate from approved vineyards. Minimum alcohol content conforms to the EEC norm of 8.5 percent.

Where do these appealing dinner wines—labeled "German Table Wines"—come from? The eleven wine-growing regions of Germany are subdivided into the four areas of the great German rivers: The Rhine and Mosel is a table wine area, as is the area on the Main, the Neckar, and the Upper Rhine. German table wine, according to German wine law, must come from one of these four areas, and the appropriate identification must appear on the label.

Just as quality wines—fine selected wines—should be kept for special occasions, light German table wines provide splendid everyday drinking and, when mixed with soda water, are refreshing and thirst-quenching.

Quality Grade: Quality Wines from Specified Regions

Quality wines are the stronger wines with typical regional flavors. Like German table wines, quality wines can only be produced by approved vineyards and must come from recognized vines. Minimum alcohol content, again in line with the EEC norm, is around 9 percent, depending on the region and variety of grape—a significant increase over table wine. Naturally, greater demands are made of quality wines. They must have the distinctive taste of their locality and a sufficiently high degree of alcohol to meet legal requirements. Quality wines have to pass a test, and the official examination number on the label acts as a guarantee to the buyer.

Quality Grade: Specially Graded Quality Wine

Five grades of highest quality, specially graded wines are allowed and mentioned on the label. A wine will only be eligible if it is fully matured and possesses a harmonious balance between sweetness and fruitness.

The "must weight" (or the grape's original sugar content) is even higher than in the ordinary quality wines, and in no circumstances may sugar be added to the juice. Each one of the five specially graded wines is checked for its time of vintage, method of harvesting, and the ripeness of the grapes. A declaration of the grade, combined with the control number, must be shown on the label.

Kabinett is an elegant, fully ripened wine, harvested at the normal time. "Normal" in Germany as a rule means October, a time when the grapes have long been gathered in the rest of Europe. It is this lengthy, slow-ripening process that increases German wine's unique characteristics.

Spätlese wines come from grapes harvested after the normal picking period. They are distinguished by a special elegance and ripeness and are appealingly "round and delicious."

Auslese wines are produced from fully ripe grapes that are specially sorted from the rest and pressed separately. Auslese wines reveal their elegance through a ripeness and full bouquet, and are unquestionably ideal for a special occasion.

Beerenauslese represents a further increase in quality, where the wine is made from ripe and over-ripe berries separated by hand. This results in a wonderful, mature, fruity, and full wine that possesses an unmistakable flowery aroma and an amber color.

Trockenbeerenauslese wine represents the very finest in quality. Only grapes shrivelled like raisins are pressed, offering significant characteristics in appearance and taste.

Eiswein is a very special type of wine similar to the previous two grades. It is made from grapes whose water content has been frozen by the first frost; the inner concentration, rich in sugar and aroma, is squeezed out.

How Wine Bottles Are Allocated Their Official Examination Number

The new German wine law was first introduced in 1971. Older wines may not carry all the label information. Although German table wines are not subjected to an individual, official test, which would be impracticable, they must meet requirements laid down by the law. Quality wines and graded quality wines have to pass a unique examination that absolutely guarantees the contents and quality to the buyer. The process is in three stages:

Stage One: Declaring the Harvest. In the autumn, the "must weight" is measured. Then the winegrower has to declare his harvest—for instance, his Spätlese—at the mayor's office. Subsequently, official inspectors carry out examinations in the grower's vineyard and wine cellar.

Stage Two: Analysis. When the wine in the cellar is ready and has been drawn off, the official quality examination follows. Specially sanctioned laboratories deliver three sample bottles along with an analysis certificate, to the examination authorities.

Stage Three: The Taste Test. Experts from the wine industry and from teaching and research institutes taste the wine and mark it on a 20-point system. Color, clarity, bouquet, and taste are individually marked. Only if the wine achieves the minimum prescribed score in all categories is it allowed to carry the coveted quality grade on its label and receive the official examination number as authentication.

The Wine's Birth Certificate

According to German wine law, quality wines and graded quality wines should show that they come from one of eleven particular wine regions referred to earlier in this booklet. As an additional declaration, the label on quality wine can also show its origin from the district or parish where it originated.

With specially graded wine, it is necessary to indicate its special area. If the wine comes from an even more restricted district, the parish is also shown or even more precise information may be displayed.

The German wine law also dictates that the origin of German table wine from one of the four table wine growing areas—Rhine and Mosel, Main, Neckar, or Upper Rhine—should be stated on the label. In addition, the district or parish may be named, but this is not compulsory.

The Year Is Important

Good wines are produced in Germany every year, but weather conditions inevitably influence results, especially with quality and graded quality wines. "Great" years are rare: 1971 was one. And the connoisseur speaks with rapture of the even rarer "Century Wines" like 1921 and 1953. The year of the wine can be a useful buyer's guide.

Another Insurance: Who the Wine Comes From

The experience and ability of the vintner can be measured in every bottle of wine when he vouches for the contents under the wording *Erzeugerabfüllung* or *Aus Eigenem Lesegut*. The supplier and bottler can also assume responsibility for this guarantee by adding the phrase *Abfüller*, in line with the existing regulations.

The Three Types of Wine

Germany distinguishes between three types of wine. These are:

- White wine made from white wine grapes.
- Red wine, from red wine grapes, pressed red.
- Rosé wine, from red wine grapes, pressed to a light color. As a quality wine, Rosé is made from only one type of vine grape and is called Weissherbst.

Sekt (German Sparkling Wine)

German Sekt (Sparkling Wine) is produced by a second fermentation that occurs when carbon dioxide is kept in the bottle. Sparkling German Sekt has the special taste and flavor of the German white wines and makes a delicate and refreshing party or celebration drink.

Sekt should have a particular level of carbonic acid. Also, Sekt and quality sparkling wine must be recorded as having been stored for at least nine months and must carry the official examination number. Sekt or quality sparkling wine from specified German wine regions must originate 100 percent from the named area and reflect all the freshness and elegance of typical wines produced in that region.

Wine Crystals

Sometimes, when uncorking a very good bottle of wine that has been stored a long time, tiny white glittering crystals can be seen around the cork or in the glass. These crystals are the best proof of the quality of the wine. Only very old wines, which once had a high proportion of fruit, produce these tartar crystals. Pour the wine carefully, so that as little of the tartar as possible gets into the glass.

Red and Rosé Wine

German red wine gets its deep, dark color, not from the pulp of the red grapes from which it is pressed, but from their skin when the red dye is released in small quantities into the pressed-out grape juice. The "mash" is left to ferment for a few days, while the fermentation, alcohol, and warmth release the red coloring from the grape skins. Only then is the mash pressed. Red wine is bottled some months later.

Rosé wine is pressed from the same red grapes, but without letting the mash ferment first (the same process as in white wine pressing). Since the juice contains no coloring, the rosé assumes a reddish-gold glow. The complementary taste is soft and velvety. The best rosé wine is Weissherbst—so known when produced as a quality wine in specific districts. Weissherbst should be drunk lightly cooled, like a white wine.

Europe's Saucepans on One Stove: Austria's Cuisine Reflects the Diversity of the Country's History

Music lovers often speak glowingly about the "Viennese classics," mentioning the names of Mozart, Beethoven, and Haydn. It is true that these three great Masters lived in Austria's capital. And it was in Vienna that they wrote many of their unforgettable works. However, none of these three composers were born in Vienna. It is still possible today to visit Mozart's place of birth in Salzburg. Beethoven was born in the German city of Bonn, and Haydn in the little village of Rohrau, about 50 kilometers from Vienna.

As far as classics go, it is much the same in the matter of Austrian cuisine. Consider *Wiener Schnitzel*, for instance. True, this famous dish has made its way through the menus of many a gourmet restaurant through Vienna, but it was not "born" in Vienna. Most probably it came into the world in the Italian city of Milan, which belonged to the Habsburg empire in the 19th century, and was known there as "Costoletta alla milanese" and from where it was "imported" to the then imperial capital Vienna.

The history of Wiener Schnitzel, which consists of tender veal covered in a golden crust of crispy egg and breadcrumbs, is quite interesting: In the 15th century, in the homes of the northern Italian aristocracy, it was the custom to eat dishes covered in a whisper-thin layer of gold foil. The reason for this very unusual preparation lies in the medical thinking of the time, which held that gold contained miraculous properties for strengthening the heart. This luxurious extravagance took on such proportions that, in 1514, in Venice, it had to be forbidden. The legend goes that the chefs of that time came upon an excellent optical replacement; a mixture of eggs and white bread crumbs. The last little detail to this recipe was added in Vienna at the turn of the century; the cooks of this city discovered that by dipping the veal lightly in flour first, they obtained an optimal *Wiener Schnitzel*.

The history of many dishes bears a resemblance to that of the *Wiener Schnitzel*. Unlike todays neutral republic, Austria's Emperor ruled over an empire on which "the sun never set." Spain and Portugal, and their colonies, as well as the Netherlands, Czechoslovakia, Hungary, large parts of Belgium, Switzerland, Italy, Poland, Rumania, Yugoslavia, France (Burgundy), and South Germany belonged to this empire. Not only did the Habsburg rulers extend their regions of power—through adroit marriages—with other ruling families in Europe, they simultaneously brought with them the best cooks and the culinary specialties of the various countries and integrated them in the kitchens at the Viennese court.

This mixture of people and materials meant that every nation, every people, every cook contributed to the culinary melting pot of Vienna a new recipe, another nuance, new spices or herbs, new additions and combinations, and even new eating habits to Vienna. The Viennese, even in those days known throughout Europe as great gourmets, took only the best materials and improved and adapted them to their own taste.

The flaky pastry of the *apple strudel* comes from the conquered Turks, *Gulasch* and *Palatschinken* (pancakes, usually with a sweet filling) come from Hungary, while the "Bohemian Cook" in the houses of rich bourgeoisie pampered her employers with *Germknoedel* (yeast dumplings filled with prune jam). The preparation of paté was learned from the French and many delicious additions have their origins in Italian cuisine.

The cuisine of this delightful country, lying at the heart of Europe, has been enriched by more than just the possessions of the imperial monarchy. Although Austria is a small country, it has a great variety of landscape, agriculture, culture, flora, and fauna. This variety is reflected in the many dishes of Austria, from the food eaten by the mountain dwellers to give them strength for their strenuous work, to the dishes eaten on high days and holidays by the farmers, and to the bounty of fresh vegetables and fruit from the eastern regions of the country.

Who can imagine Austria without its *Salzburger Nockerl* or the hearty Tyrolean dumplings, just the right dish when pursuing winter sports? Apart from the dozens of different soups, the recipes for which would fill several cook books, there are hundreds of ways to prepare the best cuts of beef, veal, pork, lamb, chicken, and game. Austria is envied throughout Europe for its wide variety of game, abounding in its woods and which you can always find on the menu in season. The heart of a gourmet will beat faster at the culinary delights offered in the form of fresh water fish and woodland mushrooms of several varieties, which in summer come fresh to your table. As for desserts, one glance at the menu and the mouth starts to water and the guest cannot help but admire the creative talents and ideas of a cuisine whose reputation is worldwide.

But it is not only the variety that is so admirable about Austrian cuisine. The high quality of ingredients and their preparation have, year after year, won the hearts of millions of visitors from throughout the world. Add to that the well known hospitality of the "World Champion in Tourism" and it is not difficult to see why a holiday in Austria, the land of festivals, will remain unforgettable.

Sweet Temptations of Austrian Cuisine

About 15 million holiday guests visit the little republic of Austria year in and year out. There are plenty of reasons for planning a trip to this country in the heart of Europe. It is world famous for its traditions and its vivid cultural life; it's practically synonymous with music, thank to its opera houses, concert halls, festival arenas, museums, castles, and galleries. Austria's cuisine and culinary specialties are one reason for its fame. If you haven't planned your trip to Austria especially to get to know its colorful cooking, you can still find out what you might be missing. Take a closer look at *Mehlspeisen*, which literally means "dishes made with flour," but has come to represent an array of cooked desserts, much in the way that pudding in Great Britain refers to any sweet course after the main meal.

Sachertorte and *Apfelstrudel* are probably the most famous "works of art" to come from the Viennese kitchen, but are certainly not the only ones. Thumb through some local cook books—they make ideal souvenirs, by the way—and you'll notice that sweet courses, pastries, cakes, tortes, and biscuits take up even more space than the so-called main courses. This makes sense when you consider that, while in other countries the dessert is merely the last sweet morsel after a full course meal, in Austria it is sometimes the main event, following immediately after soup. It's easy to get to know the subtle and highly developed art of making "Mehlspeisen" by taking a protracted tour of coffee houses and restaurants. The friendly and multi-lingual waiters will be glad to assist you. It's sometimes a good idea to cast a glance into the lavish showcases, which hold a wealth of surprises.

Mehlspeisen enjoy a long tradition in Austria. In the

Middle Ages, a number of emperors were known for their sweet tooth. In German, we say somebody is a *Naschkatze*, or "a little cat that loves to nibble." The desserts as we know them today, however, developed mostly during the previous century. In those days, patrician houses in Vienna had their very own "dessert cook" who did nothing but spoil the family with sweets, constantly thinking up new variations of the art to delight her "gentlefolks." Most of these women came from Bohemia or Moravia, and their girth was visual proof of their skills. Today, the pastry shops have become the temples of this art and the citadels of traditional tortes, cakes, gateau, biscuits, and more. Cooked desserts, however, are best sampled in restaurants and "cafe-restaurants," the latter referring to coffee houses that specialize in serving a midday meal. Even those visitors with an eye on their caloric consumption should try a few—only in Austria are such things prepared with freshness, lightness, and sheer perfection. The next few examples illustrate the inexhaustible variety.

The most famous is *Apfelstrudel*, usually served warm. Paper-thin pastry is stuffed with sliced apples, seasoned with cinnamon and sugar, and then baked. This same "Strudel dough" is used in a variation with sweet cream cheese and called *Topfenstrudel*.

The beloved *Milchrahmstrudel* is conjured out of white bread, eggs, sugar, milk, and raisins, and then served with lashings of warm vanilla sauce.

Then there are the many varieties of *Knödel*, or dumplings, many of which are made by filling the dough with such fruits as plums, peaches, apricots, or strawberries, and then boiling them until tender. Special variations include *Topfenknödel* (made from sweet cream-cheese enriched dough) and *Germknödel*, both of which contain yeast to make the dough especially light. *Germknödel* is served with drawn butter, freshly ground poppy seeds, and powdered sugar.

Don't be surprised by the name *Mohr im Hemd* (moor in a shirt). In reality, it's chocolate cake simmered to a rich, moist consistency, and then covered with chocolate sauce.

Hardly anybody can resist *Palatschinken*, the name for a very special sort of pancake. This loose translation doesn't do justice to the Hungarian original. These light, airy crepes have to be tasted to be appreciated—the combination of eggs, flour, and milk tastes unlike any other version. They are then rolled around a stuffing of jam, chocolate, or sweet cream cheese.

A similar batter, but a lighter one, is needed for the untranslatable *Kaiserchmarren*. The batter is torn into small pieces while it is cooking, and served in a heap garnished with compote or stewed plums. It was one of the favorite dishes of the legendary Emperor Franz Joseph I.

Hardly anybody visits Salzburg without sampling the world famous sweet *Salzburger Nockerln*. It's a pyramid-shaped *soufflé*, baked golden brown in the oven, but still creamy inside.

Desserts that are served at room temperature or chilled include an inexhaustible array of tortes and cakes. Of course, there is the internationally famous *Sachertorte* (created in 1832 by the hotelier Eduard Sacher and Ann Demel). It is basically a rich chocolate torte with a layer of apricot jam in the center. *Guglhupf*, on the other hand, is much lighter and is often served for Sunday breakfast. In fact, virtually every region and city in Austria is proud of its own special sweet, many of them with colorful names of their own.

Wherever you go in Germany, you will find tortes made of nuts, poppy seeds, coffee, and chestnuts. Try a *Punschtorte*, a dense rum-flavored cake covered with pink icing. Some sweets are named after towns, like *Linzer Torte*, or *Ischler Krapferl*, while others recall a famous personality, such as *Metternichschnitten* or *Elisabethtorte*. Try each town's specialty. They will make your stay in Austria a great deal sweeter.

The Vienna "Heuriger"

In Viennese colloquial speech, these two words are virtually untranslatable: *Heuriger* and *Gemütlichkeit*. However, both expressions have acquired international meaning and belong together like Castor and Pollux, Romulus and Remus, or Punch and Judy. A *Heuriger* without *Gemütlichkeit* is unthinkable, and *Gemütlichkeit* is an essential adjunct to a *Heuriger*.

Strictly speaking, *Heuriger* in Austria has a double meaning. It refers first to the wine and second to a tavern at which it is quaffed. When a Viennese says he is going on a *Heurigen* outing, he invariably refers to both these meanings at once. So, to put it in one word, The Heuriger is a Viennese specialty that visitors to the Austrian should not fail to investigate.

Since the German adjective *heurig* indicates "of this year," it is obvious that a "Heuriger" wine must be of this—or rather, the previous—grape harvest. After fermenting its way through sweet *Most* and *Sturm* (themselves delicacies that you should try if you come at the appropriate time of year), the young, invigorating wine is served up, cellar-fresh, generally in quarter-liter mugs.

Any wine of an earlier vintage is referred to collectively in Vienna as *Alter* wine, which has naturally gained in maturity and strength—provided the wine-grower has been able to store it away, out of reach of thirsty customers. Normally, though, at a tavern, you would ask for, and get, *Heuriger* wine—youthful, sparkling clear, and with a fresh "bite." *Heuriger* wine goes a long way toward accounting for the *Gemuetlichkeit*, that indefinable but ever-present happy outlook on life that is rightly considered with such a Viennese specialty.

Following an old tradition, only "home-grown" wines are served in proper Viennese Heuriger taverns, such as can be found in the centuries-old vintner's houses in Nussdorf, Heiligenstadt, Grinzing, Sievering, Neustift am Walde, and Ottakring. It is therefore up to the individual connoisseur to do a wine-tasting tour to find just the sort that pleases the palate. Incidentally, you'll have no difficulty spotting a *Heuriger* because it will always have, hanging outside its entrance on a long pole, a bush of pine-needles that suggests good cheer, to the observant eye.

Since most of the Heuriger tavern owners are basically vintners, they are not entitled to provide all the facilities of a normal inn or restaurant. For this reason, you will usually only be able to get something cold to eat with your wine. But that something—cold roast goose, smoked ham, salami and cheese—is surely no drawback. Experienced *Heuriger* visitors bring along their own packet of cold meats, fetched in advance from one of Vienna's excellent delicatessen shops.

In summer, you sit outdoors around bare but spotless tables in the courtyard, or even beside the vineyard itself, under a bower of old vines. In winter there is always a cozy parlor. More often than not, spirited music will be playing in the background, perhaps by a typical Viennese *Schrammel* quartet.

It would not be going too far to say that the "Heuriger" tavern is a very democratic institution. Within its walls, all class distinctions seem to fall, replaced instead by heartfelt cordiality in which everyone is welcome at one of the long tables. Casual clothing is the normal wear and talk flows as freely as the wine.

Only thirty minutes by tram or a quarter of an hour by car and you are out in the country-like suburbs where the hills of the Vienna Woods begin to slope upwards. A little further on, just beyond the city boundary, you come to the delightful wine-growing centers of Gumpoldskirchen, Voeslau, and Baden. Vienna itself lies on the fringes of one of Europe's biggest and best wine areas. Ever since the Roman Emperor Probus introduced the vine to the region, wine has played a major economic and social role for Vienna. And today the Heuriger wine tavern is just as essential a part of Vienna as the tower of St. Stephen's, the Giant Wheel in the Prater, and Schoenbrunn Palace.

2

How to Say It: English to German

Numbers

0	naught, zero	null
1	one	eins
2	two	zwei
3	three	drei
4	four	vier
5	five	fünf/fuenf
6	six	sechs
7	seven	sieben
8	eight	acht
9	nine	neun
10	ten	zehn
11	eleven	elf
12	twelve	zwölf/zwoelf
13	thirteen	dreizehn
14	fourteen	vierzehn
15	fifteen	fünfzehn/fuenfzehn
16	sixteen	sechzehn
17	seventeen	siebzehn
18	eighteen	achtzehn
19	nineteen	neunzehn
20	twenty	zwanzig
21	twenty-one	einundzwanzig
22	twenty-two	zweiundzwanzig
23	twenty-three	dreiundzwanzig

30	thirty	dreissig
40	forty	vierzig
50	fifty	fünfzig/fuenfzig
60	sixty	sechzig
70	seventy	siebzig
80	eighty	achtzig
90	ninety	neunzig
95	ninety-five	fünfundneunzig/ fuenfundneunzig
100	one hundred	einhundert
200	two hundred	zweihundert
560	five hundred and sixty	fünfhundertsechzig/ fuenfhundertsechzig
1,000	one thousand	eintausend
2,000	two thousand	zweitausend
60,140	sixty thousand one hundred and forty	sechzigtausendein- hundertvierzig
500,000	five hundred thousand	fünfhunderttausend/ fuenfhunderttausend
1,000,000	one million	eine Millon

Words and Phrases

AFTER   nach
AGAIN   wieder
ALL   alle
ALL RIGHT   gut
ASHTRAY PLEASE   Einen Aschenbecher, bitte!
BAKED   gebacken
BAKED IN PARCHMENT   In Pergamentpapier gebacken
BATHROOM   das Badezimmer
BOTTLE   die Flasche
BREAKFAST   das Frühstück
CALL A DOCTOR   Rufen Sie einen Doktor
CALL AN AMBULANCE   Rufen Sie einen Krankenwagen
CALL THE POLICE!   Rufen Sie die Polizei
CHAIR   der Stuhl

CHECK der Scheck, die Rechnung
CLOSED geschlossen
COLD kalt
CUP die Tasse
CURED gepökelt
DAILY MENU die Tageskarte
DAY'S SOUP Tagessuppe
DELICIOUS köstlich
DENTIST Zahnarzt
DENTIST WHO SPEAKS ENGLISH Zahnarzt, der
  Englisch spricht?
DESSERT der Nachtisch
DESSERT OF THE DAY Tagesdessert
DINING ROOM das Esszimmer
DINNER Abendessen
DO YOU SPEAK ENGLISH? Sprechen Sie Englisch?
DO YOU UNDERSTAND? Verstehen Sie?
DOCTOR WHO SPEAKS ENGLISH? Welcher Arzt
  spricht Englisch?
DOES ANYONE SPEAK ENGLISH? Spricht jemand
  Englisch?
DRY trocken
EAT essen
EMERGENCY die Notlage, der Notfall
ERROR der Fehler
EYEGLASSES die Brille
FAST schnell
FOR LADIES für Damen
FOR MEN für Herren
FORK die Gabel
FULL-BODIED vollmundig
GLASS das Glas
GOOD AFTERNOON Guten Tag
GOOD DAY Guten Tag
GOOD EVENING Guten Abend
GOOD MORNING Guten Morgen
GOOD NIGHT Gute Nacht

GOOD-BYE   auf wiedersehen
GRILLED   gegrillt, grillen
HARD   hart
HEADWAITER   Chef
HELP!   Hilfe!
HOT   heiss
HOT DISHES   warme Gerichte
HOTTER   heisser
HOW   wie
HOW ARE YOU?   Wie geht es Dir?
HOW MANY?   Wieviele?
HOW MUCH IS THAT?   Wieviel kostet das?
HURRY (TO)   eilen
I AM HUNGRY   Ich habe Hunger
I AM SORRY   Es tut mir leid
I AM THIRSTY   Ich habe Durst
I DO NOT UNDERSTAND   Ich verstehe nicht.
I HAVE HAD ENOUGH THANKS   Danke, ich habe
   genug
I HAVE LOST MY MONEY   Ich habe mein Geld veloren
I SPEAK ONLY ENGLISH   Ich spreche nur Englisch
I'VE MADE A RESERVATION   Ich habe reservieren lassen
INSTEAD   anstatt
IS THERE A DOCTOR HERE?   Ist hier ein Doktor
IT'S VERY IMPORTANT   Es ist sehr wichtig
KNIFE   das Messer
KOSHER   koscher
LADIES   Damen
LARGE SPOON   der Suppenlöffel
LUNCH   Mittagessen
MARINATED   mariniert
MASHED   zerdrückt
MATCH   passend, Streichholz
MAY I HAVE THIS, PLEASE?   Kann ich das haben, bitte?
MEAL   Mahlzeit, Mahl
MEAL SERVED QUICKLY   Schnellimbiss, Schnellservice
MEDIUM   mittel

MEDIUM RARE   halbdurch
MEN   Männer
MENU, BILL OF FARE   Speisekarte
MID-MORNING SNACK   Brotzeit
NAPKIN   Serviette
NEED   brauchen
NO   nein
NOTHING MORE, THANKS   Nichts mehr, danke
OCCUPIED   besetzt
OPEN   geöffnet
PARDON ME!   Entschuldigen Sie!
PASTRY CART   vom Brett
PEPARED AT THE TABLE   Am Tisch zubereitet
PEPPER MILL   die Pfeffermühle
PHARMACY   die Apotheke
PITCHER   der Krug
PLATE   der Teller
PLEASE CALL THE HEADWAITER   Bitte rufen Sie den
    Chef
PLEASE!   bitte!
POACHED   pochiert
RABBIT   das Kaninchen
RARE   englisch, leicht gebraten
RAW   roh
REQUEST   Nachfrage
RESTAURANT   Retaurant
ROASTED   (im Ofen) gebraten
SANDWICH   belegtes Brot
SAUSAGE DISHES   Wurstgerichte
SAUTÉED   geschwenkt
SEASONING   Würze
SMALL   klein
SMOKED   geräuchert
STEAMED   gedämpft
STEWED   geschmort
SWEET   süss
TABLE   der Tisch

TABLESPOON   Esslöffel
TAXI   das Taxi
TEASPOON   Teelöffel
THANK YOU   Danke
THANK YOU VERY MUCH   Danke vielmals
THAT IS BAD   Das ist schlecht
THERE   dort
THIRSTY   durstig,-er,-e,-es
TOASTED   getoastet
TOOTHPICK   Zahnstocher
TO YOUR HEALTH   Deine Gesundheit
UNDERDONE (RARE)   englisch, leicht gebraten
URGENT   dringend
VERY DRY   sehr trocken
WAITER!   Herr Ober!
WAITRESS!   Fräulein!
WARM DISHES   warme Gerichte
WELL-DONE   gut durch
WHAT TIME IS IT, PLEASE?   Bitte, wie spät ist es?
WHEN   wann
WHERE CAN I FIND A GOOD RESTAURANT (NOT TOO
   EXPENSIVE)?   Wo ist hier ein gutes (nicht zu teures)
   Restaurant?
WHERE IS THE RESTROOM?   Wo ist die Toilette?
WINE AND SNACK TAVERN   Weinstube
WINE GLASS   Weinglas
WINE LIST   Weinkarte
WITH   mit
WITHOUT   ohne
WRONG   falsch
YES   ja
YES, THAT'S RIGHT   Ja, das ist richtig
YOU   Sie, Du
YOU ARE WELCOME   Bitte sehr
YOU SEE?   Sehen Sie?
ZERO   null

Food and Drink

ALMOND   Mandel
ANCHOVY   Sardelle
APERITIF   Aperitif
APPETIZER   Vorspeise
APPLE   Apfel
APPLESAUCE   Apfelmus, Apfelsosse
APRICOT   Aprikose
ARTICHOKE   Artischoke
ASPARAGUS   Spargel
ASSORTED CHEESES   Auswahl an Käse
AVOCADOS   Avocados
BACON   Speck
BACON AND EGGS   Speck und Eier
BANANAS   Bananen
BASKET OF FRUIT   Schale mit Früchten
BEANS   Bohnen
BEEF   Beef, Rindfleisch
BEEFSTEAK   Beefsteak, Rindersteak
BEER   Bier
BEER BOTTLED   Flaschenbier
BEER DARK   dunkles Bier
BEER DRAFT   Fassbier
BEER LIGHT   helles Bier
BISCUIT   Bisquit
BOILED EGGS   gekochte Eier
BOILED POTATOES   gekochte Kartoffeln
BRAISED   gedünstet
BRANDY   Weinbrand
BREAD   Brot
BREAKFAST SAUSAGE   Frühstückswurst
BROCCOLI   Broccoli
BURGUNDY   Burgunder
BUTTER   Butter
CABBAGE   Kohl

CAKE   Kuchen
CANDY   Bonbon
CARP   Karpfen
CARROT   Karotte
CAULIFLOWER   Blumenkohl
CELERY   Sellerie
CEREAL COLD   kaltes Müsli
CEREAL HOT   warmes Müsli
CHAMPAGNE   Sekt
CHEESE   Käse
CHERRIES   Kirschen
CHICKEN   Huhn, Hühnchen
CHICKEN FRICASSEE   Hühnerfricassee
CHICKEN FRIED   Backhuhn
CHICKEN ROAST   Brathuhn
CHICKEN SOUP   Hühnersuppe
CHIPS (POTATO)   Kartoffelchips
CHOCOLATE   Schokolade
CHOCOLATE BAR   eine Tafel Schokolade
CHOP   hacken
CHOPPED STEAK   Hackbraten
CLAMS   Muscheln, Venusmuscheln
CLARET   Rotwein
COCKTAIL   Cocktail
COD   Kabeljau
COFFEE   Kaffee
COFFEE AMERICAN   Amerikanischer Kaffee
COFFEE BLACK   schwarzer Kaffee
COFFEE DECAFFEINATED   koffeinfreier Kaffee
COFFEE ICED   Eiskaffee
COFFEE INSTANT   schnellöslicher Kaffee
COFFEE WITH CREAM   Kaffee mit Sahne
COFFEE WITH HOT MILK   Kaffee mit heisser Milch
COFFEE WITH MILK   Kaffee mit Milch
COFFEE, ROLLS AND BUTTER   Kaffe, Brötchen und
   Butter
COGNAC   Kognac

COLD MILK   kalte Milch
CONTINENTAL BREAKFAST   kontinentales Frühstück
COOKED SAUSAGES   gekochte Würste
COOKIES   Plätzchen
CORN   Mais
CRABS   Krabben
CRAYFISH   Flusskrebs
CREAM   Sahne
CUCUMBER   Gurke
CUP OF COFFEE   Tasse Kaffee
CUSTARD   Eierspeise
DARK BEER   dunkles Bier
DRINK   Getränk
DRY WINE   trockener Wein
DUCK   Ente
EEL   Aal
EGGS   Eier
EGGS BOILED   gekochte Eier
EGGS BOILED FIRM   hartgekochte Eier
EGGS BOILED HARD   hartgekochte Eier
EGGS BOILED SOFT   weichgekochte Eier
EGGS FRIED   Spiegeleier
EGGS FRIED OVER   Spiegeleier
EGGS FRIED UP   Spiegeleier
EGGS FRIED WITH BACON   Spiegeleier mit Speck
EGGS FRIED WITH HAM   Spiegeleier mit Schinken
EGGS FRIED WITH POTATOES   Spiegeleier mit
   Kartoffeln
EGGS FRIED WITH SAUSAGE   Spiegeleier mit Wurst
EGGS POACHED   pochierte Eier, verlorene Eier
EGGS SCRAMBLED   Rühreier
EGGS SCRAMBLED WITH BACON   Rühreier mit Speck
EGGS SCRAMBLED WITH HAM   Rühreier mit Schinken
EGGS SCRAMBLED WITH POTATOES   Rühreier mit
   Kartoffeln
EGGS SCRAMBLED WITH SAUSAGE   Rühreier mit
   Wurst

EGGS WITH BACON   Eier mit Speck
ESPRESSO BLACK   schwarzer Espresso
ESPRESSO WEAK   schwacher Espresso
ESPRESSO WITH MILK   Espresso mit Milch
FISH   Fisch
FRIED   gebacken, gebraten
FRIED POTATOES   Bratkartoffeln
FROG LEGS   Froschschenkel
FRUIT   Obst
FRUIT COMPOTE   Kompott
FRUIT DRINK   Fruchtsaftgetränk
FRUIT JUICE   Fruchtsaft
FRUIT SALAD   Obstsalat
FULL-BODIED (WINE)   schwer
GAME   Wild
GARLIC   Knoblauch
GIN   Gin
GIN AND TONIC   Gin und Tonic
GLASS OF BEER   Glas Bier
GLASS OF LIQUEUR   Glas Likör
GLASS OF MILK   Glas Milch
GLASS OF WATER   Glas Wasser
GLASS OF WINE   Glas Wein
GOOSE   Gans
GOOSE LIVER PASTE   Gänseleberpastete
GRAPEFRUIT   Grapefruit
GRAPEFRUIT JUICE   Grapefruitsaft
GRAPES   Weintrauben
GRAVY   Sosse
GREEN BEANS   grüne Bohnen
GREEN OLIVES   grüne Oliven
GREEN PEPPER   grüner Pfeffer
GREEN SALAD   grüner Salat
GREEN VEGETABLES   grünes Gemüse
HADDOCK   Schellfisch
HALIBUT   Heilbutt
HAM   Schinken

HEN   Henne
HERRING   Hering
HONEY   Honig
HOT CHOCOLATE   heisse Schokolade
HOT MILK   heisse Milch
HOT WATER   heisses Wasser
ICE   Eis
ICE CREAM   Eis
ICE CUBES   Eiswürfel
ICE WATER   Eiswasser
JAM   Marmelade
JUICE   Saft
KETCHUP   Ketchup
KIDNEYS   Nieren
LAMB   Lamm
LAMB CHOPS   Hammelkotelett
LEMON   Zitrone
LEMONADE   Zitronenlimonade
LETTUCE   Salat
LIGHT BEER   helles Bier
LIMA BEANS   Puffbohnen
LIQUEUR   Likör
LIVER   Leber
LOAF OF BREAD   Brotlaib
LOBSTER   Hummer
LOCAL RED WINE   Landrotwein, hiessiger Rotwein
LOCAL WHITE WINE   Landweisswein, hiessiger
   Weisswein
LOCAL WINE   Landwein, hiessiger Wein
MACARONI   Nudeln, Makkaroni
MACKEREL   Makrele
MARMALADE   Apfelsinenmarmelade
MASHED POTATOES   Kartoffelpüree
MAYONNAISE   Mayonnaise
MEAT   Fleich
MEATBALLS   Fleischklösschen, Fleischklösse
MILK   Milch

MINERAL WATER Mineralwasser
MIXED SALAD gemischter Salat
MUSHROOMS Pilze
MUSSELS Muscheln
MUSTARD Senf
MUTTON Hammel
NEAT (STRAIGHT) pur, rein
NOODLES Nudeln
NUT Nuss
OATMEAL Haferflocken
OCTOPUS Oktopus
OIL Öl
OLIVE Olive
OLIVE OIL Olivenöl
OMELET Omelett
ON THE ROCKS mit Eis
ONIONS Zwiebeln
ORANGE JUICE Orangensaft
OYSTERS Austern
PANCAKES Pfannkuchen
PARMESAN CHEESE Parmesankäse
PARSLEY Petersilie
PASTRY Gebäck
PEACHES Pfirsiche
PEANUTS Erdnüsse
PEARS Birnen
PEAS Erbsen
PEPPER Pfeffer
PIE Pastete
PIGEON Tauben
PIKE Hecht
PINEAPPLE JUICE Ananassaft
PINEAPPLE Ananas
PLUM Pflaume, Zwetschge
PORK Schwein
PORK CHOPS Schweinekotelett
PORT Portwein

POTATO   Kartoffel
POTATO BOILED   gekochte Kartoffeln
POTATO FRIED   gebratene Kartoffeln, Bratkartoffeln
POTATO SALAD   Kartoffelsalat
POTATOES MASHED   Kartoffelpüree
POULTRY   Geflügel
PRAWNS   Garnelen
PRUNES   Backpflaume
RABBIT   (das) Kaninchen
RADISHES   Rettich, Radischen
RASPBERRIES   Himmbeere
RED CABBAGE   Rotkohl
RED WINE   Rotwein
RICE   Reis
ROAST BEEF   Roastbeef, Rinderbraten
ROAST CHICKEN   Hühnerbraten
ROAST PORK   Schweinebraten
ROAST VEAL   Kalbsbraten
ROLLS   Brötchen
ROSÉ WINE   Rosé
RUM   Rum
SACCHARIN   Süsstoff
SALAD   Salat
SALAD DRESSING   Salatsosse
SALAMI   Salami
SALMON   Lachs
SALT   Salz
SANDWICH   belegte Brot
SANDWICH ROLLS   belegte Brötchen
SAUCE   Sauce
SAUERKRAUT   Sauerkraut
SAUSAGE (BIG)   Wurst
SAUSAGE (SMALL)   Würstchen
SAUSAGE DISHES   Wurstgerichte
SCOTCH   Scotch, schottischer Whiskey
SCRAMBLED EGGS   Rühreier
SEA BASS   Barsch

SEAFOOD   Meeresfrüchte
SHARK   Hai
SHERRY   Sherry
SHRIMP   Krabben
SHRIMP COCKTAIL   Krabbencocktail
SNAILS   Schnecken
SODA WATER   Sprudel, Selters, Selterwasser
SOFT DRINKS   alkoholfreie Getränke
SOLE   Seezunge
SOUP   Suppe
SPAGHETTI   Spaghetti
SPARKLING   perlend, schäumend
SPICY SAUCE   scharfe Sosse
SPICY SAUSAGE   scharfe Wurst
SPINACH   Spinat
SQUID   Tintenfisch
STEAK   Steak
STEW   Braten, Schmorbraten
STRAWBERRIES   Erdbeeren
SUGAR   Zucker
SWEETS   Süssigkeiten
TEA   Tee
TEA WITH CREAM   Tee mit Sahne
TEA WITH LEMON   Tee mit Zitrone
TOAST   Toast
TOMATO JUICE   Tomatensaft
TOMATO SAUCE   Tomatensosse
TOMATOES   Tomaten
TONGUE   Zunge
TROUT   Forelle
TRUFFLE   Trüffel
TUNA   Tunfisch
TURKEY   Truthahn
VANILLA   Vanille
VEAL   Kalbfleisch
VEGETABLE SOUP   Gemüsesuppe
VEGETABLES   Gemüse

VERMOUTH   Vermouth
VINEGAR   Essig
VODKA   Wodka
WATER   das Wasser
WATERMELON   Wassermelone
WHIPPED CREAM   Schlagsahne
WHISKEY   Whisky
WHISKEY AND SODA   Whisky und Soda
WHITE WINE   Weisswein
WINE   Wein
WINE LOCAL RED   Landrotwein, hiessiger Rotwein
WINE LOCAL WHITE   Landweisswein, hiessiger
   Weisswein
WINE SPARKLING   Schaumwein
WINE VERY DRY   sehr trockener Wein
WINE VERY FULL-BODIED   blumiger Wien
YOGURT   Yoghurt

In the Restaurant: To Order or Make Requests

A TABLE BY THE WINDOW PLEASE   Einen Tisch am
   Fenster, bitte
A TABLE FOR ... PLEASE   Einen Tisch für ... Personen,
   bitte
A TABLE FOR FOUR PLEASE   Einen Tisch für vier
   Personen, bitte
A TABLE FOR THREE   Einen Tisch für drei Personen,
   bitte
A TABLE FOR TWO, PLEASE   Einen Tisch für zwei
   Personen, bitte
A TABLE OUTSIDE PLEASE   Bitte, einen Tisch im Freien
ANOTHER CHAIR PLEASE   Einen anderen Stuhl bitte
ASHTRAY PLEASE   Einen Aschenbecher, bitte
AT WHAT TIMES ARE MEALS SERVED?   Wann gibt es
   Essen?
BATHROOM   das Badezimmer (Toilette *in restaurants*)

BILL   Rechnung
BOILED   gekocht
BRING ME THE CHECK, PLEASE   Meine Rechnung, bitte
BRING ME THE WINE LIST, PLEASE   Die Weinkarte, bitte
BRING US SOME COFFEE NOW, PLEASE.   Bringen Sie
   uns jetzt Kaffee, bitte
CAN I HAVE ...?   Kann ich ... haben?
CAN WE DINE NOW?   Können wir jetzt essen?
CAN YOU HELP ME?   Können Sie mir helfen?
CAN YOU RECOMMEND A GOOD RESTAURANT?
   Können Sie mir ein gutes Restaurant empfehlen?
CAN YOU RECOMMEND A GOOD RESTAURANT, NOT
   TOO EXPENSIVE?   Können Sie mir ein gutes, nicht zu
   teueres Restaurant empfehlen?
CAN YOU TELL ME WHAT THIS IS?   Bitte, was ist das?
CHAIR   der Stuhl
CHECK   der Scheck, die Rechnung
COULD WE HAVE MORE ..., PLEASE   Bitte, können wir
   mehr von ... haben
DO YOU HAVE...?   Haben Sie...?
DO YOU HAVE A DISH OF THE DAY?   Haben Sie ein
   Tagesgericht?
DO YOU HAVE WINE BY THE GLASS?   Haben Sie ein
   Glas Wein?
DO YOU KNOW A GOOD RESTAURANT?   Kennen Sie
   ein gutes Restaurant?
DO YOU SPEAK ENGLISH?   Sprechen Sie Englisch?
DO YOU UNDERSTAND?   Verstehen Sie?
EXCUSE ME, HOW CAN I GO TO A GOOD RESTAU-
   RANT?   Verzeihung, wie komme ich zu einem guten
   Restaurant?
FAST   schnell
FOR LADIES   für Damen
FOR MEN   für Herren
FORK   die Gabel
FRIED   gebacken, gebraten
GLASS OF ..., PLEASE   Ein Glas ..., bitte

GRILLED   gegrillt

HAVE YOU A TABLE FOR ... PEOPLE?   Haben Sie einen
Tisch für ... Personen?

HAVE YOU ANY ...?   Haben Sie ...?

HAVE YOU COMPLETE DINNERS?   Haben Sie ein Menue?

HAVE YOU PRICE FIXED DINNERS?   Haben Sie ein
Tagesmenue?

HOTTER   heisser

HOW MUCH IS THAT?   Wieviel kostet das?

I AM IN A HURRY   Ich bin in Eile

I LIKE THE MEAT MEDIUM   Ich möchte das Fleisch
halbdurch gebraten

I LIKE THE MEAT MEDIUM RARE   Ich möchte das
Fleisch halbdurch gebraten

I LIKE THE MEAT RARE   Ich möchte das Fleisch leicht
(englisch) gebraten

I LIKE THE MEAT UNDERDONE (RARE)   Ich möchte
das Fleisch englisch, leicht gebraten

I LIKE THE MEAT WELL-DONE   Ich möchte das Fleisch
gut durchgebraten

I WANT A TABLE FOR ... PEOPLE AT ... O'CLOCK
Einen Tisch für ... Personen, um ... Uhr

I WANT SOMETHING SIMPLE, NOT TOO SPICY   Ich
möchte etwas Einfaches, nicht zu Scharfes

I'D LIKE A DESSERT PLEASE   Ich nehme einen
Nachtisch, bitte

I'D LIKE AN APERITIF PLEASE   Ich nehme einen
Aperitif, bitte

I'D LIKE AN APPETIZER PLEASE   Ich nehme eine
Vorspeise, bitte

I'D LIKE SOME BEEF PLEASE   Ich nehme Rindfleisch, bitte

I'D LIKE SOME FISH PLEASE   Ich nehme Fisch, bitte

I'D LIKE SOME LAMB PLEASE   Ich nehme Lamm, bitte

I'D LIKE SOME PORK PLEASE   Ich nehme Schweinefleisch, bitte

INSTEAD   anstatt

IS SERVICE INCLUDED?   Ist die Bedienung einbegriffen?

IS SERVICE NOT INCLUDED?   Ist die Bedienung nicht einbegriffen?

KNIFE   das Messer

KOSHER   koscher

LARGE SPOON   der Suppenlöffel

LAVATORY   Toilette

LEAN   mager

MAY I CHANGE THIS?   Kann ich dies umbestellen?

MAY I HAVE THE MENU?   Kann ich bitte die Speisekarte haben?

MAY I HAVE THE WINE LIST?   Kann ich bitte die Weinkarte haben?

MAY I HAVE THIS?   Kann ich das haben, bitte?

MORE BEER, PLEASE   Bitte noch etwas Bier

MORE BREAD, PLEASE   Bitte noch etwas Brot

MORE WATER, PLEASE   Bitte noch etwas Wasser

MORE, PLEASE   mehr, bitte

NO SAUCE, PLEASE   Bitte, keine Sosse

PASTRY CART   vom Brett

PEPPER MILL   eine Pfeffermühle

PLEASE BRING ME ANOTHER FORK.   Bringen Sie mir bitte eine andere Gabel

PLEASE CALL THE HEADWAITER   Bitte rufen Sie den Chef

PLEASE SERVE US QUICKLY   Bitte, servieren Sie uns schnell

SLICE OF   eine Scheibe

SMALL BOTTLE OF   eine kleine Flasche

SOMETHING LIGHT PLEASE   Etwas Leichtes, bitte

SOUP SPOON   Suppenlöffel

SPICY SAUCE   scharfe Sosse

SPOON   Löffel

TABLE   der Tisch

TABLE FOR TWO PLEASE   Tisch für zwei Personen, bitte

TAKE IT AWAY PLEASE   Bitte, nehmen Sie es weg!

THE CHECK, PLEASE   Die Rechnung, bitte

THE MENU, PLEASE   Die Speisekarte, bitte

TOASTED   getoastet

WATER   das Wasser

WE WOULD LIKE A BOTTLE OF DRY WINE   Bitte, eine Flasche trockenen Wein

WE WOULD LIKE A BOTTLE OF GOOD LOCAL WINE   Bitte, eine Flasche guten Wein von dieser Gegend

WE WOULD LIKE A BOTTLE OF RED WINE   Bitte, eine Flasche Rotwein

WE WOULD LIKE A BOTTLE OF SWEET WINE   Bitte, eine Flasche süssen Wein

WE WOULD LIKE A BOTTLE OF WHITE WINE   Bitte, eine Flasche Weisswein

WE WOULD LIKE A CARAFE OF LOCAL RED WINE, PLEASE   Bitte, eine Karaffe roten Tischwein

WE WOULD LIKE A CARAFE OF LOCAL WHITE WINE, PLEASE   Bitte, eine Karaffe weissen Tischwein

WE WOULD LIKE A GLASS OF DRY WINE   Bitte, ein Glas trockenen Wein

WE WOULD LIKE A GLASS OF RED WINE   Bitte, ein Glas Rotwein

WE WOULD LIKE A GLASS OF SWEET WINE   Bitte, ein Glas süssen Wein

WE WOULD LIKE A GLASS OF WHITE WINE   Bitte, ein Glas Weisswein

WELL-DONE   gut durch

WHAT DO YOU RECOMMEND?   Was können Sie empfehlen?

WHAT IS THAT?   Was ist das?

WHAT IS THE SPECIALTY OF THE HOUSE?   Was ist die Spezialität des Hauses?

WHAT SALADS DO YOU HAVE?   Welche Salate gibt es?

WHAT SEAFOOD DO YOU HAVE?   Was für einen Fisch (Meeresfrüchte) haben Sie?

WHAT WINE DO YOU RECOMMEND?   Welchen Wein empfehlen Sie?

WINE LIST PLEASE   Die Weinkarte, bitte

WITH (WITHOUT) ICE   mit (ohne) Eis

WITH POTATOES PLEASE   mit Kartoffeln, bitte

WITH SODA WATER PLEASE   Mit Sodawasser, bitte

Problems

COLD kalt
DIRTY schmutzig
DRY trocken
I AM IN A HURRY Ich bin in Eile
I AM LOST Ich habe mich verlaufen
I ASKED FOR .... Ich habe nach ... gefragt
I DID NOT ORDER THIS Ich habe dies nicht bestellt
I DO NOT LIKE THAT Mir gefällt das nicht
I DO NOT UNDERSTAND Ich verstehe nicht.
I HAVE LOST MY COAT Ich habe meinen Mantel
  verloren
I HAVE LOST MY MONEY Ich habe mein Geld veloren
I HAVE LOST MY PASSPORT Ich habe meinen Pass
  verloren
I THINK THE BILL IS INCORRECT Ich glaube, die
  Rechnung stimmt nicht
I THINK THERE IS A MISTAKE HERE Ich denke da ist
  ein Fehler
IS THERE ANYONE HERE WHO KNOWS FIRST AID?
  Kann jemand erste Hilfe leislen?
IT DOES NOT TASTE RIGHT Das schmeckt nicht gut
IT IS NOT GOOD Das ist nicht gut
IT ISN'T HOT ENOUGH Das ist nicht heiss genug
MAY I CHANGE THIS? Kann ich dies auswechseln?
PLEASE CALL THE HEADWAITER Bitte rufen Sie den
  Chef
RAW roh
THAT IS BAD Das ist schlecht
THE FISH IS BAD Der Fisch ist schlecht
THE MEAT IS BAD Das Fleisch ist schlecht
THE MEAT IS OVERDONE Das Fleisch ist zu sehr
  gebraten
THE MEAT IS TOO TOUGH Das Fleisch ist zu zäh
THE MEAT IS UNDERDONE Das Fleisch ist nicht
  durchgebraten

THE WINE IS CORKED   Der Kork ist in der Flasche
THIS IS COLD   Das ist kalt
THIS IS NOT CLEAN   Das ist nicht sauber
THIS IS OVERCOOKED   Das ist zu sehr gekocht
THIS IS TOO SOUR   Das ist zu sauer
THIS IS TOO SWEET   Das ist zu süss
THIS IS TOO TOUGH   Das ist zu hart
THIS IS UNDERCOOKED   Das ist nicht genügend
gekocht

To Pay

A CHARGE FOR SERVICE IS INCLUDED   10% Bedienung
ist einbegriffen
BILL   Rechnung
BRING ME THE CHECK, PLEASE   Meine Rechnung,
bitte
CHECK   der Scheck, die Rechnung
DO YOU ACCEPT AMERICAN MONEY?   Nehmen Sie
Dollars?
DO YOU ACCEPT AMERICAN EXPRESS CARDS?
Nehmen Sie American Express?
DO YOU ACCEPT DINERS CARD?   Nehmen Sie Diners
Card?
DO YOU ACCEPT MASTER CARD?   Nehmen Sie Master
Card?
DO YOU ACCEPT VISA CARDS?   Nehmen Sie Visa
Card?
HOW MUCH IS THAT?   Wieviel kostet das?
I THINK THE BILL IS INCORRECT   Ich glaube, die
Rechnung stimmt nicht
I THINK THERE IS A MISTAKE HERE   Ich denke, da ist
ein Fehler
IS EVERYTHING INCLUDED?   Ist alles einbegriffen?
IS SERVICE INCLUDED?   Ist die Bedienung einbegriffen?
IS SERVICE NOT INCLUDED?   Ist die Bedienung nicht
einbegriffen?

IS THE TIP INCLUDED?   Ist das Trinkgeld einbergriffen?
THE CHECK, PLEASE   Die Rechnung, bitte

Doctor and Dentist

CALL A DOCTOR   Rufen Sie einen Doktor!
CALL AN AMBULANCE   Rufen Sie einen Krankenwagen!
CALL THE POLICE!   Rufen Sie die Polizei!
CAN YOU RECOMMEND A DENTIST TO ME?   Können Sie mir einen Kahnarzt empfehlen?
DENTIST   Zahnarzt
DENTIST WHO SPEAKS ENGLISH   Welcher Zahnarzt spricht Englisch?
DOCTOR WHO SPEAKS ENGLISH?   Welcher Doktor sprich Englisch?
DOES ANYONE SPEAK ENGLISH?   Spricht jemand Englisch?
EMERGENCY   die Notlage, der Notfall
FIRE!   Feuer!
HEART ATTACK   der Herzanfall
HELP!   Hilfe!
I DON'T FEEL WELL   Ich fühle mich nicht gut
I HAVE PAIN   Ich habe Schmerzen
I HAVE A TOOTHACHE   Ich habe Zahnschmerzen
IS THERE A DOCTOR HERE?   Ist hier ein Doktor?
IS THERE ANYONE HERE WHO KNOWS FIRST AID?   Kann jemand erste Hilfe leisten?
IT HURTS HERE   Es tut hier weh
JUST FIX IT TEMPORARILY   Machen Sie es provisorisch
PHARMACY   die Apotheke
POLICE!   Polizei!
THERE HAS BEEN AN ACCIDENT   Es ist ein Unfall geschehen
URGENT   dringend
WHEN CAN HE COME?   Wann kann er kommen?

Telephone/Taxi

CAN I DIAL THIS NUMBER?   Kann ich diese Nummer wählen?

CAN I SPEAK TO ...?   Kann ich mit ... sprechen?

CAN YOU HELP ME GET THE LONG DISTANCE OPERATOR?   Ich brauche die Auslandsvermittlung, bitte

CAN YOU HELP ME GET THIS NUMBER?   Können Sie mich mit dieser Nummer verbinden?

DO I NEED TELEPHONE COINS?   Brauche ich Geld für das Telefon?

EXTENSION NUMBER ... PLEASE   Apperat ... bitte

HOW MUCH IS A TELEPHONE CALL TO ...?   Wieviel kostet ein Telefongespräch nach ...?

I HAVE BEEN DISCONNECTED   Ich bin unterbrochen worden

I WANT A LOCAL CALL TO NUMBER ...   Bitte, ein Ortsgespräch mit der Nummer ...

I WANT A LONG DISTANCE CALL ...   Bitte, ein Ferngespräch mit der Nummer ...

I WANT A PERSON TO PERSON CALL TO ...   Ein Gespräch von Person zu Person ...

I WANT A REVERSE CHARGE CALL TO ...   Bitte, ein R-Gespräch nach ...

I WANT NUMBER ... PLEASE   Bitte, die Nummer ...

I WOULD LIKE TELEPHONE COINS   Bitte, ich brauche Geld für das Telefon

I WOULD LIKE TO TELEPHONE ...   Ich möchte telefonieren...

INFORMATION   Auskunft

IT'S VERY IMPORTANT   Es ist sehr wichtig

MY NUMBER IS ...   Meine Nummer ist ...

NUMBER IS OCCUPIED   Die Nummer ist besetzt

OPERATOR   Auskunft

PLEASE ASK HIM (HER) TO CALL ME AT ...   Bitte, richten Sie ihm (ihr) aus, mich ... anzurufen

PLEASE RECONNECT ME   Bitte, verbinden Sie mich
   wieder
PLEASE SPEAK MORE SLOWLY   Bitte, langsam sprechen
PLEASE TELL HIM (HER) ... CALLED   Bitte, sagen Sie
   ihm (ihr) ... hat angerufen
TAXI   das Taxi
TELEPHONE   das Telephon
THIS PHONE IS NOT WORKING   Das Telefon ist kaputt
WHAT IS THE TELEPHONE NUMBER?   Wie ist die
   Telefonnummer?
WHAT KIND OF COIN DO I PUT IN?   Was für ein
   Geldstück muss ich einwerfen?
WHERE IS THE TELEPHONE BOOK?   Wo ist das
   Telefonbuch?
WHERE IS THE TELEPHONE?   Wo ist das Telefon?

How to Understand It: German to English

Appetizers

APPETITHÄPPCHEN   appetizer, canapé
APPETITSCHNITTCHEN   appetizer, canapé
AUFSCHNITTPLATTE   cold cut platter
AUSTERN GEBACKEN   fried oysters
BACHKREBS   stream crayfish
BIERRETTICH   black radish served with beer
BLÄTTERTEIGPASTETE   patty shell
BLÄTTERTEIGPASTETE MIT KREBSSCHWÄNZCHEN
   patty shell with crayfish tails in cream sauce
BLÄTTERTEIGPASTETE MIT GEFLÜGELRAGOUT   patty
   shell with diced chicken in cream sauce
BRATEN   roast meats
BRATENPLATTE   plate of cold roast meats
BRATENSÜLZE   cold roast meats in aspic
BROTZEIT-TELLER   mid-morning meat and other snacks
BÜCKLINGE ÜBERBACKEN   baked kippers
BÜNDNERFLEISCH   cured, dried beef
CREVETTENCOCKTAIL (AUS)   shrimp cocktail
FLEISCHFÜLLUNG   meat filling
FLEISCHRÖLLCHEN   cooked stuffed meat slices served
   cold
FLEISCHSÜLZE   meat in aspic
FLUSSLACHS   stream salmon
FORELLENFILET   fillet of trout

FROSCHSCHENKEL PANIERT GEBACKEN (AUS)
breaded and fried frog's legs
GÄNSELEBERPASTETE   goose liver pâté or paste
GEEISTE MELONE   chilled melon
GEFLÜGELLEBER   chicken livers
GEFLÜGELSALAT   chicken salad with mayonnaise
GEFÜLLTE TOMATEN MIT FLEISCHSALAT   tomatoes
stuffed with cold meat salad
GEFÜLLTE TOMATEN MIT GEFLÜGELSALAT   tomatoes
stuffed with chicken salad
GEMISCHTER AUFSCHNITT   mixed cold cuts
GERÄUCHERTER LACHS   smoked salmon
GERÄUCHERTER RHEINLACHS   smoked salmon from
the Rhine
HANDKÄSE MIT MUSIK   marinated strong-flavored
cheese
HAPPEN   snack
HAWAII   with pineapple
HERING NACH HAUSFRAUENART   herring fillets with
onions in sour cream
HERINGS TOAST   chopped herring salad on toast
HUMMERCOCKTAIL (AUS)   lobster cocktail
HUMMERKRABBEN   large prawns
HÜTTENKÄSE MIT FRÜCHTEN   cottage cheese with
fruit
KALBSBRATEN   cold cooked veal roast
KALBS KÄSE   veal meat loaf with cheese
KALTE VORGERICHTE   cold first courses or appetizers
KALTE VORSPEISEN   cold first courses or appetizers
KAROTTENEINTOPF MIT FLEISCHEINLAGE   carrot
casserole with meat
KASSELER SAFTRIPPE   pickled smoked pork loin chop
KATENRAUCHSPECK IN PAPRIKA   paprika covered,
cottage smoked bacon
KAVIAR   caviar
KLEIN, FEIN   small, tasty (dishes)
KNOCHEN   bone

KRABBEN IN MAYONNAISE   shrimp in mayonnaise dressing

KRABBENSALAT   shrimp salad with mayonnaise

KRÄUTERQUARK   white cheese seasoned with chopped herbs

KREBSCOCKTAIL (AUS)   crayfish cocktail

KREBSSCHWÄNZE   crayfish tails

KREBSSCHWANZSALAT   crayfish salad

LACHSBRÖTCHEN   smoked salmon sandwiches

LANGUSTE IN MAYONNAISE   crayfish with mayonnaise

LEBERKÄSE   cold or hot meat loaf of liver, pork and bacon

LEBERPRESSACK   pressed liver meat loaf

LUCULLUSEIER   eggs with goose liver, truffle in various sauces

MASTRINDFLEISCHSALAT   cold, cooked, grain-fed beef cut in strips and put into a salad with mayonnaise

MATJESHERING   young salted herring

MATJESHERING NACH HAUSFRAUEN-ART   herring fillets with apple slices, onion rings, onion sauce and sour cream

MEERRETICH   horseradish

MUSCHEL RAGOUT-FIN   mussels in a thick cream sauce

MUSCHELN GEBRATEN (AUS)   roast mussels

NORWEGISCHE EIER   poached eggs in aspic on shrimp salad with anchovy

OCHSENZUNGE   ox tongue

OCHSENZUNGENTASCHEN   cold sliced tongue rolls with horseradish sauce inside

ÖLSARDINEN   sardines in oil

PASTETE GEFÜLLT MIT FEINEM RAGOUT   patty shell filled with diced veal in mushroom and wine cream sauce

PASTETE KAPUZINERART   a delicate meat stew served in a patty shell

PFIFFERLINGE   wild mushroom like chanterelle

PÖKELZUNGE   pickled tongue

RAGOUT-FIN   diced veal, tongue, brains, in a cream
sauce with mushrooms and wine

RAHMMEERRETTICH   horseradish cream sauce

RÄUCHERAAL   smoked eel

RAUCHERHERING   smoked herring

RÄUCHERLACHS   smoked salmon

RAUCHFLEISCH   smoked meat

RAVIOLI IN TOMATENTUNKE   square pasta filled with
cheese or meat in tomato sauce

REGENSBURGER IN ESSIG UND ÖL   cold slices of beef
and pork sausage, dressed with oil and vinegar

REMOULADENSOSSE   mayonnaise sauce with mustard,
anchovies, capers, gherkins, tarragon, chervil

RESTAURATIONSBROT   bread served with cold cuts

RETTICH MIT BROT UND BUTTER   radishes with bread
and butter

RINDERMARK   beef marrow

RINDFLEISCHSALAT   beef strips with spicy vinegar sauce

RIPPCHEN   smoked rib loin pork chop

ROASTBEEFRÖLLCHEN   cold roast beef roll

ROLLMOPS   herring fillet rolled around chopped onions
and pickles

RUNDSTÜCK WARM   hot roast meat open-faced sandwich with gravy

RUSSISCHE EIER   stuffed hard-boiled egg halves with
mayonnaise

RUSSISCHER GEFLÜGELSALAT   chicken salad with
hard-boiled eggs covered with mayonnaise

SAFTIGER SCHINKEN   juicy ham

SAHNEMEERRETTICHSOSSE   horseradish cream
sauce

SALAMI   any salami-type cold sausage

SARDINE   pilchard or very small herring

SAUERGURKE   pickle

SCAMPI COCKTAIL   prawn appetizer

SCHINKENRÖLLCHEN   rolled ham slices with or without filling

SCHLEMMERSCHNITTE   slice of bread with raw ground beef, raw egg, chopped raw onions, capers, anchovies, like steak tartar

SCHNECKEN IN KRÄUTERBUTTER (AUS)   snails with herb butter

SCHNECKENRAGOUT PROVENCALES   snails stewed in tomato and onion sauce

SCHNECKENSPIESS MIT CHAMPIGNONS, SPECK, KNOBLAUCH UND BUTTER   snails with mushrooms, bacon and garlic butter, grilled

SCHWARTENMAGEN   headcheese loaf in aspic

SCHWARZ-GERÄUCHERTES   dark-smoked ham or pork pieces

SCHWARZWEISSER PRESSACK   dark and light meat pork headcheese

SCHWEDENBRÖTCHEN   small open-faced sandwiches

SCHWEDISCHE VORSPEISEN   plate with mixed appetizers

SCHWEINSLEBERKÄSE   liver, pork, bacon meat loaf

SCHWEINSSÜLZE   headcheese

SHRIMPSALAT   shrimp salad

SPARGELSPITZEN   white asparagus tips

SPROTTEN   sprats, like sardines

STADTWURSTSÜLZE   locally-made sausage in aspic

STANGENSPARGEL   asparagus spears

STEINBUTTSALAT   salad made of cold boiled turbot

STEINHUDER RÄUCHERAAL   smoked eel from Steinhuder Lake region

TEUFELSALAT   a salad with a spicy vinegar dressing

THUNFISCH AURORA   tuna fish with a tomato-flavored sauce

TIEFSEE KREBSFLEISCH   deep sea crayfish meat

TOMATEN MIT FEINER FLEISCHFÜLLUNG   tomatoes stuffed with light meat filling

VORSPEISEN   appetizer

WARME VORGERICHTE   hot first courses or appetizers

WEINBERGSCHNECKEN   vineyard snails (edible)

WEINBERGSCHNECKEN MIT KRÄUTERBUTTER snails
   with herbal butter
WEINBERGSCHNECKEN MIT KNOBLAUCHBUTTER
   snails with garlic butter
WEISSKOHLEINTOPF MIT SCHWEINSPFÖTCHEN
   cabbage casserole with pig's feet
WURSTSALAT sausage salad
ZERLASSENE BUTTER melted butter

Beer

BACK'NBIER strong-flavored beer
BIER beer
BIER DUNKLES dark beer
BIER HELLES light, lager
BOCKBIER dark malt beer
DUNKLES BIER dark beer
EXPORTBIER an aged stronger beer
HELLES BIER light beer
MALZBIER low alcohol malt beer
MÄRZENBIER beer with high alcohol
MASSKRUG beer mug holding about 1 quart
MOLLE a pint of beer
PILS beer with strong aroma of hops
RAUCHBIER smoked beer
SPEZIALBIER strong brewed beer
STARKBIER strong beer with a high malt content
VOLLBIER typical beer
WEISSBIER wheat beer

Beverages

ALKOHOLFREIE GETRÄNKE soft drinks
APFELMOST apple cider
APFELSAFT apple juice
APFELSINENSAFT orange juice
APFELWEIN apple cider with high alcoholic content

BRAUNER   coffee with milk

BRAUNER KLEINER   small cup of coffee with milk

BRAUSE   carbonated, flavored soda

BRULOT (AUS)   finger of brandy with lump sugar in a
   warmed cup, set on fire, doused with hot coffee and
   capped with whipped cream

BUTTERMILCH   buttermilk

CREME   cream

DOPPELMOCCA (AUS)   black coffee served in a large cup

EINSPÄNNER (AUS)   coffee served in a tall glass with
   lots of whipped cream and powdered sugar

EIS   ice, ice cream

EISKAFFEE   iced coffee

EXPRESSO   strong coffee served in a small cup

FRUCHTEIS   fruit ices or ice cream

FRUCHTSAFT   fruit juice

HEISSE SCHOKOLADE   hot chocolate

KAFFEE   coffee

KAFFEE CREME   coffee cream

KAFFEE HAG   caffeine-free coffee

KAFFEE KIRSCH (AUS)   cup or small jug of black coffee
   accompanied by a small glass of Kirsch or cherry-brandy

KAFFEE MIT SAHNE   coffee with cream

KAFFEE MIT SCHLAG   coffee with whipped cream

KAFFEE MIT ZUCKER   coffee with sugar

KAFFEE SCHWARZER   black coffee

KAFFEE VERKEHRT (AUS)   more milk than coffee

KAISERMELANGE (AUS)   half coffee, half hot milk, to
   which a fresh egg has been added

KAKAO   cocoa

KAPUZINER   coffee with whipped cream and grated
   chocolate

KAPUZINER (AUS)   small cup of black coffee with cream,
   producing the color dark brown

KONSUL (AUS)   black coffee with a dash of cream

LAUF (AUS)   coffee mixed with whipped cream and
   served in a tall glass

LIMONADE lemon drink

MAZAGRAN (AUS) cold, black, sweetened coffee served
with ice cubes and maraschino or rum in a tall glass

MELANGE (AUS) half coffee, half hot milk, sweetened
with sugar

MILCH milk

MILCHKAFFEE half coffee and half hot milk

MILCHMIX milk shake

MINERALWASSER mineral water

MOCCA mocha coffee

MOCCA GESPRITZT (AUS) mocha coffee with a dash of
brandy or rum

MOCCA MILCH small mocha coffee mixed with milk

MOCCA OBERS (AUS) small mocha coffee with cream

ORANGENSAFT orange juice

PFEFFERMINZTEE peppermint tea

PHARISÄER (AUS) cup of strong, sweetened coffee with
a dash of rum and topped with whipped cream

PICCOLO (AUS) black coffee with or without whipped
cream, served in a small cup

PUNSCH punch

RAHM cream

SAHNE cream

SCHWARZER (AUS) mocha, black coffee

SODAWASSER soda water

SPRUDELWASSER soda water

TEE tea

TEE MIT MILCH tea with milk

TEE MIT ZITRONE tea with lemon

TOMATENSAFT tomato juice

TRAUBENSAFT grape juice

TÜRKISCHER KAFFEE (AUS) finely ground coffee brought
to a boil with sugar, served foaming in a small cup

WIENER EISKAFFEE (AUS) tall glass half filled with
vanilla ice to which cold, strong black coffee is added,
topped with whipped cream

ZITRONENSAFT lemonade

Bread

BAUERNBROT   rye or wholemeal bread
BELEGTE BROTE   bread served with cold cuts
BLÄTTERTEIGPASTETE   patty shell
BREZEN   pretzels
BRIES, BRIESCHEN, BRIESEL   sweet bread
BROT   bread
BRÖTCHEN   sweet breads, rolls
BUTTERBISKUIT   butter biscuit, used in soup
BUTTERBROT   bread and butter
BUTTERHÖRNCHEN   butter crescents
DRESDNER STOLLEN   Dresden Christmas fruit bread
GERÖSTETES BROT   toast
GIPFEL   crescent-shaped roll
GRAUBROT   brown or black bread
HÖRNCHEN   crescent-shaped roll
HUTZELBROT   bread made of prunes and other dried fruit
INGWERBROT   gingerbread
KIPFEL   crescent-shaped roll
KLABEN   white bread filled with currants and almonds
LAUGENBREZEL   a round twisted roll (pretzel)
LAUGENWECKERL   a long roll (pretzel)
MAISGEBACK   baked cornmeal
MOHNBRÖTCHEN   poppyseed rolls
MUSTEWECKE   bread filled with chopped pork
ROGGENBROT   rye bread
ROGGENBRÖTCHEN   rye roll
RÖMER   caraway rolls
ROSTEN BROT   toast
SCHWARZBROT   whole-grained dark bread
SEMMEL   roll
SEMMELBRÖSEL   bread crumbs
SEMMELKLÖSSE OHNE EI   bread dumplings without egg
SEMMELKNÖDEL MIT EI   bread dumplings made with eggs
SEMOLINA   flour of hard durum wheat

TOASTBROT   toast
WECKKLÖSSCHEN   bread dumplings
WEISSBROT   white bread
WEISSBROT MIT KÜMMEL   white bread with caraway
   seeds
WEIZEN   wheat
ZWIEBACK   extra dry toast

Cakes and Pastries

ANISBROT   anice-flavored cake or biscuit
ANISSCHEIBEN   anise drops
ANISSTRIEZEL   anise coffee cake
APFELPFANNKUCHEN   apple fritters
APFELKUCHEN   apple cake
APFELKÜCHLE   deep-fried apple cookies
APFELSCHNITTEN   sliced apple fritters
APFELSINENKUCHEN   orange coffee cake
APFELSTRUDEL   apple strudel, apple pastry dessert
ARME RITTER   sweet fritter
BACKWERK   cakes, cookies, pastries, etc.
BANANEN IN WEINTEIG (AUS)   banana fritters
BERLINER PFANNKUCHEN   jam-filled doughnut with
   sprinkled sugar
BIENENSTICH   cake with honey and almonds
BIERKUCHEN   loaf beercake
BIRNENSPALTEN (AUS)   sliced pear fritters
BISCHOFSBROT   fruit-nut cake
BISKOTTENTORTE (AUS)   cake with finger biscuits
BISKUIT LISETTE   spongecake of butter, egg yolks, sugar,
   coffee extract, chopped almonds
BISKUITROLLE   jelly and butter-cream roll
BLÄTTERTEIGGEBÄCK   puff pastry
BLÄTTERTEIGPASTETCHEN   small pastry shell
BLÄTTERTEIGPASTETE   pastry shell
BLITZKUCHEN   quick coffee cake

BRAUNSCHWEIGER KUCHEN   cake with almonds and fruit

BRIES, BRIESCHEN, BRIESEL   sweet bread

BUNDKUCHEN   sweet yellow cake

BUTTERKUCHEN   butter cake

BUTTERPLÄTZCHEN   butter cookies with vanilla and sugar

CREMEFÜLLUNG   creme filling

CREMESCHNITTEN (AUS)   Napoleons

DOBOSCHTORTE   seven-layer cake with mocha cream

ENGLISCHER KUCHEN   loaf cake

ERDBEERKNÖDEL (AUS)   strawberry dumplings

ERDBEERTORTE (AUS)   strawberry cream cake

FASTNACHTSSCHERBEN   potato flour doughnuts

FEINGEBÄCK   delicate pastry or cookies

FLORENTINER   almond cookies with candied orange peel, honey, heavy cream, chocolate

FRÜCHTE IN BACKTEIG (AUS)   fruit fritters

FRUCHTKNÖDEL (AUS)   fruit dumplings

FRUCHTPASTETEN   fruit pies

GEBÄCK   pastry

GEWÜRZKUCHEN   spice cake

GITTERTORTE   almond cake or tart with a raspberry topping

GLASUREN   icings

GRIESSTORTE   farina layer cake with almonds

GUGELHUPF   coffee cake with almonds and raisins

GUGLHUPF (AUS)   light chocolate torte with center of apricot jam

HAFERFLOCKENMAKRONEN   baked oat macaroons

HASELNUSSBÄLLCHEN   hazelnut balls

HASELNUSSTORTE   hazelnut torte

HASELNUSSMAKRONEN   hazelnut macaroons

HASELNUSSRING   hazelnut ring

HASELNUSS-SCHNITTEN   baked hazelnut strips

HASELNUSSTORTE   hazelnut torte

HASENOHREN   a puff pastry
HEFEKRANZ   ring-shaped cake
HEIDELBEERSCHNITTEN   blueberry pie
HEIDELBEERSTRUDEL   blueberry strudel
HEIDESAND   baked brown butter cookies
HIMBEERBRÖTCHEN   baked raspberry mounds
HIMBEERTORTE   raspberry tart
HOBELSPÄNE   deep-fried crisp twists of rum-flavored
   dough
HONIGKUCHEN   honey cake
HONIGLEBKUCHEN   baked honey spice cake
INGWERBROT   gingerbread
KAFFEEKUCHEN   coffee cake
KAFFEECREMEROLLE   coffe cream roll
KAFFEECREMETORTE   coffee cream cake
KAFFEEROULADE   coffee cream roll
KÄSEFLÄDLE   pastry flavored with sage
KÄSEKUCHEN   white cheese or cream cheesecake
KÄSETORTE   cheesecake
KEKS   biscuit or cookie
KIRSCHKNÖDEL (AUS)   cherry dumplings
KIRSCHSTRUDEL (AUS)   cherry strudel
KIRSCHKUCHEN (AUS)   cherry cake
KIRSCHTORTE   cherry tart
KLABEN   white bread filled with currants and almonds
KLEINGEBÄCK   small fine pastries
KOKOSMAKRONEN   coconut macaroons
KÖNIGSKUCHEN   loaf cake with raisins, almonds and
   rum
KRANZKUCHEN   ring-shaped cake
KRAPFEN   fritter, jelly donut
KUCHEN   cake
LEBKUCHEN   gingerbread
LEBKUCHENHÄUSCHEN   gingerbread house
LECKERLI   honey-flavored ginger biscuit
LINZER TORTE   hazelnut or almond cake or tart with
   raspberry jam

MAISGEBÄCK   pastry with cornmeal
MAKRONE   macaroon
MAKRONENTORTE   baked macaroon tart
MANDELBOGEN   baked almond rainbows
MANDELCREMETORTE   almond cream cake
MANDELHALBMONDE   baked almond half-moons
MANDELKRÄNZCHEN   almond wreaths
MANDELMAKRONEN   baked almond macaroons
MANDELSCHNECKEN   baked snail-shaped almond pastry
MANDELTORTE   almond torte
MARMORKUCHEN   marble cake
MARZIPAN   almond paste
MARZIPANKRANZ   baked almond-shaped cookies with
   raisins and icing
MERINGE   meringue
MOHNSTRIEZEL   poppy seed yeast cake
MOHNTORTE   poppy seed cake
MOHR IM HEMD (AUS)   moist chocolate cake covered
   with chocolate sauce
MOHRENKOPF   individual white cakes filled with
   custard or whipped cream and covered with chocolate
MOKKACREMETORTE   mocha or coffee cream torte
MOKKATORTE   coffee-flavored cake
MÜRBTEIG   dessert pastry
NAPFKUCHEN   yeast cake made with raisins
NOUGATTORTE   nougat torte
NÜRNBERGER LEBKUCHEN   baked spice cake
NUSSKIPFEL   nut crescent cakes
NUSSKUCHEN   nut cake
NUSSLEBKUCHEN   baked nut spice cake
NUSS-STRUDEL   nut strudel
NUSSTORTE   nut torte
OBSTKUCHEN   pastry or tart baked with fruit
OBSTTORTE   mixed fruit tart
OFFENE TORTE   open pastry tart
ORANGENBISKUIT   orange biscuit made with cognac
   orange jelly, and egg whites

PASTETCHEN   small puff pastry patty shells
PASTETE   pastry or pie
PFEFFERKUCHEN   very spicy gingerbread
PFEFFERNUSS   gingerbread nut
PFEFFERNÜSSE   cookies made of gingerbread dough
   shaped like nuts
PFEFFERNUSSKUCHLEIN   spice cookies
PFEFFERNUSSPLÄTZLE   spice cookies
PFIRSICHKNÖDEL (AUS)   peach dumplings
PFLAUMENKUCHEN   plum cake
PLÄTZCHEN   cookie, biscuit or fancy cake
POMERANZENBRÖTCHEN   baked orange or lemon rolls
POWIDLTASCHERL (AUS)   tartlets filled with plum jam
PRINTE   honey-flavored cookie
PRINZREGENTENTORTE   layer cake with chocolate
   butter-cream covered with chocolate
PUNSCHTORTE   dense rum-flavored cake covered with
   pink icing
ROSINENBRÖTCHEN   baked raisin rolls
ROSINENKUCHEN   raisin cake
RUMKUCHEN SCHWÄBISCHER BUND   baked rum
   cake with raisins, almonds, lemon juice, lemon icing,
   toasted almonds, candied fruit
SACHERTORTE   chocolate layer cake with jam filling
SANDTORTE   pound cake
SCHAUMROLLE   puff-pastry filled with whipped cream
   or custard
SCHICHTTORTE   layer cake
SCHILLERLOCKE   pastry cone with vanilla cream filling
SCHLOTFEGER MIT SAHNE   a long pastry tube with
   whipped cream and chocolate
SCHNECKEN   round small pastries
SCHOKOLADENBREZELN   chocolate pretzels
SCHOKOLADENCREMETORTE   chocolate cream layer
   cake
SCHOKOLADENMUSCHELN   baked chocolate shells
SCHOKOLADENNUSSTORTE   chocolate nut torte

SCHWARZWÄLDER KIRSCHTORTE   Black Forest cherry cake with whipped cream

S-GEBÄCK   butter cookies shaped as letter S

SPEKULATIUS   spiced cookie

SPITZBUBEN   cookie sandwiches with almonds, jelly or jam

SPRINGERLE   anise-flavored cookies

SPRITZGEBÄCK   pressed hazelnut cookies

STOLLEN   loaf cake with raisins, almonds, nuts and candied lemon peel

STRAUBEN   deep-fried dough curls with cinnamon and sugar

STREUSELKUCHEN   coffee crumb cake with topping made of butter, sugar, flour, cinnamon

STRIEZEL   braided coffee cake

STRUDEL   thin layers of pastry filled with apple slices, nuts, raisins, jam

TASCHERL   pastry turnover with meat, cheese or jam filling

TEEBLATT   oval flake pastry with sugar sprinkled on top

TEEGEBÄCK   tea cakes or petit fours

TOPFENKNÖDEL   white cheese dumplings

TOPFENOBERSTORTE   white cheese cheesecake

TOPFENSTRUDEL   baked flaky pastry filled with vanilla-flavored white cheese

TOPFENKUCHEN   cake made with white cheese and raisins

TÖRTCHEN   small pastry dessert or tart

TORTE   layer cake, usually rich

TORTENBODEN   baked tart crust layers spread with cream

VOM BRETT   from a pastry cart

WEISSGEBÄCK   a type of pastry

WIENER FASCHINGSKRAPFEN (AUS)   Viennese jam filled doughnuts

WIENER APFELSOUFFLÉ   Viennese apple soufflé

WINDBEUTEL   baked cream puff

ZIMTKUCHEN   cinnamon coffee cake
ZIMTSTERNE   cinnamon star cookies
ZWETSCHKENKNÖDEL (AUS)   plum dumplings
ZWETSCHKENSTRUDEL (AUS)   plum strudel

Cereal

BIRCHERMÜSLI   uncooked oats with raw fruit, chopped
   nuts in milk or yogurt
BREI   porridge
GRIESS   semolina
HAFERBREI   oatmeal, porridge
HAFERFLOCKEN   rolled oats, oatmeal
HAFERSCHLEIMSUPPE   boiled oats like porridge
HIRSE   millet
MAHLZEIT   meal
PERLGRAUPE   pearl barley
SEMOLINA   flour of hard durum wheat
WEIZEN   wheat

Cheese

ALLGÄUER BERGKÄSE   hard cheese from Bavaria
   resembling Emmentaler
ALLGÄUER RAHMKÄSE   mild and creamy Bavarian
   cheese
ALTENBURGER   mild, soft goat's milk cheese
APPENZELLER KÄSE   full-flavored, slightly bitter cheese
BACKSTEINKÄSE   strong-smelling and tasting cheese
CHESTERSTANGEN   cheddar cheese straws with soup
DOTTERKÄSE   skimmed milk cheese
EMMENTALER KASE   semi-hard Swiss cheese
FONDUE, NEUCHATELER ART   fondue neuchatel, with
   garlic, eggs, white wine, Swiss cheese, cherry brandy
FRÜHSTÜCKSKÄSE   a young strong cheese with smooth
   texture
GERÖSTETE KÄSESCHNITTEN (AUS)   Welsh rarebits

GREYERZER   Gruyère cheese

HALBER HAHN   cheese sandwich on whole wheat roll

HANDKÄSE   cheese from sour milk

HANDKÄSE MIT MUSIK   marinated strong-flavored cheese

HÜTTENKÄSE MIT FRÜCHTEN   cottage cheese with fruit

KÄSE   cheese

KÄSEPASTETCHEN   baked cheese accompaniment, with eggs, sour cream, grated cheese

KÄSEPLATTE   cheese platter

KÄSESALAT (AUS)   cheese salad

KÄSESPÄTZLE   cheese with spätzle

KÄSESTANGEN   cheese sticks using pastry dough, served with soup

KRÄUTERQUARK   white cheese seasoned with chopped herbs

LIMBURGER KÄSE   semi-soft, strong-smelling whole-milk cheese

MAINAUER KÄSE   semi-hard, full-cream round cheese

MONDSEER KÄSE   whole-milk yellow cheese with moist texture

QUARGEL   slightly acid and salty round cheese

QUARK (TOPFEN)   fresh white cheese, farmer's cheese

QUARKAUFLAUF   white cheese soufflé

QUARKKLÖSSE   sweet dumplings made with white cheese

REIBEKÄSE   grated cheese

SAHNEKÄSE   cream cheese

SCHICHTKÄSE   fresh white cheese

SCHMELZKÄSE   soft and pungent cheese, usually for spreading on bread

SCHMIERKÄSE   a soft, odorous cheese

SCHWEIZER KÄSE   Swiss cheese

STEINBUSCHER KÄSE   semi-hard creamy cheese; strong and slightly bitter

STREICHKÄSE   soft cheese spread

TASCHERL   pastry turnover with meat, cheese or jam
    filling
TILSITER KÄSE   semi-hard cheese, mildly pungent
TOPFEN (QUARK)   fresh white cheese, farmer's cheese
WEISSKÄSE   fresh white cheese
WILSTERMARSCHKÄSE   semi-hard cheese, similar to
    Tilsiter

Croquettes

APFELPFANNKUCHEN   apple filled pancakes, fritters
APFELSCHMARRN   egg pancake with diced apples
APFELSCHNITTCHEN   apple fritters
APFELSCHNITTEN   sliced apple fritters
ARMER RITTER   sweet fritter
BANANEN IN WEINTEIG (AUS)   banana fritters
BAYRISCHE KUCHERL (AUS)   Bavarian fritters stuffed
    with jam
BIRNENSPALTEN (AUS)   sliced pear fritters
EIERKUCHEN   pancake
EIERPFANNKUCHEN   egg pancakes
EIERPFANNKUCHEN MIT ÄPFELN   egg pancakes with
    stewed apples, sprinkled with sugar and cinnamon
EIERPFANNKUCHEN MIT KOMPOTT   egg pancakes
    with stewed fruit
EIERPFANNKUCHEN MIT SPECK   egg pancakes with
    bacon
FISCHKRUSTELN (AUS)   fish croquettes
FLADEN   pancake
FLÄDLE   thin strips of pancake added to soup
FRIKADELLE(N)   meat, fowl or fish dumpling(s) or
    croquette(s)
FRÜCHTE IN BACKTEIG (AUS)   fruit fritters
GEFÜLLTE EIERPFANNKUCHEN   filled egg pancake
GEFÜLLTE PFANNKUCHEN   filled pancakes
INDIANERKRAPFEN (AUS)   fritters with whipped cream

KAISERSCHMARREN   sweet dessert omelette served in cut up pieces

KAISERSCHMARREN MIT KOMPOTT   sweet dessert omelette served in cut up pieces with applesauce or stewed fruit

KAISERSCHMARRN   sweet dessert omelette served in cut up pieces

KARTOFFELCROQUETTEN (AUS)   potato croquettes

KARTOFFELKROKETTEN   potato croquettes

KARTOFFELKÜCHLEIN   potato pancakes

KARTOFFELPUFFER   potato fritter

KARTOFFELPUFFER MIT APFELMUS   potato pancakes with applesauce

KIRSCHPFANNKUCHEN   cherry pancakes

KRAPFEN   fritter, jelly donut

KROKETTEN   croquettes

KUCHERL   Austrian word for fritters

MANDELKROKETTEN   croquettes of potatoes and almonds

MARMELADEPALATSCHINKEN (AUS)   pancakes with jam

MAZEDONISCHE HÜHNERCROQUETTEN   chicken croquettes, gravy and mushrooms

MEHLSPEISEN   flour-based dishes like noodles, dumplings, omelette-pancakes and sweet desserts

PALATSCHINKEN   pancake filled with jam or cheese, served with hot chocolate

PFANNENGERICHTE   pan-fried pancakes

PFANNKUCHEN   pancake

PFANNKUCHEN KRAPFEN   fritters

PFANNKUCHEN MIT ANANASSCHEIBEN (AUS)   small pancakes with pineapples

PFANNKUCHEN MIT FRÜCHTEN (AUS)   small pancakes with fruit

PFANNKUCHEN MIT HASELNUSSCREME (AUS)   small pancakes with hazelnut cream

PFANNKUCHEN MIT KÄSE   pancake with cheese

PFANNKUCHEN MIT ORANGEN (AUS)   small pancakes
   with oranges
PFANNKUCHEN MIT SCHOKOLADENCREME (AUS)
   small pancakes with chocolate cream
PFANNKUCHEN MIT SPECK   pancake with bacon
PFANNKUCHEN NATUR   plain egg pancake
REIBEKUCHEN   fried potato pancakes
REISSCHMARREN   rice pancakes
RIEVKOOCHE   fried potato pancakes
SIRUP   syrup
SPECKPFANNKUCHEN   flat pancake with pieces of
   chopped bacon
SPINATPFANNKUCHEN   spinach pancakes
TRUTHAHNKROKETTEN   turkey croquettes
WAFFELN   waffles

Desserts

APFELAUFLAUF   apple soufflé
APFELBETTELMANN   apple and pumpernickel crumb
   dessert
APFELCHARLOTTE   baked apples with sliced French
   rolls, lemon juice, cinnamon, sugar, raisins
APFELKUCHEN   apple cake
APFELPFANNKUCHEN   apple-filled pancakes
APFELREIS MIT SCHNEEHAUBE   apple-rice with lemon
   peel, raisins, topped with sweetened whipped egg
   whites
APFELSTRUDEL   apple strudel, apple pastry dessert
ARMER RITTER   sweet fritter
BACKOBSTKOMPOTT   dried fruit compote
BANANEN ÜBERBACKEN MIT SCHLAGOBERS (AUS)
   banana flambé with cream
BANANEN ÜBERBACKEN MIT SCHOKOLADENSAUCE
   (AUS)   banana flambé with chocolate sauce
BANANEN ÜBERBACKEN MIT VANILLEEIS (AUS)
   banana flambé on vanilla ice

BAUMSTAMMEIS   ice cream roll dessert

BERLINER LUFT   dessert of eggs, lemon, with raspberry juice

BERLINER PFANNKUCHEN   jam filled doughnut with sprinkled sugar

BIRNE HELEN   pear poached in syrup and served with vanilla ice cream and chocolate sauce

BIRNEN ÜBERBACKEN MIT ERDBEERSAUCE (AUS)   pear flambé with strawberry sauce

BIRNENSCHNITTEN   sliced pear fritters

BISKOTT-TORTE (AUS)   cake with finger biscuits

BISKUIT LISETTE   spongecake of butter, egg yolks, sugar, coffee extract, chopped almonds

BORKENSCHOKOLADE   chocolate cut into squares and used for dessert toppings

BROTPUDDING   bread pudding

BUTTERPLÄTZCHEN   baked butter cookies with vanilla and sugar

CREME   cream or custard

CREMECARAMEL   caramel custard

CREMENESSELRODE   Madeira wine cream

CREMEPATISSIERE   cream pastry

CREMESCHNITTE   Napoleon, custard slice

CREMESCHNITTEN (AUS)   Napoleons

CREMESPEISE   custard

CREPES SUCHARD   thin dessert pancakes with chocolate sauce and chopped almonds,

CREPES SUZETTE   dessert pancakes with orange butter cream, flamed with liqueur

DAMPFNUDEL   sweet dessert dumpling with vanilla sauce

DOBOSCHTORTE   seven-layer cake with mocha cream

EIERCREME   egg custard

EIERSCHAUM   beaten egg yolks and sugar cooked together and then flavored with sweet wine

EIERSPEISE   custard

EISBOMBE   ice cream dessert

EISBECHER   ice cream dessert, may have liquor, fruit or whipped cream

EISCREME   ice cream

EISCHNEE   whipped, sweetened, egg white dessert

EISSPEZIALITÄTEN   ice cream specialties

EISTORTE   ice cream cake made with fruit, over liqueur-soaked cookies, then topped with meringue and candied fruit

ENGLISCHER KUCHEN   loaf cake

ERDBEERCREME   strawberry cream custard dessert

ERDBEEREN "ROMANOV"   strawberries with port or liqueur, covered with whipped cream

ERDBEERTORTE (AUS)   strawberry cream cake

FLAMMERI   rice or semolina pudding with stewed fruit or vanilla sauce

FLÜSSIGE SAHNE   thick cream

FRANZÖSISCHES NOUGAT   French-style nougat candy

FRÜCHTEBECHER   fruit cup with ice cream or liqueur

FRÜCHTECREME   custard made with fruit

FRUCHTEIS   fruit ices or ice cream

FRUCHTPASTETEN   fruit pies

FRUCHTPUDDING   fruit pudding

FRUCHTSAUCE   fruit sauce

FÜRST-PÜCKLER-EIS   chocolate, strawberry and vanilla ice cream with strawberries and whipped cream

GEEIST   chilled or iced

GEFRORENES   ice-cream

GEFÜLLTE ÄPFEL   apples stuffed with raisins, sugar, cinnamon, nuts, white wine

GEFÜLLTER APFEL FLAMBIERT (AUS)   stuffed apple flambé

GEFÜLLTE ÄPFEL AUS DEM ROHR (AUS)   oven-cooked stuffed apples

GEFÜLLTER KRAPFEN   filled doughnut

GELEE   aspic, jelly, jam

GERMKNÖDEL (AUS)   light yeast dumplings with butter, freshly ground poppy seeds and powdered sugar

GITTERTORTE   almond cake or tart with a raspberry topping

GLACE   ice cream

GÖTTERSPEISE   fruit jello dessert

GRIESSAUFLAUF   farina pudding

GRIESSFLAMMERI   semolina pudding

GRIESSTORTE   farina layer cake with almonds

GRÜTZE   cooked fruit or berry pudding

GUGELHUPF   coffee cake with almonds and raisins

GUGLHUPF (AUS)   light chocolate torte with center of apricot jam

HALBGEFRORENES   frozen whipped cream or ice cream dessert

HASELNUSSTORTE   hazelnut torte

HASELNUSSEIS   hazelnut ice cream

HASELNUSSCREME   hazelnut cream pudding

HASELNUSSKUCHEN MIT SCHLAG   hazelnut cake with whipped cream

HAWAII-ANANAS ÜBERBACKEN (AUS)   pineapple flambé

HEIDELBEERSCHNITTEN (AUS)   blueberry pie

HEIDELBEERSTRUDEL (AUS)   blueberry strudel

HEXENSCHNEE   chilled dessert of applesauce, apricot preserves, rum, lemon juice

HIMBEERSCHNEE   raspberry snow, a frozen dessert

HIMBEERSOUFFLE   raspberry soufflé

HIMBEERTORTE   raspberry tart

INDIANERKRAPFEN (AUS)   fritters with whipped cream

INGWERCREME   ginger cream

JOGHURT   yogurt

KAFFEECREMEROLLE   coffee cream roll

KAFFEECREMETORTE (AUS)   coffee cream cake

KAFFEEROULADE (AUS)   coffee cream roll

KAISERSCHMARREN   sweet dessert omelette served in cut up pieces

KAISERSCHMARREN MIT KOMPOTT   sweet dessert omelette served in cut up pieces with applesauce or stewed fruit

KAISERSCHMARRN   sweet dessert omelette served in cut up pieces

KANDIERTE FRÜCHTE   candied fruit

KARAMELCREME   caramel custard

KARAMELSAUCE   caramel sauce

KARTOFFELKLÖSSE MIT PFLAUMENMUS   potato dessert dumplings with prune butter filling

KÄSEKUCHEN   white cheese cheesecake

KÄSETORTE   cheesecake

KASTANIENCREME   chestnut cream

KIRSCHEN ÜBERBACKEN MIT SCHOKOLADECREME (AUS)   cherry flambé on chocolate sauce

KIRSCHSTRUDEL (AUS)   cherry strudel

KIRSCHKUCHEN (AUS)   cherry cake

KIRSCHPUDDING   cherry pudding

KIRSCHSOSSE   cherry sauce

KIRSCHTORTE   cherry tart

KOMPOTT   stewed fruit in syrup

KONDITOREI   confectioner's or pastry shop

KÖNIGSKUCHEN   loaf cake with raisins, almonds and rum

LINZER TORTE   hazelnut or almond cake or tart with raspberry jam

MANDELCREME   almond cream custard dessert

MANDELCREMETORTE (AUS)   almond cream cake

MANDELFLAMMERI   almond pudding

MANDELSAUCE   almond sauce

MARILLEN ÜBERBACKEN MIT VANILLEEIS (AUS)   apricot flambé on vanilla ice

MEHLPUT   stewed pears and dumplings

MEHLSPEISEN   flour-based dishes like noodles, dumplings, omelette-pancakes and sweet desserts

MERINGE   meringue

MILCHRAHMSTRUDEL (AUS)   white bread, eggs, sugar, milk, raisins and warm vanilla sauce

MOHNSTRIEZEL   poppy seed cake

MOHNTORTE (AUS)   poppy seed cake

MOHR IM HEMD (AUS)   moist chocolate cake covered with chocolate sauce

MOHRENKOPF   individual white cakes filled with custard or whipped cream and covered with chocolate

MÜRBTEIG   dessert pastry

NACHSPEISE, NACHTISCH   sweet dessert

NACHSPEISEN   desserts

NACHTISCH   desserts

NOUGAT   almond and chocolate paste

NOUGAT EISTORTE   an ice cream cake made with an almond and chocolate paste

NUDELAUFLAUF   noodle pudding

NUSSAUFLAUF   nut pudding soufflee

NUSS-STRUDEL   nut strudel

NUSSTORTE (AUS)   nut torte

OBSTKUCHEN   pastry or tart baked with fruit

OBSTTORTE   mixed fruit tart

ORANGENSOUFFLÉ   orange soufflé

PALATSCHINKEN   pancake filled with jam or cheese, served with hot chocolate

PARFAIT   dessert of ice cream, fruit, or syrup and whipped cream

PASTETCHEN   puff pastry patty shells

PASTETE   pastry or pie

PFEFFERNÜSSEKÜCHLEIN   spice cookies

PFIRSICH CARDINAL   poached peach in syrup with ice cream and pureed strawberry

PFIRSICH MELBA   Peach halves poached in syrup, served over vanilla ice cream, topped with raspberry sauce and whipped cream

PFIRSICHE ÜBERBACKEN MIT HASELNUSSPARFAIT (AUS)   peach flambé with hazelnut ice cream

PLÄTZCHEN   cookie, biscuit or fancy cake

POWIDLTASCHERL (AUS)   tartlets filled with plum jam

PRINZREGENTENTORTE   layer cake with chocolate butter-cream covered with chocolate

PUNSCHTORTE (AUS)   dense rum-flavored cake covered with pink icing

QUARKAUFLAUF   white cheese soufflé

RAHMCREME   creamy rum filling

RAHMSTRUDEL   cream strudel

RAUHREIF   apple and cream dessert

REIS TRAUTMANNSDORFF   fruit rice with rum, whipped cream, and stewed fruits

REISAUFLAUF MIT ÄPFELN   rice pudding with apples

ROTE GRÜTZE   fruit jelly served with cream

SACHERTORTE   chocolate layer cake with jam filling

SALZBURGER NOCKERLN   dessert of sweet dumplings, poached in milk with hot vanilla sauce

SANDDORN   flavoring from small berry

SCHAUMROLLE   puff-pastry filled with whipped cream or custard

SCHAUMSPEISE   frozen dessert with whipped cream and mousse

SCHAUMTORTE   meringue torte

SCHILLERLOCKE   pastry cone with vanilla cream filling

SCHLAGOBERS   whipped cream

SCHLAGRAHM   whipped cream

SCHLAGSAHNE   whipped cream

SCHLOTFEGER MIT SAHNE   a long pastry tube with whipped cream and chocolate

SCHOKOLADE   chocolate

SCHOKOLADECREMETORTE (AUS)   chocolate cream cake

SCHOKOLADENCREME   chocolate cream

SCHOKOLADENCREMETORTE   chocolate cream layer cake

SCHOKOLADENEIS   chocolate ice cream

SCHOKOLADENFLAMMERI   chilled chocolate pudding

SCHOKOLADENPUDDING   steamed chocolate pudding

SCHOKOLADENSAUCE   chocolate sauce

SCHOKOLADENTORTE   chocolate torte

SCHOKOLADENAUFLAUF   chocolate soufflé

SCHOKOLADENSOUFFLE (AUS) Viennese chocolate soufflé

SCHWARZWÄLDER KIRSCHTORTE Black Forest cherry cake with whipped cream

SCHWEIZER REIS sweet rice dessert

SCHWEIZER SAHNEREIS cream rice pudding

SEMMELAUFLAUF soufflé made of thin sliced rolls with almond or poppy seed

SIRUP syrup

SORBET flavored ice sherbet

SPEISEEISE ice cream or ices

SÜSSE SAUCEN sweet sauces

SÜSSIGKEIT sweet, candy

SÜSSPEISEN desserts, sweet dishes or dessert of the day

TAGESDESSERT dessert of the day

TEEBLATT oval flake pastry with sugar sprinkled on top

TOPFENOBERSTORTE (AUS) white cheese cheesecake

TÖRTCHEN small pastry dessert or tart

TRAUBENZUCKER grape sugar, dextrose

TUTTI FRUTTI mixed fruit

VANILLERAHMEIS vanilla ice cream

VANILLESOSSE vanilla sauce

VANILLEZUCKER vanilla confectioners' sugar

VANILLECREME vanilla custard with whipped cream

VANILLEEISCREME vanilla ice cream

VANILLEPUDDING vanilla pudding

VANILLESOSSE vanilla cream sauce

VOM BRETT from a pastry cart

WALNUSSTORTE walnut torte

WEINGELEE MIT FRÜCHTEN wine jelly with fruit

WEINSCHAUMCREME wine cream

WIENER ÄPFELSOUFFLÉ Viennese apple soufflé

WIENER FASCHINGSKRAPFEN (AUS) Viennese jam-filled doughnuts

WINDBEUTEL baked cream puff

ZIMT UND ZUCKER cinnamon sugar

ZITRONENCREME   lemon cream dessert
ZITRONENPUDDING   lemon pudding
ZITRONENREIS   rice pudding with lemon juice, lemon
    peel, stewed fruits
ZITRONENSOUFFLÉ   soufflé of baked egg white with
    lemon
ZUCKERMELONE   sweet melon
ZWETSCHKENSTRUDEL (AUS)   plum strudel

Dumplings

BAYERISCHE LEBERKNÖDEL   dumpling containing
    chopped liver, bacon, onion
BAYERISCHE SEMMELKNÖDEL   Bavarian bread
    dumplings
BÖHMISCHE KNÖDEL   flour dumplings cooked in salt water
DAMPFNUDEL   sweet dessert dumpling with vanilla sauce
ERDBEERKNÖDEL (AUS)   strawberry dumplings
FISCHKLÖSSE   fish dumplings
FLEISCHKLOSS   meat dumpling
FRÄNKISCHE LEBERKLÖSSE IN SPECKSAUCE   liver
    dumplings in bacon sauce
FRIKADELLE   meat, fowl or fish dumpling or croquette
FRUCHTKNÖDEL (AUS)   fruit dumplings
GEKOCHTE KARTOFFELKLÖSSE   dumplings made
    from cooked potatoes
GERMKNÖDEL (AUS)   light yeast dumplings with butter,
    freshly ground poppy seeds and powdered sugar
GRIESSKLÖSSCHEN   small semolina dumplings
GRIESSKLÖSSE   semolina dumplings
HEFEKLÖSSE   yeast dumplings
KARTOFFELKLÖSSE MIT PFLAUMENMUS   potato
    dessert dumplings with prune butter filling
KARTOFFELKLÖSSE   potato dumplings
KARTOFFELKNÖDEL   potato dumplings
KIRSCHENKNÖDEL (AUS)   cherry dumplings
KLOSS   dumpling

KLÖSSCHEN   small meat and dough dumplings
KNÖDEL   dumplings
LEBERKLÖSSE   liver dumplings
LEBERKNÖDEL   chopped liver dumplings
MARKKLÖSSCHEN   small beef marrow dumplings
MARKKLÖSSE   beef marrow dumplings
MEHLNOCKERL   small dumpling
MEHLPUT   stewed pears and dumplings
MEHLSPEISEN   flour based dishes like noodles, dumplings, omelette-pancakes and sweet desserts
NOCKERL   small dumpling
PFIRSICHKNÖDEL (AUS)   peach dumplings
PFLAUMENKNÖDEL   plum dumplings
QUARKKLÖSSE   sweet dumplings made with white cheese
SCHWEMMKLÖSSCHEN   flour dumplings
SEMMELKNÖDEL   meat and bread dumplings
SEMMELKNÖDEL MIT EIER   bread dumplings made with eggs
SEMMELKNÖDEL OHNE EI   bread dumplings without egg
SERVIETTENKNÖDEL   large bread dumpling, cooked in a napkin, flavored with onion and parsley
SPÄTZLE   small boiled flour dumplings
SPECKKNÖDEL   dumpling made with bacon
TIROLER KNÖDEL   dumplings made with bacon fat, basil, parsley, cooked in salted water
TOPFENKNÖDEL (AUS)   white cheese dumplings
WECKKLÖSSCHEN   bread dumplings
ZWETSCHGENKNÖDEL   sweet plum dumplings
ZWETSCHKENKNÖDEL (AUS)   sweet plum dumplings

Eggs

AAL MIT EIER   eggs with eel
BAUERNFRÜHSTÜCK   boiled potatoes, fried with scrambled eggs and ham

BAUERN HOPPEL-POPPEL   peasant breakfast with veal
  instead of ham or bacon
BAUERNOMELETTE   omelette with chopped bacon,
  potatoes and onions
EI   egg
EIDOTTER   egg yolk
EIER   eggs
EIER GEBACKENE   fried eggs basted in butter
EIER GEFORMTE   poached eggs in a mold
EIER GEFÜLLTE   stuffed eggs
EIER GEKOCHTE   boiled eggs in the shell
EIER HARTGEKOCHTE   hard-boiled eggs
EIER IN SENFSOSSE   eggs in mustard sauce
EIER MIT CHAMPIGNONS   eggs with mushrooms
EIER MIT EDELPILZEN   eggs with fine mushrooms
EIER MIT PFIFFERLINGEN   eggs with mushrooms
EIER MIT RÄUCHERAAL   eggs with smoked eel
EIER MIT SCHINKEN   eggs with ham
EIER MIT SPINAT   eggs with spinach
EIER NACH BAUERN ART   eggs with bacon, potatoes
  and onions
EIER NAPFEN   baked shirred eggs
EIER UND SPECK   bacon and eggs
EIER VERLORENE   poached eggs
EIER WACHSWEICHE   medium-boiled (5-6 min.)
EIER WEICHGEKOCHTE   soft-boiled (3-4 min.)
EIERAUFLAUF   egg soufflé
EIERPFANNKUCHEN   egg pancakes
EIERPFANNKUCHEN MIT ÄPFELN   egg pancakes with
  stewed apples, sprinkled with sugar and cinnamon
EIERPFANNKUCHEN MIT KOMPOTT   egg pancakes
  with stewed fruit
EIERPFANNKUCHEN MIT SPECK   egg pancakes with
  bacon
EIERSALAT   egg salad
EIERSPEISEN   egg dishes
EIERSTICH   egg cubes, used in soup

EIHÜLLE   egg-covered or batter-dipped

EINLAUF   with egg in it

EISCHNEE   beaten egg white

EIWEISS   egg white

GABACKENE EIER   eggs fried and basted in butter

GEFÜLLTE EIER   stuffed hard-cooked eggs with ham, anchovy, onion

GEKOCHTE EIER   boiled eggs

HARTGEKOCHT   hard-boiled

HOPPELPOPPEL   eggs with bacon, onions and potatoes

KAISERSCHMARREN   sweet dessert omelette served in cut up pieces

KAISERSCHMARREN MIT KOMPOTT   sweet dessert omelette served in cut up pieces with applesauce or stewed fruit

KAISERSCHMARRN   sweet dessert omelette served in cut up pieces

KALBSHIRN MIT RÜHREI   scrambled eggs with calves' brains

KRÄUTEROMELETTE   omelette with green herbs

KRÄUTEROMELETTE MIT CHAMPIGNONS   omelette with green herbs and mushrooms

LUCULLUS EIER   eggs with goose liver, truffle in various sauces

MATROSENBROT   hard, chopped egg and anchovy sandwich

MIT EIER   with egg

NORWEGISCHE EIER   poached eggs in aspic on shrimp salad with anchovy

OMELETT   omelette (German spelling)

OMELETTE   omelette (Austrian spelling)

OMELETTE GEFÜLLT   stuffed omelette

OMELETTE MIT EDELCHAMPIGNONS IN RAHM   omelette with mushrooms in cream sauce

OMELETTE MIT FEINEN KRÄUTERN   omelette with chopped parsley, chervil, tarragon and chives

OMELETTE MIT GEFLÜGELLEBER   chicken liver omelette

OMELETTE MIT GEFLÜGELRAGOUT   omelette with diced chicken in a cream sauce

OMELETTE MIT KALBFLEISCHRAGOUT   omelette with diced veal in cream sauce

OMELETTE MIT KÄSE   omelette with cheese

OMELETTE MIT KONFITÜRE   omelette with preserves

OMELETTE MIT LEBER   omelette with chopped liver

OMELETTE MIT NIEREN   omelette with sautéed kidneys

OMELETTE MIT NUDELN   omelette with noodles and a butter and cheese sauce

OMELETTE MIT PILZEN   mushroom omelette

OMELETTE MIT SAUREN NIEREN   omelette with sautéed kidneys in sour sauce

OMELETTE MIT SCALLOPS   scallop omelette

OMELETTE MIT SCHINKEN   ham omelette

OMELETTE NACH JÄGER ART   omelette with chicken livers and mushrooms in sauce

OMELETTE NATUR   plain omelette

OMELETTE SOUFFLÉ   beaten egg whites added to yolks

OMELETTE MIT SPARGEL   asparagus omelette

OMELETTE MIT TOMATEN   tomato omelette

PANIERTE EIER   eggs cooked with bread crumbs

POCHIERTE EIER   poached eggs

POCHIERTE EIER AUF TOAST MIT SCHINKEN   poached eggs on toast with ham

RÜHREIER   scrambled eggs

RÜHREIER MIT CHAMPIGNON (AUS)   scrambled eggs with mushrooms

RÜHREIER MIT HÜHNERLEBER (AUS)   scrambled eggs with chicken livers

RÜHREIER MIT SCHINKEN (AUS)   scrambled eggs with ham

RÜHREIER MIT SPARGELSPITZEN (AUS)   scrambled eggs with asparagus tips

RÜHREIER MIT SPECK   scrambled eggs with bacon

RÜHREIER MIT TRÜFFELN (AUS)   scrambled eggs with truffle

RÜHREIER MIT ZUCKERERBSEN (AUS)   scrambled eggs with green peas

RÜHREIER NATUR (EIERSPEISE) (AUS)   plain scrambled eggs

RUSSISCHE EIER   stuffed hard-boiled egg halves with mayonnaise

SCHINKENOMELETTE   ham omelette

SCHINKENOMELETTE MIT NUDELN UND KÄSE   omelette filled with noodles, cheese and ham

SPANISCHES OMELETTE   omelette with filling of sautéed tomatoes and onions

SPARGELOMELETTE   asparagus omelette

SPECKEIER (AUS)   fried eggs with bacon

SPECKPFANNKUCHEN   flat pancake with pieces of chopped bacon

SPIEGELEI   fried egg, sunny side up

SPIEGELEIER   fried eggs, sunny side up

SPIEGELEIER MIT SCHINKEN   fried eggs with ham

SPIEGELEIER MIT SPECK   fried eggs with bacon

SPINAT UND SPIEGELEI   spinach with fried eggs, sunny side up

STIERENAUGE   fried egg, sunny side up

STRAMMER MAX   sandwich with minced pork, sausage or ham with fried eggs and onions

TOMATENOMELETTE   tomato omelette

VERLORENE EIER   poached eggs

VERLORENE EIER BENEDIKT   toast with slice of ham, then poached eggs on top, covered with cream sauce

WEICH   soft, as in soft-boiled egg

Fruits and Nuts

ANANAS   pineapples

APFEL   apple

APFELMUS   applesauce

APFELRINGE   apple rings

APFELSCHEIBEN   slices of apples

APFELSINEN   oranges
APRIKOSE   apricot
BACKOBST   dried fruit
BACKOBSTKOMPOTT   dried fruit compote
BACKPFLAUME   prune
BANANEN   bananas
BEERE   berry
BIRNE HELEN   pear poached in syrup and served with
   vanilla ice cream and chocolate sauce
BIRNEN   pears
BLAUBEERE   blueberry
BRATAPFEL   baked apple
BROMBEERE   blackberry
CANTALOUP   cantaloupe
CONFITÜRE   jam
DATTEL   date
DÖRROBST   dried fruit
EINGEMACHT   preserved
ERDBEEREN   strawberries
ERDNUSS   peanut
ERRÖTENDE JUNGFRAU   raspberries and cream
ESSKASTANIE   chestnut
FEIGE   fig
FRISCHES OBST   fresh fruit
FRUCHT   fruit
FRÜCHTE DER JAHRESZEIT   fruit in season
FRUCHTSALAT   fruit salad
GEBRANNTE MANDELN   almonds in sugar glaze
GEEISTE MELONE   chilled melon
GEFÜLLTE ÄPFEL   apples stuffed with raisins, sugar,
   cinnamon, nuts, white wine
GLASIERTE KASTANIEN   chestnuts glazed in sugar and
   butter
GRANAT-APFEL   pomegranate
HASELNUSS   hazelnut
HEIDELBEERE   blueberry

HIMBEERE raspberry
HONIGMELONE honey melon
JOHANNISBEERE redcurrant
JOHANNISBEERSOSSE redcurrant jelly sauce
KANDIERTE FRÜCHTE candied fruit
KASTANIE chestnut
KASTANIENPÜREE chestnut purée
KIRSCHE cherry
KOMPOTT stewed fruit in syrup
KONFITÜRE jam
KORINTHE currant
KRONSBEEREN cranberry
MANDARINE tangerine
MANDEL almond
MANDELSPLITTER almond chips
MARILLE apricot
MARMELADE jam
MARONE chestnut
MAULBEERE mulberry
MEHLPUT stewed pears and dumplings
MELONE melon
MIRABELLE small yellow plum
MUS stewed fruit, puree, mash
NUSS nut
OBST fruit
OBSTSALAT fruit salad
OLIVEN olives
ORANGENFILETS orange sections
PAMPELMUSE grapefruit
PFEFFERNÜSSE cookies made of gingerbread dough
    shaped like nuts
PFIRSICHE peaches
PFLAUME plum
PREISELBEERE cranberry
QUITTE quince
RIBISEL red currant

RINGE   rings, wreaths, like apple rings
ROSINEN   raisins
ROTE GRÜTZE   fruit jelly served with cream
SAUERKIRSCHEN   sour cherries
SCHWARZE JOHANNISBEERE   blackcurrant
STACHELBEERE   gooseberry
TOMATEN   tomatoes
TRAUBEN   grapes
TRAUBENZUCKER   grape sugar, dextrose
TUTTI FRUTTI   mixed fruit
WALDERDBEEREN   wild strawberries
WALNUSS   walnut
WEINGELEE MIT FRÜCHTEN   wine jelly with fruit
WEINTRAUBEN   grapes
ZITRONE   lemon
ZUCKERMELONE   sweet melon
ZWETSCHGEN   plum

Game

ELCH   elk
FALSCHE REBHÜHNER   false partridge (squab)
FASAN   pheasant
FASAN GEBRATENER (AUS)   roast pheasant
FASAN IN ROTWEIN   pheasant in red wine
FASAN IM TOPF   pheasant roasted in a covered casserole
FÖRSTEREINTOPF MIT PILZEN   stew of venison, vege-
    tables, mushrooms, forester style
FRISCHLING   young wild boar
GANS   goose
GÄNSEBRATEN   roast goose
GÄNSELEBERSCHNITZEL   goose liver cutlet
GEBRATENE ENTE   roast duckling
GEBRATENER FASAN   roast pheasant
GEDÄMPFTE REHSCHLEGEL   braised leg of venison
GEFLÜGELWILD   game bird dishes

GEFÜLLTE GANS   stuffed goose
GEFÜLLTE WACHTEL IN KASSEROLLE (AUS)   stuffed quail in casserole
GEFÜLLTER FASAN   pheasant with giblet stuffing
GEGRILLTES WILDBRETFILET   broiled venison fillets
GITZI   kid
HASE   hare, jack rabbit
HASEN   large rabbit or hare
HASENTOPF IN WEISSWEIN   casserole of hare in wine
HASENBRATEN   roast hare
HASENKEULE   leg of hare
HASENLÄUFE IN JÄGERRAHMSAUCE   hare thigh in sauce of mushrooms, shallots and wine
HASENPFEFFER   marinated hare stewed in red wine, mushrooms and onions
HIRSCH   stag
HIRSCH-SCHLEGEL   leg of venison
HIRSCH-SCHULTER   shoulder of venison
HIRSCHBRATEN   roast venison
HIRSCHKALB   stag calf
HIRSCHKEULE   leg of venison
HIRSCHRAGOUT   venison stew
HIRSCH-SCHLEGEL, GEBRATEN (AUS)   roast leg of venison
HUHN   fowl, including game birds, or chicken
JÄGERSPIESS   skewered venison, broiled or sautéed in a gravy
KANINCHEN   rabbit
KEULE   leg
MASTGANSBRATEN   grain-fed roasted goose
PIKANTES REHFILET   venison tenderloin in spiced brandy sauce
REBHUHN   partridge
REBHUHN MIT WEINTRAUBEN   roast partridges with grapes
REHSCHNITZEL MIT PILZEN   venison cutlets with mushrooms

REHKEULE   deer leg
RENTIER   reindeer
RENTIERSCHINKEN   ham from reindeer leg
SCHNEPFE   snipe or woodcock
TAUBE   pigeon or dove
WACHTEL   quail
WILDBRET   venison, game
WILDBRETBRATEN   roast venison
WILDBRETKEULE   leg or thigh of venison
WILDBRETMEDALLIONS   slices of venison loin or
   tenderloin
WILDBRETPFEFFER   jugged venison, fried and braised in
   its marinade, with sour cream
WILDBRETRAGOUT   stew of venison and vegetables
WILDBRETRÜCKEN   saddle of venison
WILDBRETRÜCKEN BADEN-BADEN   baked saddle
   of venison in brown sauce with pears and redcurrant jelly
WILDBRETRÜCKEN IN ROTWEINSOSSE   roast saddle
   of venison with red wine sauce
WILDBRETRÜCKEN JÄGERMEISTER   roasted saddle of
   venison in shallot, mushroom and wine sauce
WILDENTE   wild duck
WILDGEFLÜGEL IN BURGUNDER   game birds in
   burgundy
WILDRÜCKENSTEAK   venison steak
WILDSCHWEIN   wild boar
WILDSCHWEINBRATEN   wild boar roast
WILDSCHWEINKEULE   haunch of wild boar
WILDSCHWEINRAGOUT   stew of wild boar
WILDSCHWEINRÜCKEN   saddle of wild boar
WILDSCHWEINSCHINKEN   ham from wild boar
WILDSCHWEINSCHINKEN, GERÄUCHERTER (AUS)
   smoked boar ham
WILDSCHWEINSCHNITZEL   wild boar boneless cutlet
WILDSTEAK   venison steak
WILDTAUBE   wild pigeon

Meat

AUFLAUF   soufflé of meat, fish, fowl, fruit or vegetable, oven-browned

AUFSCHNITT   cold cuts

AUFSCHNITTPLATTE   cold cut platter

BADISCHE KRAUTWICKEL   meat stuffed cabbage rolls

BAUCHFLEISCH   boiled thick slices of pork bacon

BAUERN GERÄUCHERTES   farm-cured smoked meats

BAUERN HINTERSCHINKEN   farm-style cured ham

BAUERN HOPPEL-POPPEL   peasant breakfast with veal instead of ham or bacon

BAUERNFRÜHSTUCK   breakfast consisting of eggs, bacon and potatoes

BAUERNGESELCHTES (AUS)   mixed smoked pork

BAUERNSCHINKEN   ham cured on the farm

BAUERNSCHMAUS   sauerkraut with bacon, smoked pork, sausages, dumplings or potatoes

BAYERISCHE LEBERKNÖDEL   dumpling containing chopped liver, bacon, onion

BEEFSTEAK, DEUTSCHES   fried hamburger with fried onion rings and pan-fried boiled potatoes

BEEFSTEAK TATAR   seasoned raw beefsteak, chopped onion, raw egg

BERLINER LÖFFELERBSEN   cooked with dried peas, onion, leek, pig's ear and snout, and potatoes

BERNER PLATTE   sauerkraut or beans with pork chops, bacon and beef, sausages and boiled potatoes

BEUSCHEL   heart, kidney and liver of lamb in sour sauce

BIRNENEINTOPF   smoked ham, pears, new potatoes, baked in oven

BLÄTTERTEIGPASTETE MIT FEINEM KALBSFLEISCH-RAGOUT   patty shell with diced veal in brown cream sauce

BLUTWURST   blood sausage

BOCKWURST   boiled sausage

BOHNENEINTOPF   meat and bean stew with onion, garlic, potatoes

BRATEN   roast meats

BRATEN PLATTE   plate of cold roast meats

BRATEN SÜLZE   cold roast meats in aspic

BREMER KUCHENRAGOUT   stew of chicken, sweetbreads, meat balls, mussels, asparagus, with cream sauce

BROTZEIT-TELLER   mid-morning meat and other snacks

BRUST   breast

BRUSTSTÜCK   brisket

BULETTE   meat or fishball

BÜNDNER FLEISCH   cured, dried beef

BURGUNDERSCHINKEN   ham cooked in Burgundy wine with Madeira sauce

CHAMPIGNONSCHNITZEL (AUS)   veal escalope with mushrooms

CORDON BLEU   thin veal cutlets, a slice of ham and Swiss cheese in batter, fried in butter

CORDON ROUGE   veal or beef fillet, mushrooms, chicken livers, fried in butter

DAMPFBRATEN   beef stew

DEUTSCHES BEEFSTEAK   hamburger

DOPPELTES LENDENSTÜCK   thick beef fillet

EINGEMACHTE KALBSBRUST (AUS)   boiled breast of veal

EINGEMACHTES   veal stew

EINGEMACHTES KALBFLEISCH   pickled veal

EINGEMACHTES KALBSFLEISCH   veal stew

EINGEMACHTES LAMMFLEISCH (AUS)   lamb stew

EINTOPF   meat or vegetable stew

EINTOPFGERICHT   casserole of meat and vegetables

EISBEIN   boiled pork shanks with sauerkraut and mashed potatoes

EISBEIN ASPIK   cold pork shank in aspic

EISBEIN SAUERKRAUT   pickled pig's knuckle with sauerkraut

ENTRECOTE   boneless loin steak

ENTRECOTE MIT BEARNAISE SOSSE (AUS) sirloin
steak with sauce bearnaise

ENTRECOTE MIT ZWIEBELN UND BRATKARTOFFELN
(AUS) sirloin steak with onions and home-fried
potatoes

FALSCHER HASE false rabbit, meat loaf of beef and pork

FALSCHER WILDSCHWEINBRATEN fresh ham, made
like wild boar

FASCHIERTER BRATEN meat loaf

FASCHIERTES minced meat

FASCHIERTES LAIBCHEN meat ball

FETT fat

FILLET boneless tenderloin

FILLET STROGANOFF tenerloin beef cooked in sour
cream gravy of onions and mushrooms

FILETGULASCH cubed beef fillet with onions, browned
in butter, beef stock and wine

FILETSCHEIBEN bacon, pineapple, curry, truffle sauce
on slices of beef fillet

FILETSTEAK beef tenderloin steak

FILETSTEAK á LA MEYER beef tenderloin fried in butter
with fried onion rings

FILETSTEAK MIT KRÄUTERBUTTER steak grilled and
served with creamed seasoned butter

FISCHSCHÜSSEL bacon and fish pie

FLEISCH meat

FLEISCH MIT ZWIEBELN beef sautéed with onions

FLEISCHEINTOPF beef or veal casserole dish

FLEISCHFÜLLUNG meat filling

FLEISCHGERICHTE meat dishes

FLEISCHKÄSE seasoned meat loaf

FLEISCHKLOSS meat dumpling

FLEISCHKLÖSSE meat balls

FLEISCHKÜCHLE meat ball

FLEISCHPFLANZERL pan-fried hamburger

FLEISCHRÖLLCHEN cooked stuffed meat slices served
cold

FLEISCHSALAT   meat salad

FLEISCHSPEISEN   meat dishes

FLEISCHSÜLZE   meat in aspic

FRANKFURTER   frankfurter

FRÄNKISCHE LEBERKLÖSSE IN SPECKSAUCE   liver
dumplings in bacon sauce

FRIKADELLE(N)   pan-fried croquette(s) of meat, fowl or fish

FRIKASSEE   stew of browned meat or poultry cooked in
stock

FRÜHSTÜCKSSPECK   smoked breakfast bacon

FÜLLUNG   stuffing

GARNIERTES STEAK   garnished steak

GEBACKENE KALBSBRUST   fried breast of veal

GEBACKENE LEBER   fried liver

GEBACKENE ZUNGE   fried tongue

GEBACKENES HIRN   baked brains

GEBACKENES SCHWEINSKOTELETT   fried breaded or
unbreaded pork chop

GEBRATENE KALBSLEBER   calf's liver with apples and
onion rings

GEBRATENE LAMMKEULE   roast leg of lamb

GEBRATENE LEBER   fried liver

GEBRATENE SCHWEINSHAXE   roasted pork shank

GEBRATENES HAMMELKARREE (AUS)   roast mutton
chop

GEBRATENES LAMM   roast lamb

GEBRATENES SCHWEINSKOTELETTE MIT ÄPFELN
chops with apples

GEDÄMPFTE KALBSBRUST   breast of veal potted with
onions

GEDÄMPFTE RINDERBRUST   potted beef with natural
gravy

GEDÄMPFTER RINDSBRATEN   pot roast of beef with
wine

GEDÜNSTETE SCHWEINSKOTELETT (AUS)   braised
pork cutlet

GEDÜNSTETER PARADEISRINDSBRATEN (AUS)
  braised beef with tomatoes
GEDÜNSTETER RINDSSAFTBRATEN (AUS) braised
  beef in gravy
GEDÜNSTETES RINDSSCHNITZEL IN ROTWEIN (AUS)
  braised steak with red wine
GEFÜLLTE KALBSBRUST stuffed breast of veal
GEFÜLLTE PAPRIKA peppers stuffed with beef, pork,
  rice, in tomato sauce
GEFÜLLTE ZWIEBELN meat stuffed onions
GEFÜLLTER KRAUTKOPF cabbage stuffed with beef,
  pork and onion
GEHACKTES RINDERSCHNITZEL fried beef patties
GEKOCHTE RINDERBRUST boiled brisket of beef
GEKOCHTER SCHINKEN boiled ham
GEKOCHTES FLEISCH boiled beef
GEKOCHTES OCHSENFLEISCH boiled beef
GEKOCHTES RINDFLEISCH (AUS) boiled beef
GEKOCHTES SCHWEINEFLEISCH pork and greens
GEMISCHTER AUFSCHNITT mixed cold cuts
GEPÖKELTE RINDERBRUST MIT SAUERKRAUT boiled
  pickled beef breast with sauerkraut
GERÄUCHERTER SCHINKEN smoked ham
GERÄUCHERTES smoked meats, especially bacon and
  ham
GERÖSTET fried
GESALZENES SCHWEINEFLEISCH salt pork
GESCHMORTE SCHWEINSHAXE pot-roasted pork
  shank
GESCHNETZELTES meat cut into thin, small slices
GESCHNETZELTES IN RAHM meat cut into thin, small
  slices in cream sauce
GESCHNETZELTES NACH SCHWEIZER ART meat
  fried in brown sauce with white wine and sour cream
GESCHNETZELTES NACH ZIGEUNER ART meat fried
  in brown sauce with peppers, paprika and mushrooms

GESELCHTES   cured and smoked pork

GESPICKT   holes in meat filled with pork fat

GEWÜRZTE SCHWEINSRIPPCHEN   braised spicy pork spareribs

GLASIERT   glazed, as ham, carrots or chestnuts

GNAGI   cured pig's knuckle

GRILLHAXE   grilled shank

GRILLTELLER   plate of various cuts of grilled meats

GULASCH   meat braised in sauce with vegetables and paprika

GUT DURCHGEBRATEN   well-done

HACKBRATEN   chopped steak or meat loaf of beef and pork

HACKBRATEN MIT SPECK   meatloaf with diced smoked bacon

HACKBRATEN NACH HAUSMANNS-ART   large hamburger or slices of meat loafs

HACKFLEISCH   minced meat

HACKRAHMSTEAK   hamburger with thick brown gravy

HACKSPIESSCHEN ZIGEUNER ART   meat balls on a skewer with peppers, tomatoes and onion

HACKSTEAK   beef hamburger

HAMMEL   mutton

HAMMEL BOURGEOISE   potted mutton

HAMMELBRATEN   roast mutton

HAMMELFLEISCH   lamb and mutton meat

HAMMELFLEISCH MIT BOHNEN (AUS)   stewed mutton with beans

HAMMELFLEISCH MIT GRÜNEN BOHNEN   potted lamb and green beans

HAMMELFLEISCHEINTOPF   lamb stew with breast of lamb, potatoes, caraway seeds, bacon

HAMMELKEULE   leg of mutton

HAMMELKOTELETTEN   mutton or lamb chops

HAMMELKOTELETTEN IN ZWIEBELSOSSE   lamb chops in onion sauce

HAMMELRAGOUT   mutton ragout or stew

HAMMELREISFLEISCH IN PAPRIKASCHOTEN braised
mutton with peppers, served on rice

HAMMELSCHLEGEL thigh of mutton

HAMMELSCHULTER MIT WEISSEN RÜBEN shoulder
of mutton with red turnips

HAMMELSTEAK mutton steak

HASCHEE hash

HAUSGESELCHTES smoked pork

HAXE shank of leg

HAXE MIT SAUERKRAUT pigs' knuckles and sauerkraut

HEIDSCHNUCKENKEULE leg of lamb

HEIDSCHNUCKENKEULE IN WACHOLDERRAHM
lamb in juniper berry sauce

HERZ heart

HERZ-LEBER-NIERENSPIESSCHEN heart, liver and
kidney grilled on skewer

HIRN brains

HIRN IN BRAUNER BUTTER brains in brown butter

HIRN MIT RÜHREI calves' brains with scrambled eggs

HIRTENSTEAK veal steak

HOHE RIPPE roast ribs of beef

HOLSTEIN SCHNITZEL pan fried veal cutlet with fried
egg and anchovies

HOLSTEINER SCHNITZEL veal cutlets served with fried
eggs and anchovies

HUBERTUS SCHNITZEL butter fried veal cutlet with
wine, shallot and mushroom sauce

HÜFT STEAK top sirloin steak, beef or veal

HUSARENFLEISCH braised beef, veal and pork, sweet
peppers, onions and sour cream

JÄGER SCHNITZEL veal cutlet with wine, mushroom
and tomato sauce

JÄGEREINTOPF beef stew with onions, mushrooms,
potatoes

JÄGERSCHNITZEL MIT PFIFFERLINGEN fried veal
cutlet, sauce of mushrooms, shallots, wine, tomato

JÄGERTOPF   casserole or stew, of meat, mushrooms, tomato sauce, shallots

JUNGER SCHWEINERÜCKEN   roasted young pig's back, loin or saddle

JUNGFERNBRATEN   roast pork with bacon

KALB   veal

KALB GEGRILLTES   grilled veal

KALBFLEISCH   veal meat

KALBFLEISCH, GESHACKTES   ground veal

KALBFLEISCH NACH BERLINER-ART   veal fried in butter with onion rings and apples

KALBFLEISCH NACH JÄGERART   veal fried in butter with mushrooms, shallots, wine, tomato paste

KALBFLEISCHBÄLLCHEN   veal meat balls

KALBFLEISCHKLÖSSCHEN   veal meat balls with onions, poached in stock

KALBFLEISCHRAGOUT   pieces of veal in brown sauce

KALBFLEISCHSCHNITTE RAHMSAUCE   veal slices in gravy with cream

KALBFLEISCHVOGEL   veal scallops in anchovy cream gravy

KALBSBRATEN   cold cooked veal roast

KALBSBRATWÜRSTCHEN, ABGEBRÄUNTE   grilled or pan-fried veal sausages

KALBSBRIES   veal sweetbread

KALBSBRIES IN WEISSWEIN   calf sweetbreads poached in wine

KALBSBRUST   breast of veal

KALBSBRUST, GEFÜLLTE   breast of veal, stuffed with chicken livers or ham

KALBSBRÜSTCHEN   sweetbreads

KALBSFILLET   veal tenderloin or fillet steak

KALBSFRIKASSEE   veal fricassee

KALBSFÜSSE   calves' feet

KALBSGESCHNETZELTES   veal slices cooked in brown sauce

KALBSGOULASCH   braised pieces of veal with seasonings

KALBSGULASCH (AUS)   veal goulash

KALBSHAXE   veal hocks or shanks

KALBSHAXE, GEBRATENE   baked or roasted veal shanks or hocks

KALBSHAXE IN GEWÜRZGURKENSOSSE   veal shanks in pickle sauce

KALBSHAXE, KNUSPRIGE   crispy roasted veal shank

KALBSHERZ   broiled or baked veal heart

KALBSHIRN   calves' brains

KALBSHIRN MIT RÜHREI   scrambled eggs with calves' brains

KALBSKÄSE   veal meat loaf with cheese

KALBSKOPF   calves' head, boiled, boned, batter-dipped and deep-fried

KALBSKOTELETT, GEBACKEN, GEBRATEN, GEGRILLT (AUS)   veal cutlet, fried, roast, grilled

KALBSKOTELETTEN, NATURELL   plain veal chops

KALBSLEBER   calves' liver

KALBSLEBER, GEBRATENE   fried, breaded calves' liver

KALBSLEBER MIT SPECK   calf's liver with bacon

KALBSLEBERWURST   liverwurst made of veal

KALBSLENDCHEN   veal loin

KALBSLUNGE   calf's lungs

KALBSMEDALLIONS   veal leg slices

KALBSMILCH   sweetbreads

KALBSNIERENBRATEN   veal with kidney

KALBSNIERENSTÜCK   loin of veal

KALBSNÜSSCHEN   roasted veal sirloin

KALBSRAGOUT MIT GEMÜSE (AUS)   veal stew with vegetables

KALBSRAHMBRATEN   veal with sweet or sour cream sauce

KALBSRIPPCHEN   veal chop

KALBSROLLBRATEN   stuffed rolled veal slices
KALBSRÜCKEN   back of veal
KALBSSAFTGOULASCH   very liquid veal stew
KALBSSCHLEGEL   veal leg
KALBSSCHNITZEL   veal cutlet
KALBSSCHNITZEL, GRILLIERTES   grilled veal cutlet
KALBSSCHNITZEL MIT SARDELLEN   cutlet in sauce
   with anchovies
KALBSSCHNITZEL NATUR MIT CHAMPIGNONS UND
   RAHMSOSSE   cutlet natural, with mushrooms and
   cream sauce
KALBSSCHNITZEL PRINZESS   cutlet in mushroom sauce
   with potato croquettes and asparagus
KALBSSCHNITZEL RUSSISCH   fried cutlet with mush-
   rooms and tomatoes in cream sauce
KALBSSCHNITZEL, WIENER   cutlet breaded and fried in
   lard
KALBSSCHULTER   veal shoulder
KALBSSTEAK   veal steak
KALBSVOGERL   stuffed cutlets, pot-roasted with vege-
   tables in wine
KALDAUNEN   tripe
KALTE KALBSLENDE   cold loin of veal
KALTER AUFSCHNITT   cold cuts
KASSELER RIPPENSPEER   roasted smoked pork chops
   with sauerkraut
KASSELER RIPPESPEER   roasted smoked pork chops
   with sauerkraut
KASSELER SAFTRIPPE   pickled smoked pork loin chop
KASSLER RIPPCHEN MIT SAUERKRAUT   smoked pork
   chops with sauerkraut
KATENRAUCHSCHINKEN   country-style smoked ham
KATENRAUCHSPECK IN PAPRIKA   paprika covered,
   cottage smoked bacon
KATENSCHINKEN   cottage-cured ham
KATENWURST   country-style smoked sausage

KATZENJAMMER   cold beef slices in mayonnaise with cucumbers

KESSELFLEISCH   boiled pork served with vegetables

KESSELGOULASCH   goulash of pork meat

KEULE   leg

KIMBURGER KOTELETTE   breaded and fried ground pork and veal cutlet

KITZ   kid, young goat

KLOPS   meatball

KLUFTSTEAK   rumpsteak

KNOCHEN   bone

KNOCHENSCHINKEN   cured ham on the bone

KOHLROULADE   meat-stuffed cabbage

KOHLROULADE IN RAHMSOSSE   stuffed cabbage leaves in cream sauce

KÖNIGSBERGER KLOPS   poached meat balls in lemon and caper sauce

KOPFSÜLZE   pork head-cheese in aspic

KOTELETT IN ASPIK   smoked pork chop in aspic

KOTELETTE   veal rib chop, pork loin chop

KRAINER   spiced pork sausage

KRÄUTERSTEAK   steak topped with herb butter

KRAUTFLEISCH (AUS)   pork with sauerkraut

KRENFLEISCH   pork stew with vegetables and horse-radish

KÜCHENRAGOUT   sweetbreads stew with green peas, mussels and a cream sauce

LABSKAUS   dish of meat, fish, and potatoes

LABSKAUSE   dish of meat, fish, and potatoes

LAMMBRATEN   roast leg of lamb

LAMMCHOP, GEBRATEN, GEGRILLT (AUS)   lamb chop, roast, grilled

LAMMFLEISCH   lamb

LAMMGERICHT, IRISCHES   Irish lamb stew

LAMMGULASCH (AUS)   lamb goulash

LAMMKOTELETT VOM ROST   broiled lamb chop

LAMMKOTELETTS   lamb cutlets
LAMMKRONE   crown roast of lamb
LAMMRÜCKEN   roast shoulder of lamb
LAMMSCHLEGEL   leg of lamb
LAMMSCHULTER   shoulder of lamb
LEBER   liver
LEBER NACH BERLINER-ART   calf's liver, fried, served
   covered with fried onions and apples
LEBERKÄSE   cold or hot meat loaf of liver, pork and
   bacon
LEBERKLÖSSE   liver dumplings
LEBERKLÖSSE, FEINE   liver patties made with onion
LEBERKNÖDEL   chopped liver dumplings
LEBERPRESSACK   pressed liver meatloaf
LEBERRAGOUT BOMBAY   liver in curry sauce
LEBERSCHEIBEN   sliced liver
LEBERSPÄTZLE   thick round liver noodles
LENDEN   loin
LENDENBRATEN   roast tenderloin
LENDENGOULASCH   braised fillet in thick gravy
LENDENSCHNITTEN   tenderloin slices
LENDENSTEAK   beef tenderloin
LENDENSTEAK ESPAGÑOL   fried with onions, rice,
   stuffed tomatoes, sherry, gravy
LENDENSTEAK MIRABEAU   grilled tenderloin with
   anchovies, olives
LENDENSTEAK NATUR   plain fried steak
LENDENSTEAK VIKTORIA   sautéed steak, chicken
   croquette and fried tomato
LENDENSTEAK WESTMORELAND   braised steak in
   tomato sauce with pickles and capers
LUNGE   light (lung of an animal)
MAGER   lean or thin
MAGERER SPECK   lean bacon
MAILÄNDER SCHNITZEL   breaded veal cutlet with
   cheese, butter, fried with mushrooms and tongue

MAILÄNDER STEAK   breaded and butter-fried veal steak

MAINZER RIPPCHEN   pork chop

MAKKARONI MIT SCHINKEN   macaroni and ham

MARK   bone marrow

MARKKLÖSSE   beef marrow dumplings

MAST   grain-fed meat

MASTKALBS   grain-fed calf

MASTOCHSE   grain-fattened steer beef

MASTOCHSENLENDE   grain-fattened tenderloin or fillet

MASTOCHSENFLEISCH   boiled fattened beef

MAULTASCHE, SCHWÄBISCHE   ravioli with chopped meat, brains, spinach in a sauce

METTWURST   spiced and smoked pork sausage spread on bread

MILZWURST   sausage made of veal spleen

MÜNSTERLÄNDER TÖPFCHEN   spicy stew of calf's head

MUSTEWECKE   bread filled with chopped pork

NATURSCHNITZEL   sautéed veal chops

NIERCHEN SAUER   braised kidneys in sweet-sour sour-cream sauce

NIEREN   kidneys

NIERENBRATEN   roast loin of veal with kidneys

NIERENSTÜCK   loin

OCHSE   ox or bull

OCHSENBRATEN   roast beef

OCHSENFLEISCH   beef

OCHSENFLEISCH GEKOCHT   boiled beef

OCHSENLENDE   fillet of beef

OCHSENMARK   beef marrow

OCHSENNIERE   beef kidney

OCHSENSCHWANZ   oxtail

OCHSENSCHWANZEINTOPF   oxtail stew with vegetables

OCHSENSCHWANZRAGOUT   braised ox-tail stew

OCHSENZUNGE   ox tongue

OCHSENZUNGE IN MADEIRA   ox tongue in wine sauce

OCHSENZUNGENTASCHEN   cold sliced tongue rolls
with horseradish sauce inside

PANHAS   mixture of ground meat, buckwheat and gravy

PANIERTE KALBSSCHNITZEL   breaded veal cutlets

PANIERTE KOTELETT   breaded pork chops

PAPRIKASCHNITZEL   veal cutlet floured with paprika,
fried, with sour cream sauce

PAPRIKAGULASCH   beef goulash in sour cream sauce
with paprika

PAPRIKARAHMSCHNITZEL   veal cutlets with bell
peppers in sour cream sauce and paprika

PAPRIKASCHNITZEL   veal cutlet with bell peppers

PASTETE, GEFÜLLT MIT FEINEM RAGOUT   patty shell
filled with diced veal in mushroom and wine cream sauce

PASTETE KAPUZINERART   a delicate meat stew served
in a patty shell

PFEFFERPOTTHAST   spicy meat and onion casserole

PFEFFERSCHWEINEBRATEN   spiced or peppered pork
stew

PFEFFERSTEAK   steak fried with ground peppercorns

PFEFFERSTEAK FLAMBIERT   peppercorn fried steak
flamed with brandy

PICHELSTEINER   mixed meat and vegetable casserole

PIKANTE HAMMELSCHULTER   braised lamb shoulder
with mustard and red wine sauce

PIKANTES HERZ TÖPFLE   casserole of veal heart in
seasoned brown gravy

PIKANTES SCHNITZEL   veal cutlet in spicy sauce

PÖKELFLEISCH   marinated meat

PÖKELZUNGE   pickled tongue

PÖKELZUNGE IN MADEIRA   served hot in Madeira
sauce

PRAGER STEAK   fried veal steak, scrambled eggs and
chopped ham with brown gravy

RAGOUT DEUTSCH   beef and vegetable stew

RAGOUT-FIN   diced veal, tongue, brains, in a cream
  sauce with mushrooms and wine
RAGOUT-FIN IN MUSCHELN   stew of ox tongue, sweet-
  bread, mushrooms, anchovies, wine, grated cheese,
  baked in shells
RAHMSCHNITZEL   veal cutlet fried in lemon juice with
  sour cream sauce
RAHMHACKBRATEN   slices of meat loaf slices in brown
  gravy
RÄUBERFLEISCHSPIESS   corn-fed pork broiled on a
  skewer
RÄUCHERSCHINKEN   smoked ham
RÄUCHERSPECK   smoked bacon
RAUCHFLEISCH   smoked meat
REGENSBURGER   highly spiced and smoked sausage
REISFLEISCH   veal braised with rice
REISRAND TOULOUSER ART   stew filled rice ring with
  sweetbreads, kidneys, truffles and mushrooms
RIND, GEPÖKELT   pickled beef tongue
RIND OR RINDER   beef
RINDERBRATEN   beef roast
RINDERBRUST   brisket of beef
RINDERGULASCH   beef goulash
RINDERMARK   beef marrow
RINDERROULADE   filled beef roll
RINDERROULADE BURGUNDER ART   beef slices stuffed
  with bacon, pickle, anchovies, onions, sautéed in gravy
RINDERROULADEN   stewed beef rolls
RINDERSAFTBRATEN   beef pot roast
RINDERSCHMORBRATEN   beef pot roast
RINDERZUNGE IN MADEIRA   boiled beef tongue in
  Madeira sauce
RINDFLEISCH   beef
RINDFLEISCH À LA MODE   beef pot roast
RINDFLEISCH IN MEERRETTICHTUNKE   boiled beef
  with horseradish sauce

RINDFLEISCH IN SCHNITTLAUCHSOSSE   boiled beef with chive sauce

RINDFLEISCHSALAT   beef strips with spicy vinegar dressing

RINDFLEISCHSALAT (AUS)   beef salad

RIPPCHEN   smoked rib loin pork chop

RIPPCHEN MIT SAUERKRAUT   spareribs and sauerkraut

RIPPE   rib

RIPPENSTÜCK   ribs of beef

ROASTBEEF MIT WÜRSTCHEN   roast beef with sausages

ROASTBEEFRÖLLCHEN   cold roast beef roll

ROH   raw

ROHER SCHINKEN   uncooked ham

ROSENSPITZ   top sirloin veal steak

ROST   grill, broiler

ROSTBRATEN   rumpsteak

ROSTBRATEN HELGOLÄNDER ART   fried steak on toast with tomato strips and Hollandaise sauce

ROSTBRATEN JÄGER ART   fried steak with bacon, vegetables and wine in a sauce of pan juices

ROSTBRATEN, SCHWÄBISCHER   braised in vegetables and a brown sauce

ROSTBRATEN, WIENER   fried in butter and covered with fried onions

ROSTBRATEN, ZIGEUNER   braised with bacon and onions or fried with cabbage and potatoes

ROSTBRATWÜRSTE   pork sausages

ROULADE   thin slices of beef, stuffed, rolled and braised

ROULADEN   braised stuffed slice of meat

ROULADENFÜLLUNG   ground meat stuffing of roulade

RÜBENEINTOPF   turnip stew with breast of lamb, tomatoes and beef stock

RÜCKEN   saddle, usually mutton

RUMPSTEAK   cut from bottom round beef steak

RUMPSTEAK MIRABEAU   fried with anchovies and olives

RUMPSTEAK PROVENCIAL fried with tomatoes, mushrooms, and garlic flavored tomato sauce

RUMPSTEAK RUSSLAND with mushrooms, pickles, onions in brown sauce or horseradish

RUNDSTÜCK, WARM hot roast meat open-faced sandwich with gravy

SAFTBRATEN beef pot roast in lots of liquid

SAFTGOULASCH veal stew with lots of gravy

SAFTSCHINKEN juicy boiled ham

SAITENWURST variety of frankfurter sausage

SALZFLEISCH salted meat

SAUERBRATEN marinated pot roasted beef with herbs

SAUERBRATEN MIT ROTKOHL pot roast with red cabbage

SAUERFLEISCH sour spiced pork

SAURE LEBER liver in brown gravy

SAURE LEBER UND NIEREN liver and kidney with a sour vinegar sauce

SAURE NIEREN spiced kidneys

SCHARFER FLEISCHEINTOPF spicy casserole of veal or beef in brown gravy

SCHARFES TÖPFCHEN very spicy casserole of veal or beef

SCHASCHLIK meat, kidneys, tomatoes, onions, bacon grilled on a skewer then braised in spicy sauce

SCHASCHLIK KAUKASISCHES marinated lamb, veal or beef grilled on a skewer with onions, peppers and tomato

SCHINKEN ham

SCHINKEN IN BROTTEIG smoked ham in baked shell

SCHINKEN IN BURGUNDER ham braised in burgundy

SCHINKENBROT open-faced ham sandwich

SCHINKENFÜLLUNG chopped ham stuffing

SCHINKENHAXE ham shanks

SCHINKENPASTETE ham pie containing pork, veal, onion, Madeira wine

SCHINKENRÖLLCHEN   rolled ham slices with or without filling

SCHINKENSTREIFEN   ham strips

SCHINKENWURST   ham pieces in pork baloney filling, eaten cold

SCHLACHTPLATTE   meat, liver sausage and sauerkraut plate

SCHLEGEL   leg

SCHLESISCHES HIMMELREICH   roast pork or goose with dumplings

SCHMORBRATEN   pot roast

SCHMORBRATEN IN EIGENEM SAFT   pot roast in a rich white or brown sauce

SCHMORBRATEN MIT CHAMPIGNONS   pot roast braised with mushrooms

SCHMORBRATEN MIT KALBSBRIES, NIEREN UND TRÜFFEL   stew with calf sweetbreads, kidneys, truffles and mushrooms in brown sauce

SCHMORBRATEN MIT PILZEN   pot roast braised with mushrooms

SCHMORFLEISCH   stew meat

SCHNITZEL   cutlet

SCHNITZEL, HOLSTEINER   veal cutlets served with fried eggs and anchovies

SCHNITZEL IN SARDELLENSOSSE   butter-fried veal cutlet in anchovy sauce

SCHNITZEL NACH JÄGER ART   veal cutlet with wine, mushroom and tomato sauce

SCHNITZEL, MAILÄNDER   breaded veal cutlet with cheese, butter-fried with mushrooms and tongue

SCHNITZEL NATUR   pan-fried veal cutlet

SCHNITZEL PIKANT   veal cutlet in spicy sauce

RAHMSCHNITZEL   veal cutlet fried in lemon juice with sour cream sauce

SCHNITZEL NACH ZIGEUNER ART   veal cutlet sautéed in tomato sauce with pickled tongue, peppers, mushrooms, in a cream gravy with paprika

SCHNITZELEINTOPF   bottom round stew with onion, carrots, potatoes, cream

SCHULTER   shoulder

SCHWÄBISCHER JÄGERBRATEN   roast pork in brown sauce with mushrooms

SCHWÄBISCHES KOTELETT   simmered in sour cream sauce with little dumplings

SCHWARZ-GERÄUCHERTES   dark-smoked ham or pork pieces

SCHWARZWÄLDER SCHINKEN   Black Forest smoked ham

SCHWEIN   pork

SCHWEINEBAUCH   boiled thick bacon slices

SCHWEINEBRATEN   roast pork

SCHWEINEBRUST   pork breast

SCHWEINEFILLET   fillet of pork

SCHWEINEFLEISCH   pork meat

SCHWEINEFLEISCH IN TEIG   pork and other meats in a loaf

SCHWEINEFLEISCH MIT SAUERKRAUT   pork and sauerkraut

SCHWEINEKOTELETT   pork chop

SCHWEINEKOTELETT DREIERLEI   breaded chops

SCHWEINEKOTELETT MIT PFEFFER   spicy pork stew

SCHWEINEKOTELETT MIT SENF ODER MEERRETTICH   chops with mustard or horseradish

SCHWEINEKOTELETT NACH MÜNCHNER ART   fried or braised pork chop

SCHWEINEKOTELETT NACH ZIGEUNER ART   fried pork chop with peppers, fried onions, tomatoes, pickle, cayenne pepper in a brown sauce

SCHWEINEKOTELETT, NATUR   plain fried pork chop

SCHWEINEKOTELETT, PANIERT   fried breaded pork chop

SCHWEINEKOTELETT, UNGARISCH   fried pork chop sprinkled with paprika

SCHWEINEKOTELETT VOM ROST   broiled pork chop or cutlet

SCHWEINELEBER   pork liver
SCHWEINELEBER, SAUERE   pork liver fried with onions
   then braised in vinegar and lemon juice
SCHWEINELENDCHEN   pork tenderloin or fillet
SCHWEINELENDCHEN UNGARISCH   pork tenderloin
   browned then braised in paprika sauce
SCHWEINENACKEN   pork neck and back
SCHWEINENIEREN   pork kidneys
SCHWEINEPRESSACK   pork meat loaf
SCHWEINERAGOUT   pork ragout or stew
SCHWEINERIPPCHEN   pork spare ribs
SCHWEINERIPPCHEN MIT GEWÜRZGURKENSOSSE
   pork spareribs with pickle sauce
SCHWEINEROLLBRATEN   rolled pork roast
SCHWEINERÜCKEN   pork back
SCHWEINESCHNITZEL   pork cutlet or thin steak
SCHWEINESCHNITZEL, GEBRATENES   fried pork cutlet
SCHWEINESCHNITZEL IN SAHNESOSSE   fried pork
   cutlet in a creamy sauce
SCHWEINESCHNITZEL, PANIERTES   fried, breaded
   pork cutlet
SCHWEINESCHULTER   pork shoulder
SCHWEINESTEAK   thin pork steak or cutlet
SCHWEINESTEAK MIRABEAU   pork cutlet fried with
   anchovies and green olives
SCHWEINESTEAK NACH METZGERIN ART   pork
   cutlet buttered, coated with bread crumbs and fried
SCHWEINEWAMMERL, GESOTTENES   simmered pork
   belly slices
SCHWEINSFÜSSE   pig's feet
SCHWEINSHAXE   roast pork leg
SCHWEINSHAXE BÜRGERLICH   roasted pork leg with
   onions and carrots
SCHWEINSHIRN   pork brains
SCHWEINSKARREE   roasted pork squares
SCHWEINSKEULE   beer steamed pork leg

SCHWEINSKOTELETT À LA WESTMORELAND   fried pork chop with peppers, cauliflower, dill pickles, pearl onions, carrot, asparagus, string beans

SCHWEINSKOTELETT, KNACKWURST UND KARTOFFELN   chops with knockwurst and potatoes

SCHWEINSLEBERKÄSE   liver, pork, bacon meatloaf

SCHWEINSOHREN   pigs' ears

SCHWEINSROULADEN   pork rolls

SCHWEIZER SCHNITZEL, CORDON BLEU   pork cutlets with ham and Swiss cheese between, breaded and fried

SELCHFLEISCH   smoked pork

SELCHKARREE   smoked pork

SEMMELKNÖDEL   meat and bread dumplings

SERBISCHES REISFLEISCH   veal braised with onions, garlic, tomato puree, with rice

SERBISCHES TÖPFCHEN   beef or veal casserole with paprika

SIEDFLEISCH   boiled meat

SPANFERKEL   suckling pig

SPANFERKEL KÖPFERL   suckling pig head

SPANFERKELSPIESS   suckling pig roasted on a spit

SPANFERKELLEBER, GERÖSTETE   grilled suckling pig liver

SPANFERKELLEBERSPIESS   spit roasted suckling pig liver

SPECK   bacon

SPIESS   on a skewer

STELZE   knuckle of pork

STOTZEN   leg, haunch

SULPERKNOCHEN   pig's ears, tail, with sauerkraut and peas

SÜLZKOTELETTEN   pork chops in aspic

SUPPENFLEISCH   boiled beef, soup meat

SZEGEDINER GOULASCH   lard browned pork cubes braised in onions, then stewed with sauerkraut

TASCHERL   pastry turnover with meat, cheese or jam filling

TATAR   raw spiced minced beef

TATARENBROT   open faced sandwich of raw, spiced, minced beef

TELLERFLEISCH   boiled pork or boiled beef

TÖPFCHEN   beef or veal casserole dish

TOULOUSER SCHMORBRATEN   stew with calf sweetbreads, kidneys, truffles and mushrooms in brown sauce

TOURNEDOS   slices of steak fillet

TOURNEDOS CHATELEINE   beef fillet on stuffed artichoke bottoms in wine sauce with chestnuts and potatoes

TOURNEDOS ROSSINI   beef fillet on toast with goose liver and wine sauce

UNGARISCHE PAPRIKASCHOTEN   stuffed peppers with rice and ground beef in tomato sauce

UNGARISCHES GEPÖKELTES FLEISCH   Hungarian pickled veal

VOM HAMMEL   mutton main dishes

VOM KALB   veal main dishes

VOM LAMM   lamb main dishes

VOM RIND   beef main dishes

VOM SCHWEIN   pork main dishes

VORESSEN   meat stew

WAMMERL   home-smoked bacon

WECKEWERK   pork meat and skin mixed with bread and fried

WEISSWURST   veal sausage

WELLFLEISCH   boiled pork

WESTFÄLISCH PFEFFERPOTTHAST   beef short ribs with spicy sauce

WESTFÄLISCHER SCHINKEN   cured raw Westphalian ham

WIENER   from Vienna

WIENER GOULASCH   beef stew with onions

WIENER RAHMBEUSCHERL   calf's lung braised in cream sauce with anchovies

WIENER RAHMSCHLEGEL   pork leg with cream sauce

WIENER SCHNITZEL   breaded veal cutlet
WIENER ZWIEBELROSTBRATEN   fried steak with fried
  onions on top
WURST   sausage
WURSTPLATTE   platter of assorted sausages
WURSTSPEISEN   pork products
WURZFLEISCH   beef in spiced sour cream sauce
ZIEGE   goat
ZIGEUNERROSTBRATEN   braised ribsteak with bacon,
  cabbage and potatoes
ZIGEUNERSCHNITZEL   sautéed in tomato sauce with
  pickled tongue, peppers, mushrooms, in cream gravy
  with paprika
ZIGEUNERSPIESS   pork tenderloin broiled on a skewer
  with vegetables
ZIGEUNERSTEAK   fried beef or veal steak with mush-
  rooms, peppers, onions, pickles, chopped ham in sauce
ZUNGE   tongue
ZUNGENRAGOUT   tongue ragout or stew
ZUNGENRAGOUT MARENGO   braised tongue in oil,
  tomatoes, white wine, button mushrooms and onions
ZUNGENSTREIFEN   tongue strips
ZWIEBELFLEISCH NACH MÜNCHNER ART   thin beef
  slices sautéed in fried onions
ZWIEBELROSTBRATEN   fried club steak with fried onions

Pasta

BUTTERNUDELN   buttered noodles
EIERNUDELN   egg noodles
EIERSPÄTZLE   thick egg noodles
EIERTEIGWAREN   pastas, macaronis, spaghetti
FADENNUDEL   thin noodle
FLEISCHBRÜHE MIT MAULTASCHEN   pasta envelopes
  filled with meat in clear soup
KNÖPFLI   thick noodle
MAKKARONI   macaroni

MAKKARONI MIT SCHINKEN   macaroni and ham
MAULTASCHE   ravioli filled with meat and vegetables
MAULTASCHE SCHWÄBISCH   ravioli with chopped
 meat, brains, spinach in a sauce
MEHLSPEISEN   flour-based dishes like noodles, dump-
 lings, omelette-pancakes and sweet desserts
NUDEL   noodle
NUDELTOPF MIT HUHN UND SPARGEL   chicken and
 noodle casserole with asparagus
RAVIOLI IN TOMATENTUNKE   square pasta filled with
 cheese or meat in tomato sauce
RIEBELE   noodles
SCHNUPFNUDEL   a heavy noodle
SCHWAMMNUDELN   spongy soup noodles
SPÄTZLE   small boiled flour dumplings
TEIGGEMÜSE   macaroni dishes
TEIGWAREN   macaroni, noodles, spaghetti

Potatoes

BAUERNFRÜHSTÜCK   breakfast consisting of eggs,
 bacon and potatoes
BRATKARTOFFELN   fried potatoes
BRÜHKARTOFFELN   potatoes boiled in broth
BUTTERKARTOFFELN   buttered potatoes
DAMPFKARTOFFELN   boiled or steamed potatoes
GEBACKENE KARTOFFEL   baked potato
GEBACKENE KARTOFFELN   baked potatoes
GEBACKENE KARTOFFELSCHALE   baked potato skin
GEKOCHTE KARTOFFELKLÖSSE   boiled potato
 dumplings
GEKOCHTE KARTOFFELN   boiled potatoes
GERÖSTETE KARTOFFELN   pan-fried boiled potatoes
GRÖSTL   grated, fried potatoes with meat pieces
HERINGSAUFLAUT MIT KARTOFFELN   casserole of
 layers of herring and potatoes

HERZOGINKARTOFFELN   mashed potatoes in different shapes, oven-browned or pan-fried

KARTOFFEL   potato

KARTOFFEL UND TOMATENAUFLAUF   potato and tomato casserole

KARTOFFELBÄLLCHEN   pan-fried mashed potato balls

KARTOFFELBREI   mashed potatoes

KARTOFFELCHIPS   potato chips

KARTOFFELCROQUETTEN (AUS)   potato croquettes

KARTOFFELFÜLLE   potato stuffing

KARTOFFELGERICHTE   potato dishes

KARTOFFELKLÖSSE   potato dumplings

KARTOFFELKNÖDEL   potato dumplings

KARTOFFELKROKETTEN   potato croquettes

KARTOFFELKÜCHLEIN   potato pancakes

KARTOFFELN   potatoes

KARTOFFELN, GERÖSTETE   crisp pan-fried potatoes

KARTOFFELN IN DER SCHALE   potatoes in their jackets

KARTOFFELN, KRONPRINZESSIN   mashed potatoes breaded and deep-fried

KARTOFFELN, LYONNAISE   sliced potatoes, fried in lard with fried onions

KARTOFFELN MIT SPECK   fried potatoes with bits of bacon

KARTOFFELPASTETCHEN   potato patties, containing onion in pastry tart

KARTOFFELPUFFER   potato pancakes

KARTOFFELPUFFER MIT APFELMUS   potato pancakes with applesauce

KARTOFFELPUFFER, REIBEKUCHEN   potato pancakes

KARTOFFELPÜREE   mashed potatoes

KARTOFFELPÜREE MIT GELBEN RÜBEN   whipped potatoes and carrots

KARTOFFELPÜREE MIT SAHNE   mashed potatoes with cream

KARTOFFELSALAT   potato salad

LEICHTER KARTOFFELSALAT summer potato salad
NEUE KARTOFFELN new potatoes
PELLKARTOFFEL potato boiled in its jacket
PELLKARTOFFELN potatoes boiled in their jackets
PETERSILIENKARTOFFELN boiled potatoes with parsley
PETERSILKARTOFFELBÄLLCHEN parsley potato balls
PFANNKUCHEN AUS ROHEN GEBACKENEN
    KARTOFFELN raw potatoes fried in a skillet like a
    pancake
POMMES FONDANT baked mashed potatoes
POMMES FRITES french fries
RAHMKARTOFFELN creamed potatoes
REIBEKUCHEN fried potato pancake
RIEVKOOCHE fried potato pancakes
RISOLEEKARTOFFELN butter-sautéed boiled potatoes
RÖSTI course-grated fried potatoes
RÖSTKARTOFFEL roast potato
RÖSTKARTOFFELN raw potatoes parboiled then
    browned in butter
SALZKARTOFFELN potatoes boiled in salt water
SALZKARTOFFELN MIT KÄSE boiled potatoes with
    cheese
SAURE KARTOFFELN sour potatoes
SCHLOSSKARTOFFELN oval-shaped potatoes fried in
    butter
SCHMELZKARTOFFELN egg shaped potatoes, in a
    covered pan
SCHNEEKARTOFFELN riced boiled potatoes
SCHUPFNUDELN potato noodles
SCHWENKKARTOFFELN potatoes boiled then fried
STOCK mashed potatoes
STROHKARTOFFELN shoestring potatoes
SÜSSKARTOFFELN sweet potatoes
SÜSSKARTOFFELN, SÜDLICHE mashed sweet potatoes
    with butter, sweet cream and sherry
SÜSSKARTOFFELN, ÜBERBACKENE sweet potatoes
    baked with brown sugar

WARMER KARTOFFELSALAT MIT SPECK   hot potato
  salad with bacon
WÜRFELKARTOFFELN   fried diced potatoes

Poultry

AUFLAUF   soufflé of meat, fish, fowl, fruit or vegetable,
  oven browned
BACKHÄHNCHEN   roast chicken
BACKHENDEL   roast chicken
BACKHUHN   roast chicken
BAUERNENTE   farm grown duck
BERLINER HÜHNERFRIKASSEE   Berlin-style chicken
  fricassee
BLÄTTERTEIGPASTETE MIT GEFLÜGELRAGOUT   patty
  shell with diced chicken cream sauce
BRATHÄHNCHEN   large chicken, can be roasted, fried,
  sautéed
BRATHENDEL   roast chicken
BRATHUHN   roast chicken
BREMER KÜCHENRAGOUT   stew of chicken, sweet-
  breads, meat balls, mussels, asparagus, with cream sauce
BRUSTFLEISCH   white meat
ENTE   duck
ENTE GEFÜLLT MIT ÄPFELN UND BROT   roast duck
  with apple and bread stuffing
ENTE MIT KASTANIENFÜLLUNG   roast duck with
  chestnut filling
ENTENBRÜSTCHEN   duckling breast
FLÜGEL   wing
FRIKADELLE   meat, fowl or fish dumpling or croquette
FRIKASSEE   stew of browned meat or poultry cooked in stock
FRIKASSEEHUHN   stewing chicken
FÜLLUNG   stuffing
GANS   goose
GÄNSEBRATEN MIT ÄPFELN, ROSINEN UND NÜSSEN
  roast goose with apple, raisin and nut stuffing

GÄNSEBRATEN MIT KARTOFFELFÜLLUNG   roast goose with prune, apple, and potato stuffing
GÄNSEBRUST   breast of goose
GÄNSEKLEIN   goose giblets
GÄNSELEBER   goose liver
GÄNSELEBER MIT ÄPFELN   goose liver with apples
GÄNSELEBERPASTETE   goose liver pâté or paste
GÄNSELEBERSCHNITZEL   goose liver cutlet
GÄNSESCHMALZ   goose fat
GEBRATENE ENTE   roast duckling
GEBRATENE HÜHNERLEBER   fried chicken livers
GEBRATENER HAHN   roast chicken
GEBRATENER TRUTHAHN   roast turkey
GEFLÜGEL   fowl
GEFLÜGELFRIKASSEE   chicken fricasee
GEFLÜGELKLEIN   giblets
GEFLÜGELLEBER   chicken livers
GEFLÜGELLEBER NACH STRASSBURGER ART   chicken livers in red wine sauce with mushrooms on rice
GEFLÜGELPASTETE   poultry pot pie
GEFLÜGELRAGOUT   chicken stew
GEFLÜGELREISBOMBE   rice mold with chicken
GEFLÜGELRISOTTO   pieces of chicken in rice pilaf
GEFLÜGELSALAT   chicken salad with mayonnaise
GEFÜLLTE GANS   stuffed goose
GEFÜLLTER GÄNSEBRATEN   roast goose with potato stuffing
GEFÜLLTER GÄNSEHALS   stuffed goose neck
GESCHNETZELTE HÄHNCHENBRUST   pieces of chicken breast in cream sauce
GUGGELI   spring chicken
HAHN   rooster
HÄHNCHEN   spring chicken
HÄHNCHEN MAGEN   chicken giblets
HUHN   fowl, including game birds, or chicken
HUHN IN BURGUNDER   chicken in burgundy

HUHN MIT NOCKERLN   chicken with dumplings
HUHN MIT NUDELN   stewed chicken with noodles
HUHN MIT REIS UND SPARGEL   chicken on rice with
  asparagus
HÜHNCHEN   chicken
HÜHNERBRATEN   roast chicken
HÜHNERBRUST   breast of chicken
HÜHNERFLÜGEL   chicken wings
HÜHNERFRIKASSEE   chicken fricassee
HÜHNERKLEIN   chicken giblets
HÜHNERLEBER   chicken livers
HÜHNERLEBER, GERÖSTET (AUS)   sautéed chicken
  liver
HÜHNERPASTETE   chicken patties with grated cheese,
  truffle, cream, onion
HÜHNERRAGOUT   chicken stew
HÜHNERSALAT   chicken salad
JUNGE ENTE   duckling
JUNGE ENTE, GEBRATEN, GEDÜNSTET, GEFÜLLT (AUS)
  duckling, roasted, stewed, stuffed
JUNGES HUHN   spring chicken
KALTES GEFLÜGEL   cold poultry
KALTES HUHN (AUS)   cold chicken
KAPAUN   capon
KÖNIGINPASTETCHEN   pastry shells stuffed with
  chicken, tongue, mushrooms
KÖNIGINPASTETE GEFÜLLT MIT FEINEM RAGOUT
  patty shell filed with diced chicken in a cream sauce
  with mushrooms, wine, herbs. (Chicken a la King)
MASTENTE   grain-fed fattened duck
MASTGANSBRATEN   grain-fed roasted goose
MASTHÄHNCHEN   grain-fed chicken
MASTHUHN   fattened roasting chicken
MASTHUHN SUPREME   boned chicken breast in sauces
MASTPOULARDE   fattened roasting chicken
MASTPUTER   fattened turkey

MAZEDONISCHE HÜHNERCROQUETTEN   chicken croquettes, gravy and mushrooms
NUDELTOPF MIT HUHN UND SPARGEL   chicken and noodle casserole with asparagus
OMELETTE NACH JÄGER ART   omelette with chicken livers and mushrooms in sauce
PAPRIKAHUHN   chicken paprika with sour cream sauce
PAPRIKASAHNEHUHN   braised chicken in cream sauce with paprika
PERLHUHN   Guinea hen
POULARDE   grain-fed roasting chicken
POULET   chicken
PUTER   turkey
SCHLESISCHES HIMMELREICH   roast pork or goose with dumplings
STUBENKÜKEN   young broiler chicken
SUPPENTOPF HUHN (AUS)   chicken pot with vegetables
TAUBE   pigeon or dove
TOULOUSER GEFLÜGELPASTETE   chicken stew with mushrooms in a patty shell
TRUTHAHN   turkey
TRUTHAHN, GEFÜLLTER   turkey with stuffing
TRUTHAHN VOM ROST   roast turkey
TRUTHAHNBRATEN   roast turkey
TRUTHAHNKEULE   turkey drumstick
TRUTHAHNKROKETTEN   turkey croquettes
TRUTHAHNSCHINKEN   turkey leg
WACHTEL   quail
WIENER BACKHENDL   deep-fat fried and baked chicken
WIENER BACKHUHN   deep-fat fried and baked chicken

Rice

BUTTERREIS   buttered rice
CHAMPIGNONREIS (AUS)   rice with mushrooms
GEFLÜGELREISBOMBE   rice mold with chicken
GEFLÜGELRISOTTO   pieces of chicken in rice pilaf

GEKOCHTER REIS   boiled rice
MILCHREIS   rice in milk
NASI GORENG   rice with chicken, pork or beef
PILAFREIS (AUS)   rice pilaf
REIS   rice
REISAUFLAUF MIT ÄPFELN   rice pudding with apple
REISRAND TOULOUSER ART   stew filled rice ring with
   sweetbreads, kidneys, truffles and mushrooms
REISSOCKEL   bed of rice

Salad

BANANENSALAT   salad of bananas, french dressing and
   lettuce
BLUMENKOHLSALAT   salad of cauliflower, olive oil,
   soup stock, vinegar
BOHNENSALAT   bean salad
BOLIVIANISCHER SALAT   salad of potato and hard-
   boiled egg
BRUNNENKRESSE   watercress
BUNTER SALATTELLER   mixed salad plate
CHICORÉE   Belgian endive
CHICORÉESALAT   chicory salad
CHIKORÉE   chicory, endive
EIERSALAT (AUS)   egg salad
ENDIVIEN   endive or chicory
ENDIVIENSALAT   endive salad
ESSIG   vinegar
FISCHSALAT   fish salad
FLEISCHSALAT   meat salad
FRANZÖSISCHE RAHMMARINADE   French dressing
FRUCHTSALAT   fruit salad
GEFLÜGELSALAT   chicken salad with mayonnaise
GEFÜLLTE TOMATEN MIT FLEISCHSALAT   tomatoes
   stuffed with cold meat salad
GEFÜLLTE TOMATEN MIT GEFLÜGELSALAT   tomatoes
   stuffed with chicken salad

GEHACKTE PETERSILIE   chopped parsley
GEMISCHTER SALAT   mixed salad
GEMÜSESALAT   vegetable salad
GRÜNER SALAT   lettuce salad
GURKENKÖRBCHEN   scooped-out cucumbers filled
   with chopped tomatoes
GURKENSALAT   cucumber salad
HERINGSALAT   herring salad
HERINGSTOAST   chopped herring salad on toast
HÜHNERSALAT   chicken salad
ITALIENISCHER SALAT   veal, salami, tomatoes, anchov-
   ies, cucumber in mayonnaise
KARTOFFELSALAT   potato salad
KÄSESALAT   cheese salad
KOPFSALAT   green head lettuce salad
KRABBEN IN MAYONNAISE   shrimp in mayonnaise
   dressing
KRABBEN SALAT   shrimp salad with mayonnaise
KRÄUTERSOSSE   herb dressing
KRAUTSALAT   coleslaw
KREBSSCHWANZSALAT   crayfish salad
KRESSENSALAT   cress salad
LAUCHSALAT   leek salad
LEICHTER KARTOFFELSALAT   summer potato salad
LÖWENZAHNSALAT   dandelion green salad
MASTRINDFLEISCHSALAT   cold, cooked, grain-fed beef
   cut in strips and put into a salad with mayonnaise
MAYONNAISENSALAT   vegetables, meat, fish in
   mayonnaise
MEERESFRÜCHTESALAT (AUS)   sea food salad
MUSCHELSALAT   mussel salad
OBSTSALAT   fruit salad
OCHSENMAULSALAT   ox muzzle salad
ÖL   oil
PALMENMARK   palm hearts
PAPRIKASALAT   sweet bell pepper salad

PILZSALAT   mushroom salad with oil, vinegar, onions
RAHMMARINADE   cream dressing with mustard, sugar,
   butter, vinegar, heavy whipped cream
RETTICHSALAT   radish salad
RHEINLÄNDER MARINADE   dressing of sugar, Wor-
   cestershire, ketchup, olive oil, vinegar, mustard,
   Tabasco, lemon juice
RINDFLEISCHSALAT (AUS)   beef salad
ROHKOSTPLATTE   salad plate
ROHKOSTSALAT   raw vegetable salad
ROTER RÜBENSALAT   pickled beet salad
RUSSISCHER GEFLÜGELSALAT   chicken salad with
   hard-boiled eggs covered with mayonnaise
SALAT   salad
SALAT MIMOSA   salad of lettuce with grated egg yolk
SALAT UND BEILAGE   salad accompaniment or side
   dish
SALAT VON GERÄUCHERTEM AAL   smoked eel salad
SALATE   salads
SALATPLATTE   assorted salad plate
SALATTELLER   salad plate
SAUERKRAUTSALAT   sauerkraut, olive oil, apples,
   onions
SCHINKENSALAT (AUS)   ham salad
SCHNITTLAUCH   chive
SCHOTENSALAT   bell pepper salad
SCHWEIZER WURSTSALAT   Swiss baloney salad
SELERIE MIT ÄPFELN   celery root and apple salad
SELLERIESALAT   celery root salad
SENFGELEE   mustard relish
SHRIMPSALAT   shrimp salad
SPARGELSALAT   asparagus salad
SPECKKRAUTSALAT   cabbage salad with bacon
STANGENSELLERIE   stalk celery
STEINBUTTSALAT   salad made of cold boiled turbot
TEUFELSALAT   a salad with a spicy, vinegar dressing

TOMATENSALAT   tomato salad
TOMATENWÜRFEL   diced or cubed tomatoes
WACHSBOHNEN SALAT   wax bean salad
WARMER KARTOFFEL SALAT MIT SPECK   hot potato
    salad with bacon
WURSTSALAT   sausage salad with vegetables,
    mayonnaise
ZIGEUNERSALAT   bell pepper salad

Sandwiches

BELEGTE BRÖTCHEN   open sandwiches
BERNER BRÖTCHEN   sandwich with cooked ham, Swiss
    cheese on toast
HALBER HAHN   cheese sandwich on whole wheat roll
KÄSEBROT   open-faced cheese sandwich
LACHSBRÖTCHEN   smoked salmon sandwiches
RUNDSTÜCK WARM   hot roast meat open-faced sand-
    wich with gravy
SCHINKENBROT   open-faced ham sandwich
SCHWEDENBRÖTCHEN   small open-faced sandwiches
SCHWEDENPLATTE   tiny assorted sandwiches
STRAMMER MAX   sandwich with minced pork, sausage
    or ham with fried eggs and onions
STULLE   rye bread sandwiches with various fillings
TATARENBROT   open-faced sandwich of raw, spiced,
    minced beef
WURSTBROT   open-faced sausage sandwich

Sauces

ABGESCHMELZT   melted sauce poured over vegetables
ANSCHOVIS-SOSSE   anchovy sauce
ÄPFELMUS   applesauce
BERCY   creamy sauce of butter, shallots, wine, stock
BERNAISE   sauce of butter, egg yolks, flavored vinegar
BERNAISTUNKE   bernaise sauce

BORDELAISE SAUCE   made with stock, red wine shallots and herbs

BRATENSOSSE   gravy

BRAUNE TUNKE   brown sauce

BURGUNDER WEINSAUCE   Burgundy wine sauce

CHAMPIGNON IN RAHMSAUCE   mushroom cream sauce

CHAMPIGNON SOSSE   mushroom sauce

CHAMPIGNON TUNKE   mushroom sauce

DILLSOSSE   dill sauce

DILLRAHMSAUCE   dill flavored cream sauce

DILLTUNKE   dill sauce

FRUCHTSAUCE   fruit sauce

GEBUNDEN   sauce or soup which is thickened with flour

GEWÜRZBUTTER   seasoned butter

GRÜNE SOSSE   green herb sauce from fish poaching broth

HELLE SOSSE   basic cream sauce

HOLLÄNDISCHE SOSSE   Hollandaise sauce

INGWERSAHNESOSSE   ginger cream sauce

JOHANNISBEERSOSSE   redcurrant jelly sauce

KAPERNSOSSE   caper sauce

KARAMELSAUCE   caramel sauce

KÄSESOSSE   cheese sauce

KRÄUTERMAYONNAISE (AUS)   mayonnaise sauce with herbs

MADEIRASAUCE (AUS)   Madeira sauce

MANDELSAUCE   almond sauce

MARKSOSSE   bone marrow sauce

PAPRIKARAHMSAUCE   paprika-flavored cream sauce

PETERSILIENBUTTER   parsley butter

PETERSILIENSOSSE   parsley sauce

PIKANTE SOSSE   spicy sauce

POMERANZENSOSSE   bitter orange wine and brandy sauce

RAHMMARINADE   cream dressing with mustard, sugar, butter, vinegar, heavy whipped cream

RAHMMEERRETTICH   horseradish cream sauce
REMOULADENSOSSE   mayonnaise sauce with mustard,
   anchovies, capers, gherkins, tarragon, chervil
ROSINENSOSSE   raisin sauce
ROTWEINSOSSE   red wine sauce
SAFT   juice or gravy
SAHNEMEERRETTICHSOSSE   horseradish cream sauce
SARDELLENBUTTER   anchovy butter
SARDELLENSOSSE   anchovy sauce
SCHNITTLAUCHSAUCE   chopped chive cream sauce
SENFBUTTER   mustard flavored butter
SENFSOSSE   mustard sauce
SENFTUNKE   mustard sauce
SOSSEN   sauces
SPANISCHE SOSSE   brown sauce with herbs
SPECKSAUCE   sauce flavored with bacon or gravy
SPECKSTIPPE   sauce flavored with bacon
STIPPE   gravy or sauce
SÜSSER UND SAUERER RAHM   sweet and sour cream
TOMATENSOSSE   tomato sauce
TUNKE   sauce or gravy
VANILLESOSSE   vanilla cream sauce
WACHOLDERBEERENRAHM   juniper berry cream sauce
WEINSOSSE   wine sauce
WEINSUD   sauce made from wine and fish stock
WEISSE SOSSE   white sauce
ZWIEBELSOSSE   onion sauce

Sausages

BIERWURST   dried salami stick, eaten cold
BLUTWURST   blood sausage
BOCKWURST   boiled sausage
BRATWURST   sausage for roasting or frying
BRATWURST IN SAURER SAHNENSOSSE   bratwurst in
   sour cream sauce

BRATWURST IN SÜSS-SAURER TUNKE   sweet and sour sausage

BRATWURST SÜLZE PIKANTE   bratwurst in aspic with spices

BRIESMILZWURST   sausage of veal sweetbreads

CERVELATWURST   seasoned and smoked sausage of pork, beef and bacon

DÜRRE RUNDE   dried sausage

FLEISCHWURST   similar to baloney, served hot boiled, grilled, or cold

FRANKFURTER   frankfurter

GÄNSELEBERWURST   goose liver sausage

GRIEBENWURST   larded frying sausage

HIMMEL UND ERDE   slices of pudding made with sausages, fried onions, mashed potatoes and apple sauce

JAGDWURST   smoked pork, beef and bacon sausage

KALBSBRATWURST   grilled sausage made of veal

KALBSLEBERWURST   veal sausage

KATENWURST   country-style smoked sausage

KNACKWURST   garlic-flavored sausage

KOPFSÜLZE   pork headcheese in aspic

KRAINER   spiced pork sausage

LEBERWURST   liverwurst

LINSENEINTOPF MIT WIENERWÜRSTCHEN   lentil pot with sausages

LUFTGETROCKNETE METTWURST   air-dried, cold, cooked sausage

LYONER   like baloney, hot or cold

METTWURST   spiced and smoked pork sausage spread on bread

MILZWURST   sausage made of veal spleen

NÜRNBERGER BRATWÜRSTE   small grilled, veal and pork sausages

PFÄLZER   spicy sausage

PINKELWURST   spicy oatmeal and bacon fat sausage

PRESSACK   a pork headcheese

PRESSKOPF   headcheese from pork pieces
REGENSBURGER   highly-spiced and smoked sausage
REGENSBURGER IN ESSIG UND ÖL   cold slices of beef
  and pork sausage, dressed with oil and vinegar
RIESENBOCKWURST   spicy sausage like knockwurst
RINDSWURST   grilled beef sausage
ROASTBEEF MIT WÜRSTCHEN   roast beef with sausages
ROSTBRATWÜRSTE   pork sausages
ROT-WEISSER PRESSACK   Austrian pressed headcheese
  meatloaf
SAITENWURST   variety of frankfurter sausage
SALAMI   any salami-type cold sausage
SCHINKENWURST   ham pieces in pork baloney filling,
  eaten cold
SCHLACHTPLATTE   hot meat, liver sausage and sauer-
  kraut plate
SCHLACHTSCHÜSSEL   boiled dish of liver sausage, blood
  sausage, pork belly with sauerkraut, potatoes and
  dumplings
SCHWARTENMAGEN   headcheese loaf in aspic
SCHWARZ-WEISSER PRESSACK   dark and light meat
  pork headcheese
SCHWEINSKOPFSÜLZE   pork headcheese loaf
SCHWEINSSÜLZE   headcheese
SCHWEINSWÜRSTL   grilled pork sausages
STADTWURSTSÜLZE   locally made sausage
STREICHWURST   very soft spreadable sausage
SÜSS-SAURE BRATWURST   bratwurst in sweet-sour
  sauce
WARME WURSTSPEISEN   cooked sausage dishes
WEISSWURST   veal sausage
WIENER WÜRSTCHEN   frankfurter type of sausage
WIENER WÜRSTL   frankfurter type of sausage
WINTEREINTOPF   winter stew, made with chestnuts,
  yellow turnips, leeks, sausages
WOLLWURST   grilled mild white veal sausage
WURST IN TEIG   sausage cooked in dough

WURSTBROT   open-faced sausage sandwich
WURSTBRÖTCHEN   sausage in pastry
WÜRSTCHEN   sausages
WURSTGERICHTE   hot sausage dishes
WURSTPLATTE   platter of assorted sausages
WURSTSPEZIALITÄTEN   house specialties in hot sausages
ZUNGENWURST   ox tongue sausage
ZWIEBELWURST   liver and onion sausage

Seafood

AAL   eel
AAL ASPIK   eel in aspic
AAL BLAU   boiled eel
AAL GERÄUCHERT   smoked eel
AAL GRÜN   eel poached in wine with sauce, served cold
AAL NACH TRENTINER ART   grilled eel
AAL STEINHUDER   eel from Steinhuder Lake area
ALSE   shad fish
AUFLAUF   soufflé of meat, fish, fowl, fruit or vegetable,
   oven-browned
AUSTERN   oysters
AUSTERN GEBACKEN   fried oysters
AUSTERN HOLLÄNDISCH   oysters from Holland
BACHFORELLE   stream-raised trout
BACHKREBS   stream crayfish
BACKFORELLE   baked trout
BARSCH   perch
BASSIN   live fish tank
BISMARCKHERING   pickled herring, seasoned with
   onions
BISMARCKHERING UND PELLKARTOFFELN   herring
   and new potatoes
BLÄTTERTEIGPASTETE MIT KREBSSCHWÄNZCHEN
   patty shell with crayfish tails in cream sauce
BLAU   freshly poached fish
BLAUE FORELLE   fresh trout quickly boiled

BLAUFELCHEN   fresh water whitefish
BODENSEEFELCHEN   trout from Lake Constance
BRATFISCH   fried fish
BRATHERING   fried herring, marinated in onions, vinegar and sour cream
BÜCKLING   smoked herring
BÜCKLINGE UBERBACKEN   baked kippers
BULETTE   meat or fish ball
DONAUWALLER   catfish
DORSCH   cod
DORSCHROGEN   codfish roe
FELCHEN   lake trout
FISCHCREME   creamed fish
FISCHFRIKADELLEN   fish cakes
FISCHSCHÜSSEL   casserole of fish and diced bacon
FISCHGERICHTE   seafood
FISCHKLÖSSCHEN   fish ball
FISCHKLÖSSE   fish dumplings
FISCHKRUSTELN (AUS)   fish croquets
FISCHLEIN   little fish
FISCHRAGOUT   fish stew
FISCHROULADEN   fish rolls
FISCHSALAT   fish salad
FISCHSCHÜSSEL   bacon and fish pie
FLUNDER   flounder
FLUNDER GEBACKEN   baked founder
FLUSSKARPFEN   river carp
FLUSSLACHS   stream salmon
FORELLE   trout
FORELLE "MÜLLERIN ART"   trout prepared in Miller's wife style; dredged in flour, and fried in butter and oil
FORELLE BLAU   blue trout
FORELLE GERÄUCHERT MIT OBERSKREN (AUS)   smoked trout with horseradish cream
FORELLE IN ASPIK (AUS)   trout in aspic
FORELLE IN WEISSWEIN   trout in white wine

FORELLE IN WEISSWEINSUD   trout served in a creamed white wine sauce

FORELLE NACH MÜLLERIN ART   fried trout

FORELLEN IN ASPIK   jellied trout

FORELLENFILET   fillet of trout

FRIKADELLE   meat, fowl or fish dumpling or croquette

FROSCHSCHENKEL   frogs' legs

FROSCHSCHENKEL PANIERT GEBACKEN (AUS)   breaded and fried frog's legs

GANZ   whole, entire, as the whole fish

GARNELE   shrimp

GEBACKENE SCHOLLE   baked sole

GEBACKENE AUSTERN   oysters fried in dough case

GEBACKENER FISCH   fried or baked fish

GEBACKENER ZANDER IN WEISSWEIN   walleyed pike baked in white wine

GEBAKENER FISCH MIT KRAUT   baked fish with sauerkraut

GEBRATENE FORELLEN   pan-fried lake trout

GEBRATENER HUMMER   fried lobster

GEFÜLLTER FISCH   stuffed fish

GEGRILLTER FISCH   grilled fish

GEGRILLTER FISCH MIT MAYONNAISE   fine quality grilled fish with mayonnaise

GEGRILLTER LACHS   grilled salmon

GEKOCHTER KREBS (AUS)   boiled crayfish

GELEEHERINGE   jellied herring

GERÄUCHERTE FORELLE MIT MEERETTICH   smoked trout with horseradish cream

GERÄUCHERTER LACHS   smoked salmon

GERÄUCHERTER RHEINLACHS   smoked salmon from the Rhine

GESÜLZTE FORELLEN   jellied trout

GLATTBUTT   brill

GOLDBARSCH   red seabass, like red snapper

GOLDBARSCHFILET, GEBACKEN   baked fillet of sea bass

GOLDBUTT   flat fish similar to turbot
GRANAT   prawn
HECHT   pike
HECHT IN SAUERRAHM   pike in sour cream
HEILBUTT   halibut
HEILBUTT IN SAHNE   halibut under cream
HERING   herring
HERING BLAU   blue herring
HERING IN PERGAMENT   herring in wax paper
HERING NACH HAUSFRAUENART   herring fillets with
   onions in sour cream
HERING VOM ROST   grilled herring
HERINGSAUFLAUF   baked herring casserole
HERINGSAUFLAUF MIT KARTOFFELN   casserole of
   layers of herring and potatoes
HIESIGER DORSCH   local or native cod
HUMMER   lobster
HUMMER KALT (AUS)   cold lobster
HUMMER VOM ROST (AUS)   grilled lobster
HUMMERKRABBEN   large prawns
JAKOBSMUSCHEL   scallop
KABELJAU   codfish
KABELJAU, GEGRILLTER   codfish or haddock, grilled
   with butter, paprika and grated cheese
KABELJAU, UNGARISCHER   codfish sautéed in butter,
   onion, sour cream, paprika
KAISERGRANAT   Norway lobster, Dublin Bay prawn
KAISERKRABBEN   special shrimps
KAMMUSCHEL   scallop
KARPFEN   carp
KARPFEN GEGRILLTER   grilled carp
KARPFEN GESÜLZTER (AUS)   carp in aspic
KATERFISCH   fish with tomato sauce and pickles
KAVIAR   caviar
KIELER SPROTTEN   sprats from Kiel
KÖNIGSKRABBEN   king crabs
KRABBEN   crabs or shrimp

KRABBEN, BÜSUMER   shrimp from the North Sea coast
KRABBEN IN MAYONNAISE   shrimp in mayonnaise
   dressing
KRABBEN SALAT   shrimp salad with mayonnaise
KREBS   freshwater crayfish
KREBSSCHWÄNZE   crayfish tails
KREVETTEN   shrimps
KRUSTENTIER   shellfish
KÜMMELSUD   caraway-flavored poaching liquid
KUTTERKABELJAU   cutter, codfish
LACHS   salmon
LACHSFORELLE   salmon trout
LACHSMEDALLIONS   fillets of salmon
LANGUSTE   spiny lobster, crawfish
LANGUSTE IN MAYONNAISE   crayfish with mayonnaise
LANGUSTENSCHWÄNZE   lobster tail
LEBENSFRISCHEFORELLE   trout taken fresh and alive
   from the restaurant's fish tank
LENGFISCHFILET   ling cod fillet
MAIFISCH   shad
MAKRELE   mackerel
MAKRELEN IN ÖL (AUS)   mackerels in oil
MATJESHERING   young salted herring
MATJESHERING NACH HAUSFRAUEN ART   herring
   fillets with apple slices, onion rings, onion sauce and
   sour cream
MATJESHERINGSFILET   fillets of young herring
MEER   sea
MEERESFRÜCHTE   seafood
MEERESFRÜCHTESALAT (AUS)   seafood salad
MEERESKREBSE IN BIERTEIG GEBACKEN (AUS)   deep
   fried scampi
MIESMUSCHEL   mussel
MÜLLERIN-ART   dredged in flour and fried in butter and
   oil
MUSCHEL   mussel
MUSCHEL RAGOUT-FIN   mussels in a thick cream sauce

MUSCHELN IN SPANISCHER SHERRYWEINSOSSE
  Spanish mussels in sherry wine sauce
MUSCHELN, GEBRATENE (AUS)   roast mussels
MUSCHELSALAT   mussel salad
NORDISCHER RAUCHSALM   northern smoked salmon
ÖLSARDINEN   sardines in oil
PFAHLMUSCHEL   mussel
PLATTFISCH   plaice fish like flounder
PLATZLI   scallop
RÄUCHER HERING   smoked herring
RÄUCHERAAL   smoked eel
RÄUCHERLACHS   smoked salmon
REGENBOGENFORELLE   rainbow trout
RENKE   fresh water whitefish
RHEINLACHS   Rhine salmon
RIESENKRABBEN   giant crabs
RIESENSCAMPI   large prawn
ROCHEN   skate fish
ROGEN   codfish eggs or roe
ROLLMOPS   herring fillet rolled around chopped onions
  and pickles
ROTBARBE   red mullet or red seabass
ROTZUNGE   lemon sole
SALM   salmon
SANDMUSCHEL   clam
SARDELLE   anchovy
SARDELLENRING   rolled anchovy
SARDINE   pilchard or very small herring
SCAMPI   shrimp or prawns
SCAMPI COCKTAIL   prawn appetizer
SCAMPI KÖNIG   medium prawn
SCHALENTIER   shellfish
SCHELLFISCH   haddock
SCHILL (AUS)   pike-perch
SCHLEIE   carp fish
SCHLEIE BLAU   carp fish boiled with butter

SCHLEIE MIT SAHNEMEERRETTICH carp with creamed horseradish sauce

SCHNECKEN IN KRÄUTERBUTTER (AUS) snails with herb butter

SCHNECKENRAGOUT PROVENCALES snails stewed in tomato and onion sauce

SCHNECKENSPIESS MIT CHAMPIGNONS, SPECK, KNOBLAUCH UND BUTTER snails with mushrooms, bacon and garlic butter, grilled

SCHOLLE flat fish like flounder or plaice

SCHWÄNZE tails

SEEBARSCH (AUS) perch

SEEKRABBE crab

SEELACHS codfish called sea salmon

SEEZUNGE sole fish like plaice or flounder

SEEZUNGE COLBERT sole breaded and fried in butter, served with herbal butter and wine sauce

SEEZUNGE, GEBACKENE breaded and deep-fried sole

SEEZUNGE IN BUTTER sole fillets in butter

SEEZUNGE IN WEISSWEIN sole in white wine

SEEZUNGE MÜLLERIN sole floured and fried

SEEZUNGENRÖLLCHEN rolled fillets of sole poached in white wine served with sauce

SHRIMPSALAT shrimp salad

SOLOKREBS very large prawns

SPIESS on a skewer

SPROTTEN sprats, like sardines

STEINBEISSER sea bass

STEINBUTT turbot, similar to halibut

STEINBUTT GEKOCHT boiled turbot

STEINBUTTSALAT salad made of cold boiled turbot

STEINGARNELE prawn

STEINHUDER RÄUCHERAAL smoked eel from Steinhuder Lake region

STINT sardine-like smelt fish

STOCKFISCH dried cod fish

STÖR   sturgeon
STÖR GERÄUCHTERTER   smoked sturgeon
STÖRSTEAK   sturgeon steak
SUD   broth
TAFEL   selection or choice suitable for the table
THUNFISCH   tuna
THUNFISCH AURORA   tuna with a tomato flavored
    sauce
THUNFISCH GRIECHICHER   slices poached in with
    lemon juice and oil
TIEFSEE KREBSFLEISCH   deep sea crayfish meat
TINTENFISCH   octopus
WALLER   large catfish
WEINBERGSCHNECKEN   snails (edible)
WEINBERGSCHNECKEN IN KNOBLAUCHBUTTER
    snails in garlic butter
WEINBERGSCHNECKEN MIT KRÄUTERBUTTER   snails
    with herbal butter
WEINSUD   broth made from wine and fish stock
WEISSFISH   Whiting, a type of fish
WELS (AUS)   catfish
WITTLING   whiting
WOLFSBARSCH   bass
WURZELSUD   pickling brew
ZANDER   pike-perch
ZANDERSCHNITTE IN SENFBUTTER   fillet of walleyed
    pike with mustard butter
ZERLASSENE BUTTER   melted butter
ZITRONE   lemon

Soup

AALSUPPE   sweet-sour soup with boiled eel, prunes,
    dried fruits, wine broth and vegetables
AMSTERDAMER AUSTERNSUPPE   Dutch oyster soup
APRIKOSENKALTSCHALE   chilled fruit soup with
    apricots

BACKERBSENSUPPE balls of deep fried dough served in bouillon

BAUERNSUPPE thick soup of sliced frankfurters and cabbage

BAYRISCHE LEBERKNÖDELSUPPE Bavarian liver dumpling soup

BIERSUPPE sweet, spicy soup made with beer

BLUMENKOHLCREMESUPPE cream of cauliflower soup

BOHNENSUPPE bean soup

BOUILLABAISSE "MARSEILLER ART" Marseilles fish soup-stew

BOUILLON broth or consommé

BOUILLON MIT EI broth with beaten egg

BOUILLON MIT MARK broth with bone marrow

BOUILLON MIT MARKKLÖSSCHEN broth with marrow dumplings

BROTSUPPE broth with stale bread

BROTSUPPE MIT ROSTZWIEBEL broth with fried onions

BRÜHE broth, consomme'

BUTTERBISKUIT butter biscuit, used in soup

BUTTERKLÖSSCHEN small butter dumplings

BUTTERMILCHSUPPE buttermilk soup

CHAMPIGNONCREMESUPPE cream of mushroom soup

CHAMPIGNONRAHMSUPPE cream of mushroom soup

CHESTERSTANGEN cheddar cheese straws (with soup)

CONSOMMÉ bouillon

DOPPELTE KRAFTBRÜHE double consommé

ECHTE SCHILDKRÖTENSUPPE genuine turtle soup

EIERFLOCKENSUPPE beaten eggs in boiling soup, like egg drop soup

EIERSTICH egg cubes, used in soup

EINLAGE something added to a clear soup

EINLAUFSUPPE beaten eggs in boiling soup stirred to form long strings

ERBSENSUPPE split pea soup

ERBSENSUPPE MIT SAURER SAHNE green pea soup with sour cream

ERBSENSUPPE MIT WIENER WÜRSTCHEN   pea soup with sausages

ERDBEERENKALTSCHALE   chilled fruit soup with strawberries

FEINE KARTOFFELSUPPE MIT GURKEN   pureed potato soup with cucumber

FISCHRAHMSUPPE   creamed fish soup

FISCHSUPPE   fish soup

FLÄDLE   thin strips of pancake added to soup

FLÄDLESUPPE   bouillon with thin strips of pancake

FLEISCHBRÜHE   meat soup

FLEISCHBRÜHE MIT EI   meat broth with beaten egg

FLEISCHBRÜHE MIT LEBERKNÖDEL   meat broth with liver dumplings

FLEISCHBRÜHE MIT MARK   meat broth with marrow

FLEISCHBRÜHE MIT MARKKLÖSSCHEN   meat broth with marrow dumplings

FLEISCHBRÜHE MIT RINDERMARK   meat broth with beef marrow

FLEISCHBRÜHE NATUR   plain meat broth or bouillon

FRÄNKISCHE BROTSUPPE   soup of stock, onion, liverwurst, potatoes and rye bread

FRANZÖSISCHE FISCHSUPPE   fish soup like French bouillabaisse

FRANZÖSISCHE HUMMERSUPPE   French-style lobster soup

FRANZÖSISCHE ZWIEBELSUPPE   French onion soup

FRUCHTKALTSCHALE   chilled soup with sugar and pureed fruits added to a wine base

FRÜHLINGSSUPPE   soup with diced spring vegetables

GAISBURGER MARSCH   soup with cubes of meat, onions, potatoes, noodles

GAZPACHO   cold tomato, cucumber, vegetable soup

GEBUNDEN   sauce or soup thickened with flour

GEFLÜGELCREMESUPPE   cream of chicken soup

GELBE ERBSENSUPPE   dried yellow pea soup

GEMÜSECREMESUPPE   cream of vegetable soup

GEMÜSESUPPE   vegetable soup
GERSTENSUPPE   barley soup
GRAUPENSUPPE   barley soup
GRAUPENSUPPE MIT HÜHNERKLEIN   barley soup
   with chicken giblets
GRIESSKLOSSUPPE   bouillon with small semolina
   dumplings
GRIESSNOCKERLSUPPE   semolina dumpling soup
GRIESSSUPPE   beef soup with grits
GRÜNE KARTOFFELSUPPE   green potato soup
GRÜNKERNSUPPE   young wheat cooked in soup, like
   barley
GULASCHSUPPE   soup with meat pieces, vegetables and
   paprika
GURKENSUPPE   cucumber soup
HAFERFLOCKENSUPPE   oatmeal soup
HAIFISCHFLOSSENSUPPE   shark fin soup
HAMMELBOUILLON   clear soup made with mutton
HAUSGEMACHTE SUPPE   homemade soup
HEISSE BIERSUPPE   hot beer soup
HIRNSSUPPE   brain soup
HOCHZEITSSUPPE   rich soup with meats and vegetables
HÜHNERBOUILLON   chicken bouillon
HÜHNERBRÜHE MIT NUDELN   chicken soup with
   noodles
HÜHNERCREMESUPPE   creamed chicken soup
HÜHNERKRAFTBRÜHE   chicken consommé
HÜHNERSUPPE   chicken soup
HÜHNERSUPPE MIT REIS   chicken soup with rice
HUMMER CREMESUPPE   cream of lobster soup
HUMMER SUPPE   lobster soup
INDISCHE REISCREMESUPPE   Indian rice cream soup
JULIENNESUPPE MIT SAGO   vegetable soup with
   tapioca
KALBFLEISCHRAHMSUPPE   veal cream soup
KALBFLEISCHSUPPE   clear soup with veal
KALTE WEINSUPPE   cold wine soup

KALTSCHALE   chilled fruit soup with white wine base
KANGURUHSCHWANZSUPPE   kangaroo tail soup
KAROTTENSUPPE   carrot soup
KARTOFFELSUPPE   potato soup
KÄSESTANGEN   cheese sticks made of puff pastry
KERBELSUPPE   thick potato soup with meat and
   chopped chervil
KIRSCHENKALTSCHALE   chilled fruit soup with
   cherries
KLARE SUPPE   clear soup (broth)
KOHLSUPPE   cabbage soup
KÖNIGINSUPPE   creamed chicken soup with pieces of
   chicken breast
KRAFTBRÜHE   brothor clear soup made of beef or
   chicken
KRAFTBRÜHE MIT HÜHNERFLEISCH   chicken soup
KRAFTBRÜHE MIT EI   broth with beaten egg
KRAFTBRÜHE MIT FADENNUDELN   broth with string
   noodles
KRAFTBRÜHE MIT FLÄDLE   broth with thin strips of
   pancake
KRAFTBRÜHE MIT LEBERKNÖDEL   broth with liver
   dumplings
KRAFTBRÜHE MIT LEBERSPÄTZLE   broth with liver
   dumplings
KRAFTBRÜHE MIT MARK   broth with marrow
KRAFTBRÜHE MIT NUDELN   broth with noodles
KRAFTSUPPE   broth
KRÄUTERSUPPE   soup with chopped herbs or cabbage
KREBSSUPPE   crayfish soup
KÜMMELSUPPE   caraway soup
KÜRBISSUPPE   pumpkin soup
LAUCHCREMESUPPE   leek soup
LEBERKLÖSSUPPE   liver dumpling soup
LEBERKNOCKERLSUPPE   soup with liver, chicken,
   chopped onions, stuffed dumplings

LEBERKNÖDELSUPPE   clear soup with dumplings of
minced liver and onions
LEGIERT   thickened as soup or salad sauces
LINSENPÜREESUPPE (AUS)   lentil puree soup
LINSENSUPPE   lentil soup
LINSENSUPPE MIT WÜRSTCHEN   lentil soup with
frankfurters
MARKKLOSSUPPE   marrow dumpling soup
MEHLSUPPE   brown flour soup
MOHRRÜBENSUPPE   carrot soup
MORGENRÖTESUPPE   thick soup of meat, tapioca,
tomatoes and chicken stock
MUSCHELSUPPE   mussel soup
NUDELSUPPE   noodle soup
NUDELSUPPE MIT HUHN   chicken noodle soup
NUDELSUPPE MIT HÜHNERKLEIN   noodle soup with
chicken giblets
OCHSENSCHWANZSUPPE   oxtail soup
OCHSENSCHWANZSUPPE, GEBUNDEN MIT MADEIRA
oxtail soup with Madeira wine
OCHSENSCHWANZSUPPE MIT KLÖSSCHEN   oxtail
soup with dumplings
OCHSENSCHWANZSUPPE MIT PILZEN   oxtail soup
with mushrooms
PFANNKUCHENSUPPE   hot consommé with thin strips
of pancake added
PORREESUPPE (AUS)   leek soup
REISSUPPE   broth with rice
RIEBELE   noodles
RINDFLEISCHSUPPE   soup made from boiling beef
RUMFORDSUPPE   pea soup with barley, potatoes and
fried bacon
SAUERAMPFERSUPPE   sorrel soup
SCHILDKRÖTENSUPPE   turtle soup
SCHILDKRÖTENSUPPE LADY CURZON   turtle soup
with curry powder and whipped cream garnish

SCHNECKENSUPPE MIT RAHMCURRY snail cream soup flavored with curry

SCHOKOLADENSUPPE chocolate soup

SCHOTTISCHE KRAFTBRÜHE Scotch mutton broth

SCHWALBENESTERSUPPE bird's nest soup

SCHWAMMNUDELN spongy soup noodles

SCHWARZBROTSUPPE dark bread soup

SELLERIECREMESUPPE cream of celery soup

SPARGELCREMESUPPE cream of asparagus soup

SPARGELSUPPE asparagus soup

SPINATCREMESUPPE cream of spinach soup

SUPPE soup

SUPPE NACH WAHL soup of your choice

SUPPENEINLAGEN something added to a clear soup

SUPPENFLEISCH boiled beef, soup meat

SUPPENHUHNTOPF chicken soup casserole

SUPPENMAKRONEN baked almonds and macaroons added to soups

TERRINE large bowl

TOMATENCREMESUPPE cream of tomato soup

TOMATENKRAFTBRÜHE consommé flavored with tomatoes

TOMATENSUPPE tomato soup

TRAPANGSUPPE smoked fried sea cucumber boiled in broth

TRÜFFELKRAFTBRÜHE consommé with truffles

WALSUPPE whale soup

WEINSUPPE soup made of a liquid base of wine

WEISSE WINDSORSUPPE cream soup with rice and veal seasonings

WIENER ERBSENSUPPE pea soup

ZWIEBELSUPPE onion soup

ZWIEBELSUPPE, FRANZÖSISCHE French onion soup

Spices

ANIS aniseed

BASILIKUM basil

FENCHEL fennel
GEWÜRZNELKE clove
GEWÜRZE spice
GEWÜRZT spiced
INGWER ginger
KATCHUP catsup
KERBEL chervil, an herb in the parsley family
KNOBLAUCH garlic
KRÄUTER herbs
KRÄUTERBUTTER herb butter
KREN horse-radish
KÜMMEL caraway
MEERRETICH horseradish
MOHN poppy
MOHNSAMEN poppyseeds
MUSKAT nutmeg
NELKE clove
OEL oil
ÖL oil
PETERSILIE parsley
PFEFFER pepper
PRISE pinch (of salt)
ROSMARIN rosemary
SAFRAN saffron
SALBEI sage
SALZ salt
SCHNITTLAUCH chive
SENF mustard
THYMIAN thyme
WÜRZE spice, seasoning, pickled
ZERLASSENE BUTTER melted butter
ZIMT cinnamon

Vegetables

ANANASKRAUT pineapple sauerkraut
ÄPFELBLAUKRAUT red cabbage with apples

ÄPFELROTKOHL   red cabbage with apples
ÄPFELROTKRAUT   red cabbage cooked with apples
ARTISCHOCKE   artichoke
ARTISCHOCKENBODEN   artichoke bottom
ARTISCHOCKENHERZEN   artichoke hearts
AUBERGINE   eggplant
AUBERGINE, GEFÜLLT MIT SCHINKEN, ÜBERBACKEN
   eggplant with ham stuffing browned in broiler
AUFLAUF   soufflé of meat, fish, fowl, fruit or vegetable,
   oven browned
BADISCHE KRAUTWICKEL   meat-stuffed cabbage rolls
BAMBUSSPROSSEN   canned bamboo shoots
BAUERNSCHMAUS   sauerkraut with bacon, smoked
   pork, sausages, dumplings or potatoes
BAYERISCHER LINSENTOPF MIT GERÄUCHERTEM
   Bavarian lentil casserole with smoked pork
BAYERISCHES KRAUT   cooked cabbage with apples and
   juniper berries
BERLINER LÖFFELERBSEN   cooked dried peas, onion,
   leek, pig's ear and snout, and potatoes
BERNER PLATTE   sauerkraut or beans with pork chops,
   bacon and beef sausages, and boiled potatoes
BETE   beet
BIERRETTICH   black radish served with beer
BLATTSPINAT   leaf spinach
BLAUKRAUT   red cabbage
BLUMENKOHL   cauliflower
BLUMENKOHL MIT SENFSOSSE   cauliflower with mus-
   tard sauce
BLUMENKOHL POLNISCH   cooked cauliflower with
   butter and breadcrumbs
BLUMENKOHL UBERBACKEN   baked cauliflower
BOHNEN   beans
BOHNENAUFLAUF   baked beans casserole
BOHNENSALAT   bean salad
BRAUNKOHL   kale
BRECHBOHNEN   pieces of string beans

BROKKOLI   broccoli
BRUNNENKRESSE   watercress
BRÜSSELER ENDIVIE   endive, chicory
BÜCHSENSTANGENSPARGEL   white asparagus spears
BUTTERBOHNEN   buttered string beans
BUTTERERBSEN   buttered peas
BUTTERKAROTTEN   buttered carrots
CHAMPIGNON   mushroom
CHICORÉE   Belgian endive
CHICORÉE MIT SCHINKEN UND KÄSE ÜBERBACKEN
   endive baked with ham and cheese
CORNICHON   small pickle
DICKE BOHNEN   broad beans
EDELPILZE   fine quality mushrooms
EIERSCHWAMM   chanterelle mushroom
EINGEMACHT   preserved
EINTOPF   meat or vegetable stew
ERBSEN   peas
ERBSENBREI   puree of green peas
ERBSENPÜREE   mashed peas
ERBSPÜREE   yellow pea puree with bacon
ERDBIRNEN   potatoes
ESSIGGURKEN   pickles
GEBACKENER BLUMENKOHL   fried cauliflower
GEBACKENER SPARGEL   deep-fried asparagus
GEDÜNSTETES SAUERKRAUT   steamed spiced
   sauerkraut
GEFÜLLTE AUBERGINE   stuffed eggplant
GEFÜLLTE TOMATEN   stuffed tomatoes
GEFÜLLTE TOMATEN MIT FLEISCHSALAT   tomatoes
   stuffed with cold meat salad
GEFÜLLTE ZWIEBELN   meat-stuffed onions
GELBERÜBE   carrot
GEMÜSEBEILAGE   vegetables or other side dishes
GEMÜSEPLATTE   vegetable plate
GEMÜSESALAT   vegetable salad
GERSTE   barley

GEWÜRZGURKE pickle, gherkin
GLASIERT glazed, as ham, carrots or chestnuts
GRÜNE BOHNEN French bean, green bean
GRÜNE ERBSEN green peas
GRÜNE GURKEN cucumber
GRÜNKOHL kale, a dark green leafy vegetable
GRÜNKOHL MIT KARTOFFELN baked kale with
  potatoes
GURKE cucumber
HOPPELPOPPEL eggs with bacon, onions and potatoes
HÜLSENFRÜCHTE legumes
JUNGES GEMÜSE young vegetables
KAISERSCHOTEN small peas
KAPERN capers
KARFIOL cauliflower
KAROTTEN carrots
KAROTTENEINTOPF MIT FLEISCHEINLAGE carrot
  casserole with meat
KARTOFFELN potatoes
KARTOFFELPÜREE MIT GELBRÜBEN whipped
  potatoes and carrots
KARTOFFEL UND TOMATENAUFLAUF potato and
  tomato casserole
KNOBLAUCH garlic
KOHL cabbage
KOHLRABI kohlrabi
KOHLRABI IN RAHMSOSSE kohlrabi with sour cream
KOHLRÄBCHENGEMÜSE young kohlrabi
KOHLRABIGEMÜSE kohlrabi
KOHLRÜBEN turnips
KRAUSKOHL kale
KRAUT cabbage
KRAUTSALAT coleslaw
KRAUTSTIEL white beet, Swiss chard
KRAUTWICKEL stuffed cabbage
KREN horse-radish
KRESSE cress

KUKURUZ   corn
KÜMMELKRAUT   cabbage with caraway seeds
KÜRBIS   pumpkin
LAUCH   leek
LAUCH GRATIN   leeks with sharp cheddar cheese
LAUCHRAHMSOSSE   leek gravy with sour cream
LEIPZIGER ALLERLEI   mixed vegetable dish
LINSEN   lentils
LINSENEINTOPF   lentil pot
LINSENEINTOPF MIT WIENER WÜRSTCHEN   lentil pot
   with sausages
MAÏS   corn
MANGOLD   root or beet, only the leafy tops are eaten;
   somewhat like spinach
MISCHGEMÜSE   mixed vegetables
MISCHPILZE   mixed mushrooms
MÖHRE, MOHRRÜBE   carrot
MORCHEL   morel mushroom
PALMENMARK   palm hearts
PAPRIKASCHOTE   sweet pepper, yellow, red or green
PARADIESAPFEL   tomato
PERLZWIEBELN   pearl onions
PFEFFERSCHOTE   hot pepper
PFIFFERLINGE   wild mushroom like chanterelle
PFIFFERLINGE MIT SPECK   sautéed mushrooms with
   bacon
PICHELSTEINER   mixed meat and vegetable casserole
PILZAUFLAUF MIT NUDELN   baked mushrooms with
   noodles
PILZE   mushrooms
PILZE GLAS   mushroom entree with white bread, sherry,
   cream sauce
PILZE MIT SPECK   sautéed wild mushroom with bacon
PILZE MIT TOMATEN UND SPECK   mushrooms with
   tomatoes and bacon
PORREE   leek
PRINZESSBOHNEN   thick string beans

PUFFBOHNEN   lima beans

RADIESCHEN   radish

RAHMSPINAT   creamed spinach

RETTICH   white radish

RETTICH MIT BROT UND BUTTER   radishes with bread
and butter

RHABARBER   rhubarb

ROHKOST   uncooked vegetables, vegetarian food

ROHKOSTSALAT   raw vegetable salad

ROSENKOHL   brussels sprout

ROSENKOHL MIT SCHINKEN UND TOMATEN
brussels sprouts with ham and tomatoes

RÖSTZWIEBELN   crisp fried onions

ROTE BETE   red beets

ROTE RÜBE   beetroot

ROTE RÜBEN   beetroots

ROTE RÜBEN IN BUTTER   red beets in butter

ROTKOHL   red cabbage

ROTKOHL MIT ÄPFELN   red cabbage with apples

ROTKRAUT   red cabbage

RÜBEN   turnips

RÜBENEINTOPF   turnip stew with breast of lamb, tomatoes and beef stock

SALZGURKE   pickled cucumber

SAUBOHNE   broad bean

SAUERAMPFER   sorrel

SAUERGURKE   pickle

SAUERKRAUT MIT ANANAS   sauerkraut with
pineapple

SCHALOTTE   shallot, a milder type of onion

SCHALOTTEN   shallots

SCHMINKBOHNEN   kidney beans

SCHMORGURKEN IN SAUREM DILLRAHM   stewed
cucumbers with sour cream and dill

SCHNITTBOHNE   sliced French bean

SCHNITTLAUCH   chive

SCHWAMM   sponge mushroom

SCHWETZINGER SPARGEL asparagus
SELLERIE celery
SENFGURKEN mustard pickles
SPARGEL asparagus
SPARGELGERICHT ÜBERBACKEN baked asparagus
  with potatoes, ham, parsley, cheese, nutmeg
SPARGELSPITZEN white asparagus tips
SPECKBOHNEN string beans with bacon
SPECKKRAUT cabbage with bacon
SPINAT spinach
SPROSSENKOHL brussels sprout
STANGENBOHNEN pole or string beans
STANGENSELLERIE stalk celery
STANGENSPARGEL asparagus spears
STAUDENSELLERIE stalk celery
STECKRÜBE turnip
STEINPILZE wild yellow mushrooms
SÜSS-SAURE ROTE RÜBEN pickled beets
TAFELPILZE select mushrooms
TELTOWER RÜBCHEN baby turnips cooked in sugar
TOMATEN tomatoes
TOMATEN MIT FEINER FLEISCHFÜLLUNG tomatoes
  stuffed with light meat filling
TOMATENSCHEIBEN tomato wedges
TOMATENWÜRFEL diced or cubed tomatoes
TRÜFFEL flavorful mushroom-like plant that grows
  underground
TÜRKENKORN corn or maize
ÜBERBACKENER BLUMENKOHL baked cauliflower
UNGARISCHE PAPRIKASCHOTEN stuffed peppers
  with rice and ground beef in tomato sauce
WACHSBOHNEN yellow wax beans
WALDPILZE forest mushrooms
WEIN-SAUERKRAUT sauerkraut cooked in white wine,
  may have apples
WEIN-WEISSKRAUT white cabbage braised with apples
  and simmered in wine

WEISSKOHL   white cabbage
WEISSKOHLEINTOPF MIT SCHWEINSPFÖTCHEN
   cabbage casserole with pig's feet
WEISSKRAUT   white cabbage
WEISSKRAUT MIT SPECK   cooked cabbage with bacon
WEISSE BOHNEN   white dried beans
WEISSE RÜBEN   turnips
WELSCHKORN   corn
WESTFÄLISCHES BLINDHUHN   beans with fruit and
   vegetables
WINTEREINTOPF   winter stew, made with chestnuts,
   yellow turnips, leeks, sausages
WINTERKOHL   winter cabbage
WIRSING   savoy cabbage
WURZEL   root
ZUCCINI   Italian zucchini squash
ZUCKERERBSEN   young green peas
ZWIEBEL   onions
ZWIEBELRINGE   onion rings, usually fried

Wines and Liquor

ABFÜLLUNG   bottled wine bought from the grower
ABZUG   wine bottled at the vineyard where grown
AHR-WEIN   red wine from the Ahr River region
ALKOHOL   alcohol, hard liquor
APRIKOSENLIKÖR   apricot liqueur
AUSLESE   wine produced from choice grapes
BADEN-WEIN   a variety of delicious and full-bodied
   wines from the Baden region
BEERENAUSLESE   dessert wine
BOWLE   wine cup
BRANNTWEIN   brandy
BRULOT (AUS)   finger of brandy with lump sugar in a
   warmed cup, set on fire, doused with hot coffee and
   capped with whipped cream

DANZIGER GOLDWASSER   caraway liqueur with gold leaves
DOPPELKORN   grain spirit
DORNKAAT   grain spirit, flavored with juniper berries
EIERLIKÖR   egg liqueur
ENZIAN   gentian root liquor (schnaps)
FISTERNOLLEKEN   corn brandy
FLASCHE   bottle
FRANKEN-WEIN   strong, dry, high-quality, robust, fruity white wine
GESÜSSTER WEIN   sweetened wine
GETRÄNKE   drinks, liquor
GEZUCKERT   sugar added, sweetened
GLÜHWEIN   mulled wine
HESSISCHE BERGSTRASSE   fruity, elegant, fragrant, mild wine
HIMBEERGEIST   spirit distilled from raspberries
KABINETT   wine of high quality
KIRSCHWASSER   cherry brandy
KLOSTERLIKÖR   herb liqueur made in monastery
KOGNAK   cognac
KORNBRANNTWEIN   whiskey distilled from grain
KÜMMELBRANNTWEIN   caraway flavored spirit
LIKÖR   liqueur or cordial
MARASCHINO   cherry liqueur
MITTELRHEIN-WEIN   fresh and dry wine
MOSEL-SAAR-RUWER-WEIN   fresh, delicate wine with a fine fruity flavor
MOSELWEIN   a white wine
MOST   young wine
NAHE-WEIN   fragrant, fruity, lively wine
NATURWEIN   unblended, unsweetened wine
PERLWEIN   white, semi-sparkling wine
PFLÜMLIWASSER   liquor distilled from plums
PORTWEIN   port wine
PUNSCH   punch

RHEIN-WEIN   country's best white wines

RHEINGAU-WEIN   good dessert wine, fruity taste with character and elegance

RHEINHESSEN-WEIN   smooth, mild wine

RHEINPFALZER WEIN   mild, aromatic, round and full-bodied, strong wine

ROTWEIN   red wine

SCHAUMWEIN   champagne

SCHILLERWEIN   rose wine

SCHNAPS   brandy

SCHOPPENWEIN   wine from a keg (1/4 liter, 1/2 pint) sold by the glass

SEKT   champagne

SPÄTLESE   full-bodied wine

STEINHÄGER   juniper-flavored spirit

SÜSSE WEINE   dessert wine

SÜSSWEIN   dessert wine

TROCKEN   dry

UNGEZUCKERT   unsweetened

VIERTEL LITER WEIN   about 1/2 pint of wine

WACHSTUM   grower name on a wine label guarantees wines

WEIN   wine

WEINBRAND   brandy distilled from wine

WEISSWEIN   white wine

WERMUT   vermouth liqueur

WÜRTTEMBERGISCHER WEIN   wine that is strikingly fruity, with a distinctive after-taste

ZWETSCHGENWASSER   spirit distilled from plums

What It Means: A Complete Aphabetical Dictionary of German Food and Drink

A

AAL   eel
AAL ASPIK   eel in aspic
AAL BLAU   boiled eel
AAL GERÄUCHERT   smoked eel
AAL GRÜN   eel poached in wine with sauce, served cold
AAL MIT EIERN   eel with eggs
AAL NACH TRENTINER ART   grilled eel
AAL, STEINHUDER   eel from Steinhuder Lake area
AALSUPPE   sweet and sour soup with boiled eel, prunes, dried fruits, wine broth, and vegetables
ABENDBROT   evening meal, supper
ABENDESSEN   dinner
ABFÜLLUNG   bottled wine bought from the grower
ABGEBRÄUNT   browned quickly or grilled
ABGEBRÄUNTE KALBSBRATWÜRSTCHEN   grilled or pan-fried veal sausages
ABGESCHMECKT   taste tested
ABGESCHMELZT   melted sauce poured over vegetables
ABZUG   wine bottled at the vineyard where grown
AHR-WEIN   red wine from the Ahr River region
ALKOHOL   alcohol, hard liquor
ALKOHOLFREIE GETRÄNKE   soft drinks

ALLERLEI   all sorts of

ALLGÄUER BERGKÄSE   hard cheese from Bavaria resembling Emmentaler

ALLGÄUER RAHMKÄSE   mild and creamy Bavarian cheese

ALSE   shad fish

ALTENBURGERKÄSE   mild, soft goat's milk cheese

AMSTERDAMER AUSTERNSUPPE   Dutch oyster soup

ANANAS   pineapples

ANANASKRAUT   sauerkraut with pineapple

ANANAS-SAUERKRAUT   pineapple sauerkraut

ANCHOVIS-SOSSE   anchovy sauce

ANGEMACHT   prepared, ready to serve

ANIS   aniseed

ANISBROT   cake or biscuit with anise

ANISSCHEIBEN   anise drops

ANISSTRIEZEL   anise coffee cake

ÄPFEL   apples

APFELAUFLAUF   apple soufflé

APFELBETTELMANN   apple and pumpernickel crumb dessert

APFELBLAUKRAUT   red cabbage with apples

APFELCHARLOTTE   baked apples with sliced French rolls, lemon juice, cinnamon, sugar, raisins

APFELKUCHEN   apple cake

APFELKÜCHLE   batter-dipped, deep-fried apple rings

APFELMOST   apple cider

APFELMUS   applesauce

APFELNPFANNKUCHEN (AUS)   small pancakes with apples

APFELPFANNKUCHEN   apple filled pancakes

APFELREIS MIT SCHNEEHAUBE   apple-rice with lemon peel, raisins, topped with sweetened whipped egg whites

APFELRINGE   apple rings

APFELROTKOHL   red cabbage cooked with apples

APFELROTKRAUT   red cabbage cooked with apples
APFELSAFT   apple juice
APFELSCHEIBEN   slices of apples
APFELSCHMARRN   egg pancake with diced apples
APFELSCHNITTCHEN   apple fritters
APFELSCHNITTEN   sliced apple fritters
APFELSINEN   oranges
APFELSINENKUCHEN   orange coffee cake
APFELSINENSAFT   orange juice
APFELSTRUDEL   apple strudel, apple pastry dessert
APPENZELLER KÄSE   full-flavored, slightly bitter cheese
APPETITHÄPPCHEN   appetizer, canapé
APPETITSCHNITTCHEN   appetizer, canapé
APRIKOSE   apricot
APRIKOSENKALTSCHALE   chilled fruit soup with
   apricots
ARMER RITTER   sweet fritter
ART DES HAUSES   homemade
ARTISCHOCKE   artichoke
ARTISCHOCKENBODEN   artichoke bottom
ARTISCHOCKENHERZEN   artichoke hearts
AUBERGINE   eggplant
AUBERGINE, GEFÜLLT MIT SCHINKEN ÜBERBACKEN
   eggplant with ham stuffing browned in broiler
AUFLAUF   soufflé of meat, fish, fowl, fruit or vegetable,
   oven browned
AUFSCHNITT   cold cuts
AUFSCHNITTPLATTE   cold cut platter
AUSGANG   exit
AUSGEBACKEN (AUS)   fried
AUSKUNFT   information
AUSLESE   wine produced from choice grapes
AUSTERN   oysters
AUSTERN GEBACKEN   fried oysters
AUSTERN HOLLÄNDISCH   oysters from Holland
AUTOBAHN   highway

B

BACHFORELLE   stream raised trout
BACHKREBS   stream crayfish
BACK'NBIER   strong flavored beer
BACKERBSENSUPPE   balls of deep-fried dough served in
   bouillon
BACKFORELLE   baked trout
BACKHÄHNCHEN   roasted chicken
BACKHENDEL   roasted chicken
BACKHUHN   roasted chicken
BACKOBST   dried fruit
BACKOBSTKOMPOTT   dried fruit compote
BACKPFLAUME   prune
BACKSTEINKÄSE   strong-smelling and tasting cheese
BACKTEIG, IM (AUS)   deep fried
BACKWERK   cakes, cookies, pastries, etc.
BADEN-WEIN   a variety of delicious and full-bodied wines
BADISCHE KRAUTWICKEL   meat stuffed cabbage rolls
BAHNHOFSGASTSTÄTTE   railway station restaurant
BAMBUSSPROSSEN   canned bamboo shoots
BANANEN   bananas
BANANEN IN WEINTEIG (AUS)   banana fritters
BANANEN ÜBERBACKEN MIT SCHLAGOBERS (AUS)
   banana flambé with cream
BANANEN ÜBERBACKEN MIT SCHOKOLADESAUCE
   (AUS)   banana flambé with chocolate sauce
BANANEN ÜBERBACKEN MIT VANILLEEIS (AUS)
   banana flambé on vanilla ice
BANANENSALAT   salad of bananas, french dressing and
   lettuce
BARSCH   perch
BASILIKUM   basil
BASSIN   live fish tank
BAUCHFLEISCH   boiled thick slices of pork bacon
BAUERN...   farm-style
BAUERNBROT   rye or wholemeal bread

BAUERNENTE   farm-grown duck
BAUERNFRÜSTÜCK   boiled potatoes, fried with
   scrambled eggs and ham
BAUERNGERÄUCHERTES   farm cured smoked meats
BAUERNGESELCHTES (AUS)   mixed smoked pork
BAUERNHINTERSCHINKEN   farm-style cured ham
BAUERN-HOPPEL-POPPEL   peasant breakfast with veal
   instead of ham or bacon
BAUERNOMELETTE   omelette with chopped bacon,
   potatoes and onions
BAUERNSCHMAUS   sauerkraut with bacon, smoked
   pork, sausages, dumplings or potatoes
BAUERNSCHINKEN   ham cured on the farm
BAUERNSUPPE   thick soup of sliced frankfurters and
   cabbage
BAUMSTAMMEIS   ice cream roll dessert
BAYERISCHE LEBERKNÜDEL   dumpling containing
   chopped liver, bacon, onion
BAYERISCHE SEMMELKNÜDEL   Bavarian bread
   dumplings
BAYERISCHER LINSENTOPF MIT GERÄUCHERTEM
   Bavarian lentil casserole with smoked pork
BAYERISCHES KRAUT   cooked cabbage with apples and
   juniper berries
BAYRISCHE KUCHERL (AUS)   Bavarian fritters stuffed
   with jam
BAYRISCHE LEBERKNÜDELSUPPE   Bavarian liver
   dumpling soup
BECHER   goblet (dessert dish)
BEDIENUNG   service
BEDIENUNG EINBEGRIFFEN   service included
BEDIENUNG NICHT EINBEGRIFFEN   service not
   included
BEEFSTEAK, DEUTSCHES   fried hamburger with fried
   onion rings and pan-fried, boiled potatoes
BEERE   berry
BEERENAUSLESE   dessert wine

BEFSTEAKTATAR   seasoned raw beefsteak, chopped onion, raw egg

BEI NÄSSE GLATT   slippery when wet

BEILAGE   side dish

BEILAGEN   side dishes of vegetables, salads or starches

BELEGTE BRÖTCHEN   open sandwiches

BELEGTE BROTE   bread served with cold cuts

BERCY   creamy sauce of butter, shallots, wine, stock

BERLINER ART   cooked Berlin style

BERLINER HÜHNERFRIKASSE   Berlin style chicken fricassee

BERLINER LÖFFELERBSEN   cooked dried peas, onion, leek, pig's ear and snout, and potatoes

BERLINER LUFT   dessert of eggs, lemon, with raspberry juice

BERLINER PFANNKUCHEN   jam filled doughnut sprinkled with sugar

BERNAISE   sauce of butter, egg yolks, flavored vinegar

BERNAISTUNKE   bernaise sauce

BERNER BRÖTCHEN   sandwich with cooked ham, Swiss cheese on toast

BERNER PLATTE   sauerkraut or beans with pork chops, bacon and beef, sausages and boiled potatoes

BESETZT   occupied

BETE   beet

BEUSCHEL   heart, kidney and liver of lamb in sour sauce

BIENENSTICH   cake with honey and almonds

BIER   beer

BIER, DUNKLES   dark beer

BIER, HELLES   light, lager beer

BIERKUCHEN   loaf beercake

BIERRETTICH   black radish served with beer

BIERSTUBE   beer parlors

BIERSUPPE   sweet, spicy soup made with beer

BIERTEIG GEBACKEN, IM (AUS)   deep-fried in beer batter

BIERWURST   dried salami stick, eaten cold

BIRCHERMÜSLI   uncooked oats with raw fruit, chopped nuts in milk or yogurt

BIRNE HELENE   pear poached in syrup and served with vanilla ice cream and chocolate sauce

BIRNEN   pears

BIRNEN ÜBERBACKEN MIT ERDBEERSAUCE (AUS)   pear flambé with strawberry sauce

BIRNEN-EINTOPF   smoked ham, pears, new potatoes, baked in oven

BIRNENSCHNITTEN   sliced pear fritters

BIRNENSPALTEN (AUS)   sliced pear fritters

BISCHOFSBROT   fruit-nut cake

BISKOTTENTORTE (AUS)   cake with finger biscuits

BISKUIT LISETTE   sponge cake of butter, egg yolks, sugar, coffee extract, chopped almonds

BISKUITROLLE   jelly and butter-cream roll

BISMARCKHERING   pickled herring, seasoned with onions

BISMARCKHERING UND PELLKARTOFFELN   herring and new potatoes

BLÄTTERTEIGGEBÄCK   puff pastry goods

BLÄTTERTEIGPASTETCHEN   round flaky potato cookies with jelly

BLÄTTERTEIGPASTETE   pastry shell

BLÄTTERTEIGPASTETE KREBSSCHWÄNZCHEN   pastry shell with crayfish tails in cream sauce

BLÄTTERTEIGPASTETE MIT FEINEM KALBSFLEISCH-RAGOUT   patty shell with diced veal in brown cream sauce

BLÄTTERTEIGPASTETE MIT GEFLÜGELRAGOUT   pastry shell with diced chicken cream sauce

BLATTSPINAT   leaf spinach

BLAU   freshly poached fish

BLAUBEERE   blueberry

BLAUE FORELLE   fresh trout quickly boiled

BLAUFELCHEN   fresh water whitefish

BLAUKRAUT   red cabbage

BLITZKUCHEN   quick coffee cake
BLUMENKOHL   cauliflower
BLUMENKOHL MIT SENFSOSSE   cauliflower with
   mustard sauce
BLUMENKOHL POLNISCH   cooked cauliflower with
   butter and breadcrumbs
BLUMENKOHL ÜBERBACKEN   baked cauliflower
BLUMENKOHLCREMSUPPE   cream of cauliflower soup
BLUMENKOHLSALAT   salad of cauliflower, olive oil,
   soup stock, vinegar
BLUTWURST   blood sausage
BOCKBIER   dark malt beer
BOCKWURST   boiled sausage
BODENSEEFELCHEN   trout from Lake Constance
BÖHMISCHE KNÖDEL   flour dumplings cooked in salt
   water
BOHNEN   beans
BOHNENAUFLAUF   casserole-baked beans
BOHNENEINTOPF   meat and bean stew with onion,
   garlic, potatoes
BOHNENSALAT   bean salad
BOHNENSUPPE   bean soup
BOLIVIANISCHER SALAT   salad of potato and hard-
   boiled egg
BORDELAISESAUCE   made with stock, red wine shallots
   and herbs
BORKENSCHOKOLADE   chocolate cut into squares and
   used for dessert toppings
BOUILLABAISSE "MARSEILLER ART"   Marseilles fish
   soup-stew
BOUILLON   broth or consommé
BOUILLON MIT EI   broth with beaten egg
BOUILLON MIT MARK   broth with bone marrow
BOUILLON MIT MARKKLÖSSCHEN   broth with
   marrow dumplings
BOWLE   spiced wine
BRANNTWEIN   brandy

BRATAPFEL   baked apple
BRATEN   roast meats
BRATENPLATTE   plate of cold roast meats
BRATENSOSSE   gravy
BRATENSÜLZE   cold roast meats in aspic
BRATFISCH   fried fish
BRATHÄHNCHEN   large chicken, can be roasted, fried,
   sauteed
BRATHENDEL   roast chicken
BRATHERING   fried herring, marinated in onions,
   vinegar and sour cream
BRATHUHN   roast chicken
BRATKARTOFFELN   fried potatoes
BRATWURST   sausage
BRATWURST IN SAURER SAHNENSOSSE   bratwurst in
   sour-cream sauce
BRATWURST SÜSS-SAURER TUNKE   bratwurst in sweet
   and sour sauce
BRATWURSTSÜLZE, PIKANTE   bratwurst in aspic with
   spices
BRAUNE BUTTER   browned butter
BRAUNE TUNKE   brown sauce
BRAUNER   coffee with milk
BRAUNER, KLEINER   small cup of coffee with milk
BRAUNKOHL   kale
BRAUNSCHWEIGER KUCHEN   cake with almonds and
   fruit
BRAUSE   carbonated flavored soda
BRECHBOHNEN   pieces of string beans
BREI   porridge, purée
BREMER KÜCHENRAGOUT   stew of chicken, sweet-
   breads, meat balls, mussels, asparagus, with cream
   sauce
BREZEN   pretzels
BRIES, BRIESCHEN, BRIESEL   sweet bread
BRIESMILZWURST   sausage of veal sweetbreads
BROKKOLI   broccoli

BROMBEERE   blackberry
BROT   bread
BRÖTCHEN   sweetbreads, rolls
BROTPUDDING   bread pudding
BROTSUPPE   broth with stale bread
BROTSUPPE MIT RÖSTZWIEBEL   broth with fried onions
BROTZEITTELLER   mid-morning meat and other snacks
BRÜHE   broth, consommé
BRÜHKARTOFFELN   potatoes boiled in broth
BRULOT (AUS)   finger of brandy with lump sugar in a warmed cup, set on fire, doused with hot coffee and capped with whipped cream
BRUNNENKRESSE   watercress
BRÜSSELER ENDIVIE   endive, chicory
BRUST   breast
BRUSTFLEISCH   white meat
BRUSTSTÜCK   brisket
BÜCHSENSTANGENSPARGEL   canned white asparagus spears
BÜCKLING   smoked bloater fish
BÜCKLINGE ÜBERBACKEN   baked kippers
BULETTE   meat or fishball
BUNDKUCHEN   sweet yellow cake
BÜNDNERFLEISCH   cured, dried beef
BUNTER SALATTELLER   mixed salad plate
BURGUNDERSCHINKEN   ham cooked in Burgundy wine with Madeira sauce
BURGUNDERWEINSAUCE   Burgundy wine sauce
BUTTERBISKUIT   butter biscuit, used in soup
BUTTERBOHNEN   buttered string beans
BUTTERBROT   bread and butter
BUTTERERBSEN   buttered peas
BUTTERHÖRNCHEN   butter crescents
BUTTERKAROTTEN   buttered carrots
BUTTERKARTOFFELN   buttered potatoes
BUTTERKLÖSSCHEN   butter soup balls

BUTTERKUCHEN   coffee cake
BUTTERMILCH   buttermilk
BUTTERMILCHSUPPE   buttermilk soup
BUTTERNUDELN   buttered noodles
BUTTERPLÄTZCHEN   baked butter cookies with vanilla and sugar
BUTTERREIS   buttered rice

C

CANTALOUP   cantaloupe
CERVELATWURST   seasoned and smoked sausage of pork, beef and bacon
CHAMPIGNON   mushroom
CHAMPIGNON IN RAHMSAUCE   mushroom cream sauce
CHAMPIGNONCREMESUPPE   cream of mushroom soup
CHAMPIGNONRAHMSUPPE   cream of mushroom soup
CHAMPIGNONREIS (AUS)   rice with mushrooms
CHAMPIGNONSCHNITZEL (AUS)   veal escalope with mushrooms
CHAMPIGNONSOSSE   mushroom sauce
CHAMPIGNONTUNKE   mushroom sauce
CHESTERSTANGEN   cheddar cheese straws with soup
CHICORÉE   chicory, Belgian endive
CHICORÉE MIT SCHINKEN UND KÄSE ÜBERBACKEN   endive baked with ham and cheese
CHICORÉESALAT   chicory salad
CONFITÜRE   jam
CONSOMMÉ   bouillon
CORDON BLEU   thin veal cutlets, a slice of ham and Swiss cheese in batter, fried in butter
CORDON ROUGE   veal or beef fillet, mushrooms, chicken livers, fried in butter
CORNICHON   small pickle
CREME   cream
CREME, CARAMEL   caramel custard

CREME NESSELRODE   Madeira wine cream
CREME PATISSERIE   pastry cream
CREMEFÜLLUNG   frosting
CREMESCHNITTEN (AUS)   Napoleons
CREMESPEISE   custard
CREPES SUCHARD   thin dessert pancakes with chocolate
   sauce and chopped almonds,
CRÊPES SUZETTE   dessert pancakes with orange butter
   cream, flamed with liqueur
CREVETTENCOCKTAIL (AUS)   shrimp cocktail

D

DAMEN   ladies
DAMPFBRATEN   beef stew
DAMPFKARTOFFELN   boiled or steamed potatoes
DAMPFNUDEL(N)   sweet dessert dumpling(s) with
   vanilla sauce
DANZIGER GOLDWASSER   caraway liqueur with gold
   leaves
DATTEL   date
DAZU   in addition
DELIKATESSE: KALTER AUFSCHNITT   cold cuts
DEUTSCHES BEEFSTEAK   hamburger
DICKE BOHNEN   broad beans
DICKE SCHEIBE   thick slice
DIENST   service
DILLRAHMSAUCE   dill flavored cream sauce
DILLSOSSE   dill sauce
DILLTUNKE   dill sauce
DIVERSES   various, several, mixed
DOBOSCHTORTE   seven-layer cake with mocha cream
DONAUWALLER   catfish
DOPPELKORN   grain spirit
DOPPELMOCCA (AUS)   black coffee served in a large cup
DOPPELTE KRAFTBRÜHE   double consommé
DOPPELTES LENDENSTÜCK   thick beef fillet

DORNKAAT   grain spirit, flavored with juniper berries
DÖRROBST   dried fruit
DORSCH   cod
DORSCHROGEN   codfish roe
DOSE   can or tin
DOTTERKÄSE   skimmed milk cheese
DRESDNER STOLLEN   Dresden christmas fruit bread
DUNKEL GERÄUCHERTES   dark-smoked ham or pork
  pieces
DUNKLES BIER   dark beer
DURCHGEBRATEN   well-done
DÜRRE RUNDE   dried sausage

E

ECHTE   genuine
ECHTE SCHILDKRÖTENSUPPE   genuine turtle soup
EDEL   fine quality
EDELPILZE   fine quality mushrooms
EI   egg
EIDOTTER   egg yolk
EIER   eggs
EIER, GEBACKENE   fried eggs basted in butter
EIER, GEFORMTE   poached eggs in a mold
EIER, GEFÜLLTE   stuffed eggs
EIER, GEKOCHTE   boiled eggs in the shell
EIER, HARTGEKOCHTE   hard-boiled eggs
EIER IN SENFSOSSE   eggs in mustard sauce
EIER MIT CHAMPIGNONS   eggs with mushrooms
EIER MIT EDELPILZEN   eggs with fine mushrooms
EIER MIT PFIFFERLINGEN   eggs with mushrooms
EIER MIT RÄUCHERAAL   eggs with smoked eel
EIER MIT SCHINKEN (AUS)   ham and eggs
EIER MIT SCHINKEN   eggs with ham
EIER MIT SPINAT   eggs with spinach
EIER NACH BAUERNART   eggs with bacon, potatoes
  and onions

EIER UND SPECK   bacon and eggs
EIER, VERLORENE   poached eggs
EIER, WACHSWEICHE   medium-boiled eggs (5–6 min.)
EIER, WEICHGEKOCHTE   soft-boiled eggs (3–4 min.)
EIERAUFLAUF   egg soufflé
EIERCREME   egg custard
EIERFLOCKENSUPPE   beaten eggs in boiling soup, like
   egg drop soup
EIERKUCHEN   pancake
EIERLIKÖR   egg liqueur
EIERNAPFEN   baked shirred eggs
EIERNUDELN   egg noodles
EIERPFANNKUCHEN   egg pancakes
EIERPFANNKUCHEN MIT ÄPFELN   egg pancakes with
   stewed apples, sprinkled with sugar and cinnamon
EIERPFANNKUCHEN MIT KOMPOTT   egg pancakes
   with stewed fruit
EIERPFANNKUCHEN MIT SPECK   egg pancakes with
   bacon
EIERSALAT (AUS)   egg salad
EIERSCHAUM   beaten egg yolks and sugar cooked
   together and then flavored with sweet wine
EIERSCHWAMM   chanterelle mushroom
EIERSPÄTZLE   thick egg noodles
EIERSPEISE   custard
EIERSPEISEN   egg dishes
EIERSTICH   egg cubes, used in soup
EIERTEIGWAREN   pastas, macaronis, spaghetti
EIHÜLLE   egg covered or batter dipped
EINGANG   entrance
EINGELEGT   pickled
EINGEMACHT   preserved
EINGEMACHTE KALBSBRUST (AUS)   boiled breast of veal
EINGEMACHTES   stew
EINGEMACHTES KALBFLEISCH   veal stew
EINGEMACHTES LAMMFLEISCH (AUS)   lamb stew

EINLAGE   something added to a clear soup

EINLAUF   with egg in it

EINLAUFSUPPE   beaten eggs in boiling soup stirred to form long strings

EINSPÄNNER (AUS)   coffee served in a tall glass with lots of whipped cream and powdered sugar

EINTOPF   meat or vegetable stew

EINTOPFGERICHT   casserole of meat and vegetables

EIS   ice

EISBECHER   ice cream dessert, may have liquor, fruit or whipped cream

EISBEIN   boiled pork shanks with sauerkraut and mashed potatoes

EISBEIN ASPIK   cold pork shank in gel

EISBEIN MIT SAUERKRAUT   pickled pig's knuckle with sauerkraut

EISBOMBE   ice cream dessert

EISCHNEE   whipped, sweetened egg-white dessert

EISCREME   ice cream

EISKAFFEE   iced coffee

EISSPEZIALITÄTEN   ice cream specialties

EISTORTE   ice cream cake made with fruit, over liqueur soaked cookies, then topped with meringue and candied fruit

EIWEISS   egg white

ELCH   elk

EMMENTALER KÄSE   semi-hard Swiss cheese

ENDIVIE   endive

ENDIVIENSALAT   endive salad

ENG   narrow

ENGLISCHER KUCHEN   loaf cake

ENTE   duck

ENTE GEFÜLLT MIT ÄPFELN UND BROT   roast duck with apple and bread stuffing

ENTE MIT KASTANIENFÜLLUNG   roast duck with chestnut filling

ENTENBRÜSTCHEN   duckling breast
ENTRECOTE   boneless loin steak
ENTRECOTE MIT SOSSE BEARNAISE (AUS)   sirloin
steak with sauce bearnaise
ENTRECOTE MIT ZWIEBELN UND BRATKARTOFFELN
(AUS)   sirloin steak with onions and home-fried potatoes
ENZIAN   gentian root liqueur
ERBSEN   peas
ERBSENBREI   purée of green peas
ERBSENPÜREE   mashed peas
ERBSENSUPPE   split pea soup
ERBSENSUPPE MIT SAURER SAHNE   green pea soup
with sour cream
ERBSENSUPPE MIT WIENER WÜRSTCHEN   pea soup
with sausages
ERBSPÜRÉE   yellow pea puree with bacon
ERDBEERCREME   strawberry cream custard dessert
ERDBEEREN "ROMANOV"   strawberries with port or
liqueur, covered with whipped cream
ERDBEEREN   strawberries
ERDBEERENKALTSCHALE   chilled fruit soup with
strawberries
ERDBEERKNÖDEL (AUS)   strawberry dumplings
ERDBEERTORTE (AUS)   strawberry cream cake
ERDBIRNEN   potatoes
ERDNUSS   peanut
ERDNUSSKONFEKT   peanut candy
ERLESEN   first class or choice
ERRÖTENDE JUNGFRAU   raspberries and cream
ESSIG   vinegar
ESSIGGURKEN   pickles
ESSKASTANIE   chestnut
EXPORTBIER   an aged stronger beer
EXPRESSO   strong coffee served in a small cup
EXTRAAUFSCHLAG   extra charge or supplementary
charge

F

FADENNUDEL thin noodle

FALSCHE REBHÜHNER false partridge (squab)

FALSCHER HASE false rabbit, meat loaf of beef and pork

FALSCHER WILDSCHWEINBRATEN fresh ham, made like wild boar

FARBSTOFF artificial coloring

FASAN pheasant

FASAN, GEBRATENER (AUS) roast pheasant

FASAN IM TOPF pheasant roasted in a covered casserole

FASAN IN ROTWEIN pheasant in red wine

FASCHIERTER BRATEN meat loaf

FASCHIERTES minced meat

FASCHIERTES LAIBCHEN meatball

FASTNACHTSSCHERBEN potato flour doughnuts

FEIGE fig

FEIN fine

FEINE KARTOFFELSUPPE MIT GURKEN pureed potato soup with cucumber

FEINGEBÄCK delicate pastry or cookies

FELCHEN lake trout

FENCHEL fennel

FERTIGE SPEISEN ready main dishes

FESTER PREIS fixed price

FETT fat

FILET boneless tenderloin

FILET STROGANOFF tenderloin beef cooked in sour cream gravy of onions and mushrooms

FILETGULASCH cubed beef fillet with onions, browned in butter, beef stock and wine

FILETSCHEIBEN bacon, pineapple, curry, truffle sauce on slices of beef fillet

FILETSTEAK beef tenderloin steak

FILETSTEAK MIT KRÄUTERBUTTER steak grilled and served with creamed seasoned butter

FILETSTEAK Á LA MEYER   beef tenderloin fried in
  butter with fried onion rings
FISCHCREME   creamed fish
FISCHFRIKADELLEN   fish cakes
FISCHGERICHTE   seafood
FISCHKLÖSSCHEN   small fish dumplings
FISCHKLÖSSE   fish dumplings
FISCHKRUSTELN (AUS)   fish croquettes
FISCHLEIN   little fish
FISCHRAGOUT   fish stew
FISCHRAHMSUPPE   creamed fish soup
FISCHROULADEN   fish rolls
FISCHSALAT   fish salad
FISCHSCHÜSSEL   casserole of fish and diced bacon
FISCHSUPPE   fish soup
FISTERNOLLEKEN   corn brandy
FLÄDLE   thin strips of pancake added to soup
FLÄDLESUPPE   bouillon with thin strips of pancake
FLAMBIERT   flambé, food flamed with brandy
FLAMMERI   rice or semolina pudding with stewed fruit
  or vanilla custard
FLASCHE   bottle
FLECK   spot or stain
FLEISCH   meat
FLEISCH MIT SAUERKRAUT (AUS)   pork with
  sauerkraut
FLEISCHBRÜHE   meat soup
FLEISCHBRÜHE MIT EI   meat broth with beaten egg
FLEISCHBRÜHE MIT LEBERKNÖDEL   meat broth with
  liver dumplings
FLEISCHBRÜHE MIT MARK   meat broth with marrow
FLEISCHBRÜHE MIT MARKKLÖSSCHEN   meat broth
  with marrow dumplings
FLEISCHBRÜHE MIT MAULTASCHEN   meat stock with
  pasta envelopes filled with meat
FLEISCHBRÜHE MIT RINDERMARK   meat broth with
  beef marrow

FLEISCHBRÜHE NATUR   plain meat broth or bouillon
FLEISCHEINTÖPF   beef or veal casserole dish
FLEISCHFÜLLUNG   meat filling
FLEISCHGERICHTE   meat dishes
FLEISCHKÄSE   seasoned meat loaf
FLEISCHKLOSS   meat dumpling
FLEISCHKLÖSSE   meat balls
FLEISCHKÜCHLE   meat dumplings
FLEISCHPFLANZERL   pan-fried hamburger
FLEISCHRÖLLCHEN   cooked stuffed meat slices served
   cold
FLEISCHSALAT   meat salad
FLEISCHSPEISEN   meat dishes
FLEISCHSÜLZE   meat in aspic
FLEISCHWURST   similar to baloney, served hot boiled,
   grilled, or cold
FLORENTINER   almond cookies with candied orange
   peel, honey, heavy cream, chocolate
FLÜGEL   wing
FLUNDER   flounder
FLUNDER, GEBACKEN   baked founder
FLÜSSIGE SAHNE   thick cream
FLUSSKARPFEN   river carp
FLUSSLACHS   stream salmon
FONDANTNÜSSE   nut fondant
FONDUE, NEUCHATELER ART   fondue neuchatel, with
   garlic, eggs, white wine, Swiss cheese, cherry brandy
FORELLE "MÜLLERIN-ART"   trout prepared in Miller's
   wife style; dredged in flour, and fried in butter and oil
FORELLE   trout
FORELLE BLAU   steamed trout
FORELLE GERÄUCHERT MIT OBERSKREN (AUS)
   smoked trout with horseradish cream
FORELLE IN ASPIK (AUS)   trout in aspic
FORELLE IN WEISSWEIN   trout in white wine
FORELLE IN WEISSWEINSUD   trout served in a creamed
   white wine sauce

FORELLE, LEBENSFRISCHE   trout taken fresh and alive
   from the restaurant's fish tank
FORELLE NACH MÜLLERIN-ART   fried trout
FORELLEN IN ASPIK   jellied trout
FORELLENFILET   fillet of trout
FÖRSTER   gamekeeper
FÖRSTEREINTOPF MIT PILZEN   stew of venison,
   vegetables, mushrooms, forester style
FRANKEN   strong, dry, high quality, robust, fruity white
   wine
FRANKFURTER   frankfurter
FRÄNKISCHE BROTSUPPE   soup of stock, onion,
   liverwurst, potatoes and rye bread
FRÄNKISCHE LEBERKLÖSSE IN SPECKSAUCE   liver
   dumplings in bacon sauce
FRANZÖSISCHE FISCHSUPPE   fish soup like French
   bouillabaisse
FRANZÖSISCHE HUMMERSUPPE   French-style lobster
   soup
FRANZÖSISCHE RAHMMARINADE   French dressing
FRANZÖSISCHE ZWIEBELSUPPE   French onion soup
FRANZÖSISCHES NOUGAT   French-style nougat candy
FREI   free
FRIKADELLE(N)   meat, fowl or fish dumpling(s) or
   croquette(s)
FRIKASSEE   stew of browned meat or poultry cooked in
   stock
FRIKASSEEHUHN   stewing chicken
FRISCH   fresh
FRISCHES OBST   fresh fruit
FRISCHLING   young wild boar
FRITTIEREN   to fry foods
FROSCHSCHENKEL   frogs' legs
FROSCHSCHENKEL PANIERT, GEBACKEN (AUS)
   breaded and fried frog's legs
FRUCHT   fruit

FRUCHTBECHER fruit cup with ice cream or liqueur
FRUCHTCREME custard made with fruit
FRÜCHTE DER JAHRESZEIT fruit in season
FRÜCHTE IN BACKTEIG (AUS) fruit fritters
FRUCHTEIS fruit ices or ice cream
FRUCHTKALTSCHALE chilled soup with sugar and
  pureed fruits added to a wine base
FRUCHTSAUCE fruit sauce
FRÜHLINGSSUPPE soup with diced spring vegetables
FRÜHSTÜCK breakfast
FRÜHSTÜCKSKÄSE a young strong cheese with smooth
  texture
FRÜHSTÜCKSSPECK smoked breakfast bacon
FÜLLUNG stuffing
FÜRST-PÜCKLER-EIS chocolate, strawberry and vanilla
  ice cream with strawberries and whipped cream

G

GABACKENE EIER eggs fried and basted in butter
GABEL fork
GABELFRÜHSTÜCK brunch
GAISBURGER MARSCH soup with cubes of meat,
  onions, potatoes, noodles
GANS goose
GANSBRATEN roast goose
GÄNSEBRATEN MIT ÄPFELN, ROSINEN UND NÜSSEN
  roast goose with apple, raisin and nut stuffing
GÄNSEBRATEN MIT KARTOFFELFÜLLUNG roast
  goose with prune, apple, and potato stuffing
GÄNSEBRUST breast of goose
GÄNSEKLEIN goose giblets
GÄNSELEBER goose liver
GÄNSELEBER MIT ÄPFELN goose liver with apples
GÄNSELEBERPASTETE goose liver pâté or paste
GÄNSELEBERSCHNITZEL goose liver cutlet

GÄNSELEBERWURST   goose liver sausage
GÄNSESCHMALZ   goose fat
GANZ   whole, entire, as the whole fish
GARNELE   shrimp
GARNIERT   garnish surrounding a dish
GARNIERTES STEAK   garnished steak
GARNITUR   garnish
GASTHAUS   a restaurant
GASTHOF   country word for restaurant serving drinks and meals
GASTSTÄTTE   restaurant
GAZPACHO   cold tomato, cucumber, vegetable soup
GEBÄCK   pastry
GEBACKENE AUSTERN   batter-fried oysters
GEBACKENE KALBSBRUST (AUS)   fried breast of veal
GEBACKENE KARTOFFEL   baked potato
GEBACKENE KARTOFFELN   baked potatoes
GEBACKENE KARTOFFELSCHALE   baked potato skin
GEBACKENE LEBER   fried liver
GEBACKENE SCHOLLE   baked sole
GEBACKENE ZUNGE   small fried tongue
GEBACKENER BLUMENKOHL   fried cauliflower
GEBACKENER FISCH   fried or baked fish
GEBACKENER FISCH MIT KRAUT   baked fish with sauerkraut
GEBACKENER SPARGEL   deep-fried asparagus
GEBACKENER ZANDER IN WEISSWEIN   walleyed pike baked in white wine
GEBACKENES HIRN   baked brains
GEBACKENES SCHWEINEKOTELETT   fried breaded or unbreaded pork chop
GEBEIZT   pickled
GEBRANNTE MANDELN   almonds in sugar glaze
GEBRATEN   roasted or fried
GEBRATENE ENTE   roast duckling
GEBRATENE FORELLE   pan-fried trout
GEBRATENE HÜHNERLEBER   fried chicken livers

GEBRATENE KALBSLEBER   calf's liver with apples and onion rings

GEBRATENE LAMMKEULE   roast leg of lamb

GEBRATENE LEBER   fried liver

GEBRATENE SCHWEINSHAXE   roasted pork shank

GEBRATENER FASAN   roast pheasant

GEBRATENER HAHN   roast chicken

GEBRATENER HUMMER   fried lobster

GEBRATENER TRUTHAHN   roast turkey

GEBRATENES HAMMELKARREE (AUS)   roast mutton chop

GEBRATENES LAMM   roast lamb

GEBRATENES SCHWEINSKOTELETTE MIT ÄPFELN   pork chops with apples

GEBUNDEN   sauce or soup which is thickened with flour

GEDÄMPFT   steamed or sometimes braised

GEDÄMPFTE KALBSBRUST   breast of veal potted with onions

GEDÄMPFTE REHSCHLEGEL   braised leg of venison

GEDÄMPFTE RINDERBRUST   potted beef with natural gravy

GEDÄMPFTER RINDSBRATEN   pot roast of beef with wine

GEDECK   set price meal

GEDÜNSTET   braised or steamed

GEDÜNSTETER PARADIESRINDSBRATEN (AUS)   braised beef with tomatoes

GEDÜNSTETER RINDERSAFTBRATEN (AUS)   braised beef in gravy

GEDÜNSTETES RINDERSCHNITZEL IN ROTWEIN (AUS)   braised steak with red wine

GEDÜNSTETES SAUERKRAUT   steamed sauerkraut

GEDÜNSTETES SCHWEINSKOTELETT (AUS)   braised pork cutlet

GEFLÜGEL   fowl

GEFLÜGELCREMESUPPE   cream of chicken soup

GEFLÜGELFRIKASÉE   chicken fricasee

GEFLÜGELKLEIN giblets
GEFLÜGELLEBER chicken livers
GEFLÜGELLEBER STRASSBURGER-ART chicken livers in red wine sauce with mushrooms on rice
GEFLÜGELPASTETE poultry pot pie
GEFLÜGELRAGOUT chicken fricassé
GEFLÜGELREISBOMBE rice mold with chicken
GEFLÜGELRISOTTO pieces of chicken in rice pilaf
GEFLÜGELSALAT chicken salad with mayonnaise
GEFLÜGELWILD game bird dishes
GEFROREN chilled or iced
GEFRORENES ice cream
GEFÜLLTE ÄPFEL apples stuffed with raisins, sugar, cinnamon, nuts, white wine
GEFÜLLTE ÄPFEL AUS DEM ROHR (AUS) oven-cooked stuffed apples
GEFÜLLTE ÄPFEL FLAMBIERT (AUS) stuffed apples flambé
GEFÜLLTE AUBERGINE stuffed eggplant
GEFÜLLTE EIER stuffed hard-cooked eggs with ham, anchovy, onion
GEFÜLLTE EIERPFANNKUCHEN filled egg pancake
GEFÜLLTE GANS stuffed goose
GEFÜLLTE KALBSBRUST stuffed breast of veal
GEFÜLLTE PAPRIKA peppers stuffed with beef, pork, rice, in tomato sauce
GEFÜLLTE PFANNKUCHEN filled pancakes
GEFÜLLTE TOMATEN (AUS) stuffed tomatoes
GEFÜLLTE TOMATEN MIT FLEISCHSALAT tomatoes stuffed with cold meat salad
GEFÜLLTE TOMATEN MIT GEFLÜGELSALAT tomatoes stuffed with chicken salad
GEFÜLLTE WACHTEL IN KASSEROLLE (AUS) stuffed quail in casserole
GEFÜLLTE ZWIEBELN stuffed onions
GEFÜLLTER FASAN stuffed pheasant
GEFÜLLTER FISCH stuffed fish or chopped fish

GEFÜLLTER GÄNSEBRATEN   roast goose with potato stuffing

GEFÜLLTER GÄNSEHALS   stuffed goose neck

GEFÜLLTER KRAPFEN   baked apple tart

GEFÜLLTER KRAUTKOPF   cabbage stuffed with beef, pork and onion

GEGRILLT   grilled

GEGRILLTER FISCH MIT MAYONNAISE   fine quality fried or boiled fish with mayonnaise

GEGRILLTER LACHS   grilled salmon

GRILLIERTES KALBSSCHNITZEL   grilled veal cutlet

GEGRILLTES WILDBRETFILET   broiled venison fillets

GEHACKT   minced or chopped

GEHACKTE PETERSILIE   chopped parsley

GEHACKTES RINDERSCHNITZEL   fried beef patties

GEHOBELT   shredded

GEKOCHT   cooked, boiled

GEKOCHT KREBSE (AUS)   boiled crayfish

GEKOCHTE EIER   boiled eggs

GEKOCHTE KARTOFFELKLÖSSE   potato dumplings

GEKOCHTE KARTOFFELN   boiled potatoes

GEKOCHTE RINDERBRUST   boiled brisket of beef

GEKOCHTER REIS   boiled rice

GEKOCHTER SCHINKEN   boiled ham

GEKOCHTES FLEISCH   boiled beef

GEKOCHTES OCHSENFLEISCH   boiled beef

GEKOCHTES RINDFLEISCH (AUS)   boiled beef

GEKOCHTES SCHWEINEFLEISCH   boiled pork

GELBE ERBSENSUPPE   dried yellow pea soup

GELBE RÜBE   carrot

GELEE   aspic, jelly, jam

GELEEHERINGE   jellied herring

GEMISCHT   mixed or varied

GEMISCHTER AUFSCHNITT   mixed cold cuts

GEMISCHTER SALAT   mixed salad

GEMÜSE BEILAGE   vegetables or other side dishes

GEMÜSE PLATTE   vegetable plate

GEMÜSE SALAT   vegetable salad
GEMÜSECREMESUPPE   cream of vegetable soup
GEMÜSESUPPE   vegetable soup
GEPÖKELT   pickled
GEPÖKELTE RINDERBRUST MIT SAUERKRAUT   boiled
   pickled beef breast with sauerkraut
GERÄUCHERT   smoked
GERÄUCHERTE FORELLE MIT MEERETTICH   smoked
   trout with horseradish cream
GERÄUCHERTER LACHS   smoked salmon
GERÄUCHERTER RHEINLACHS   smoked salmon from
   the Rhine
GERÄUCHERTER SCHINKEN   smoked ham
GERICHT   dish or meal course
GERIEBEN   ground or grated
GERIEBENER KÄSE   grated cheese
GERMKNÖDEL (AUS)   light yeast dumplings with butter,
   freshly-ground poppy seeds and powdered sugar
GERÖSTET   roast
GERÖSTETE KARTOFFELN   pan-fried boiled potatoes
GERÖSTETE KÄSESCHNITTEN   Welsh rarebits
GERÖSTETES BROT   toast
GERSTE   barley
GERSTENSUPPE   barley soup
GESALZEN   salted
GESALZENES VOM SCHWEIN   salt pork
GESCHLOSSEN   closed
GESCHMORT   stewed, braised
GESCHMORTE SCHWEINSHAXE   pot roasted pork
   shank
GESCHNETZELTE HÄHNCHENBRUST   pieces of
   chicken breast in cream sauce
GESCHNETZELTES   meat cut into thin, small slices
GESCHNETZELTES IN RAHM   in cream sauce
GESCHNETZELTES NACH SCHWEIZER ART   meat
   fried in brown sauce with white wine and sour cream

GESCHNETZELTES NACH ZIGEUNER ART   meat fried in brown sauce with peppers, paprika and mushrooms
GESELCHTES   cured and smoked pork
GESOTTEN   simmered, boiled
GESPICKT   holes in meat filled with pork fat
GESÜLZTE FORELLEN   jellied trout
GESÜSSTER WEIN   sweetened wine
GETRÄNKE   drinks, liquor
GEWÜRZBUTTER   seasoned butter
GEWÜRZE   spice
GEWÜRZGURKE   pickle, gherkin
GEWÜRZKUCHEN   spice cake
GEWÜRZNELKE   clove
GEWÜRZT   spiced
GEWÜRZTE SCHWEINSRIPPCHEN   braised, spiced pork spareribs
GEZUCKERT   sugar added, sweetened
GIPFEL   crescent shaped roll
GITTERTORTE   almond cake or tart with a raspberry topping
GITZI   kid
GLACÉ   ice cream
GLAS   glass
GLASIERT   glazed, as ham, carrots or chestnuts
GLASIERTE KASTANIEN   chestnuts glazed in sugar and butter
GLASUREN   icings
GLATTBUTT   brill
GLÜHWEIN   mulled wine
GNAGI   cured pig's knuckle
GOLDBARSCH   red seabass, like red snapper
GOLDBARSCHFILET, GEBACKEN   baked fillet of sea bass
GOLDBUTT   flat fish similar to turbot
GÖTTERSPEISE   fruit jello dessert
GRANAT   prawn

GRANATÄPFEL   pomegranate
GRATINIERT   oven-browned with bread crumbs and cheese
GRAUBROT   brown or black bread
GRAUPENSUPPE   barley soup
GRAUPENSUPPE MIT HÜHNERKLEIN   barley soup with chicken giblets
GREYERZER   Gruyere cheese
GRIEBENWURST   larded frying sausage
GRIESS   semolina
GRIESSAUFLAUF   farina pudding
GRIESSFLAMMERI   semolina pudding
GRIESSKLÖSSCHE(N)   semolina dumpling(s)
GRIESSKLOSSUPPE   bouillon with small semolina dumplings
GRIESSNOCKERLSUPPE   semolina dumpling soup
GRIESSSUPPE   beef soup with semolina
GRIESSTORTE   farina layer cake with almonds
GRILLGERICHTE   dishes from the grill
GRILLHAXE   grilled shank
GRILLTELLER   plate of various cuts of grilled meats
GROSS   large
GRÖSTL   grated, fried potatoes with meat pieces
GRÜN   green
GRÜNE BOHNEN   French bean, green bean
GRÜNE ERBSEN   green peas
GRÜNE GURKEN   cucumber
GRÜNE KARTOFFELSUPPE   green potato soup
GRÜNE SOSSE   green herb sauce from fish poaching broth
GRÜNER SALAT   lettuce salad
GRÜNKERNSUPPE   young wheat cooked in soup, like barley
GRÜNKOHL   kale, a dark green leafy vegetable
GRÜNKOHL MIT KARTOFFELN   baked kale with potatoes
GRÜTZE   cooked fruit or berry pudding

GUGELHUPF   coffee cake with almonds and raisins
GUGGELI   spring chicken
GUGLHUPF (AUS)   light chocolate torte with center of
   apricot jam
GULASCH   meat braised in sauce with vegetables and
   paprika
GULASCHSUPPE   soup with meat pieces, vegetables and
   paprika
GURKE   cucumber
GURKENKÖRBCHEN   scooped out cucumbers filled
   with chopped tomatoes
GURKENSALAT   cucumber salad
GURKENSUPPE   cucumber soup
GUT DURCHGEBRATEN   well-done

H

HACKBRATEN   chopped steak or meat loaf of beef and
   pork
HACKBRATEN MIT SPECK   meat loaf with diced
   smoked bacon
HACKBRATEN NACH HAUSMANN'S-ART   large
   hamburger or slices of meat loaf
HACKFLEISCH   minced meat
HACKRAHMSTEAK   hamburger with thick brown gravy
HACKSPIESSCHEN ZIGEUNER ART   meat balls on a
   skewer with peppers, tomatoes and onion
HACKSTEAK   beef hamburger
HAFERBREI   oatmeal, porridge
HAFERFLOCKEN   rolled oats, oatmeal
HAFERFLOCKENMAKRONEN   baked oat macaroons
HAFERFLOCKENSUPPE   oatmeal soup
HAFERSCHLEIMSUPPE   boiled oats like porridge
HAHN   rooster
HÄHNCHEN   spring chicken
HÄHNCHENMAGEN   chicken giblets
HAIFISCHFLOSSENSUPPE   shark fin soup

HALB   half
HALB GAR   rare, underdone
HALB ROH   rare
HALBER HAHN   cheese sandwich on whole wheat roll
HALBGEFRORENES   frozen whipped cream or ice-cream
   dessert
HALT   stop
HÄMMCHEN   pigs' knuckles and sauerkraut
HAMMEL   mutton
HAMMEL BOURGEOISE   potted mutton
HAMMEL-REISFLEISCH IN PAPRIKASCHOTEN
   braised mutton with peppers, served on rice
HAMMELBOUILLON   clear soup made with mutton
HAMMELBRATEN   roast mutton
HAMMELFLEISCH   lamb and mutton meat
HAMMELFLEISCH MIT BOHNEN   stewed mutton with
   beans
HAMMELFLEISCH MIT GRÜNEN BOHNEN   potted
   lamb and green beans
HAMMELFLEISCHEINTOPF   lamb stew with breast of
   lamb, potatoes, caraway seeds, bacon
HAMMELKEULE   leg of mutton
HAMMELKOTELETTEN   mutton or lamb chops
HAMMELKOTELETTEN IN ZWIEBELSOSSE   lamb
   chops in onion sauce
HAMMELRAGOUT   mutton ragout or stew
HAMMELSCHLEGEL   thigh of mutton
HAMMELSCHULTER MIT WEISSEN RÜBEN   shoulder
   of mutton with red turnips
HAMMELSTEAK   mutton steak
HANDKÄSE   cheese from sour milk
HANDKÄSE MIT MUSIK   marinated strong flavored
   cheese
HAPPEN   snack
HARTGEKOCHT   hard-boiled
HASCHEE   hash
HASE   hare, jack rabbit

HASELHUHN   local grouse
HASELNUSS   hazelnuts
HASELNUSSBÄLLCHEN   hazelnut balls
HASELNUSSCREME   hazelnut cream pudding
HASELNUSSEIS   frozen hazelnut ice cream dessert
HASELNUSSKUCHEN MIT SCHLAG   hazelnut torte
   with whipped cream
HASELNUSSMAKRONEN   hazelnut macaroons
HASELNUSSRING   hazelnut ring
HASELNUSSSCHNITTEN   baked hazelnut strips
HASELNUSSTORTE   hazelnut tart
HASELNUSSTORTE   hazelnut torte
HASEN   large rabbit or hare
HASENBRATEN   roast hare
HASENKEULE   leg of hare
HASENLÄUFE IN JÄGERRAHMSAUCE   hare thighs in
   sauce of mushrooms, shallots and wine
HASENOHREN   a puff pastry
HASENPFEFFER   marinated hare stewed in red wine,
   mushrooms and onions
HASENTOPF IN WEISSWEIN   casserole of hare in wine
HAUPTGERICHTE   main courses
HAUSGEBEIZT   home cured
HAUSGEM.   house or homemade (abbreviation)
HAUSGEMACHT   homemade
HAUSGEMACHTE SUPPE   homemade soup
HAUSGEPÖKELT   home pickled or home cured
HAUSGERÄUCHERTES   smoked home style
HAUSGESELCHTES   smoked pork
HAUSMACHER   homemade
HAUSMANNSKOST   plain food
HAWAII   with pineapple
HAWAII-ANANAS ÜBERBACKEN (AUS)   pineapple
   flambé
HAXE   shank of leg
HAXE MIT SAUERKRAUT   pigs' shank and sauerkraut
HAZELNUSS   hazelnut

HECHT   pike
HECHT IN SAUERRAHM   pike in sour cream
HEFEKLÖSSE   yeast dumplings
HEFEKRANZ   ring-shaped cake
HEIDELBEERE   blueberry
HEIDELBEERSCHNITTEN (AUS)   blueberry pie
HEIDELBEERSTRUDEL (AUS)   blueberry strudel
HEIDESAND   baked brown butter cookies
HEIDSCHNUCKENKEULE   leg of lamb
HEIDSCHNUCKENKEULE IN WACHOLDERRAHM
    lamb in juniper berry sauce
HEILBUTT   halibut
HEILBUTT IN SAHNE   halibut with cream
HEISS   hot or warm
HEISSE BIERSUPPE   hot beer soup
HEISSE SCHOKOLADE   hot chocolate
HELLE SOSSE   basic cream sauce
HELLES BIER   light beer
HERING   herring
HERING BLAU   blue herring
HERING IN PERGAMENT   herring in wax paper
HERING NACH HAUSFRAUEN-ART   herring fillets
    with onions in sour cream
HERING VOM ROST   grilled herring
HERINGS TOAST   chopped herring salad on toast
HERINGSALAT   herring salad
HERINGSAUFLAUF   baked herring casserole
HERINGSAUFLAUT MIT KARTOFFELN   casserole of
    layers of herring and potatoes
HERZ   heart
HERZ-LEBER-NIERENSPIESSCHEN   heart, liver and
    kidney grilled on skewer
HERZOGINKARTOFFELN   mashed potatoes in different
    shapes, oven-browned or pan-fried
HESSISCHE BERGSTRASSE-WEIN   fruity, elegant,
    fragrant, mild wine

HEXENSCHNEE   chilled dessert of applesauce, apricot preserves, rum, lemon juice

HIESIG   native or local

HIESIGER DORSCH   local or native cod

HIMBEERBRÖTCHEN   baked raspberry mounds

HIMBEERE   raspberry

HIMBEERGEIST   spirit distilled from raspberries

HIMBEERSOUFFLE   raspberry soufflee

HIMBEERTORTE   raspberry tart

HIMMEL UND ERDE   slices of pudding made with sausages, fried onions, mashed potatoes and apple sauce

HIRN   brains

HIRN IN BRAUNER BUTTER   brains in brown butter

HIRN MIT RUHREI   calves' brains with scrambled eggs

HIRNSUPPE   brain soup

HIRSCH   stag, venison

HIRSCHBRATEN   roast venison

HIRSCHKALB   stag calf

HIRSCHKEULE   leg of venison

HIRSCHRAGOUT   venison stew

HIRSCHSCHLEGEL   leg of venison

HIRSCHSCHLEGEL GEBRATEN (AUS)   roast leg of venison

HIRSCHSCHULTER   shoulder of venison

HIRSE   millet

HIRTENSTEAK   veal steak

HOBELSPÄNE   deep-fried crisp twists of rum flavored dough

HOCHZEITSSUPPE   rich soup with meats and vegetables

HOHE RIPPE   roast ribs of beef

HOLLÄNDISCHE SOSSE   Hollandaise sauce

HOLSTEIN SCHNITZEL   pan-fried veal cutlet with fried egg and anchovies

HOLSTEINER SCHNITZEL   veal cutlets served with fried eggs and anchovies

HOLZBRETT   wooden plank
HOLZTELLER   wooden plate
HONIGKUCHEN   honey cake
HONIGLEBKUCHEN   baked honey spice cake
HONIGMELONE   honey melon
HOPPELPOPPEL   eggs with bacon, onions and potatoes
HÖRNCHEN   crescent-shaped roll
HUBERTUSSCHNITZEL   butter fried veal cutlet with
   wine, shallot and mushroom sauce
HÜFTSTEAK   top sirloin steak, beef or veal
HUHN   fowl, including game birds, or chicken
HUHN IN BURGUNDER   chicken in burgundy
HUHN MIT NOCKERLN   chicken with dumplings
HUHN MIT NUDELN   stewed chicken with noodles
HUHN MIT REIS UND SPARGEL   chicken on rice with
   asparagus
HÜHNCHEN   chicken
HÜHNERBOUILLON   clear chicken broth
HÜHNERBRATEN   roast chicken
HÜHNERBRÜHE MIT NUDELN   chicken soup with
   noodles
HÜHNERBRUST   breast of chicken
HÜHNERCREMESUPPE   creamed chicken soup
HÜHNERFLEISCHKRAFTBRÜHE   chicken soup
HÜHNERFLÜGEL   chicken wings
HÜHNERFRIKASEE   chicken fricassee
HÜHNERKLEIN   chicken giblets
HÜHNERKRAFTBRÜHE   chicken consommé
HÜHNERLEBER   chicken livers
HÜHNERLEBER, GERÖSTET (AUS)   sautéed chicken liver
HÜHNERPASTETE   chicken patties with grated cheese,
   truffle, cream, onion
HÜHNERRAGOUT   chicken stew
HÜHNERSALAT   chicken salad
HÜHNERSUPPE   chicken soup
HÜHNERSUPPE MIT REIS   chicken soup with rice
HÜLSENFRÜCHTE   legumes

HUMMER   lobster
HUMMER, KALT (AUS)   cold lobster
HUMMER VOM ROST (AUS)   grilled lobster
HUMMERCOCKTAIL (AUS)   lobster cocktail
HUMMERCREMESUPPE   cream of lobster soup
HUMMERKRABBEN   large crabs
HUMMERSUPPE   lobster soup
HUSARENFLEISCH   braised beef, veal and pork, sweet
   peppers, onions and sour cream
HÜTTENKÄSE MIT FRÜCHTEN   cottage cheese with
   fruit
HUTZELBROT   bread made of prunes and other dried
   fruit

I

IMBISS   snack
INDIANERKRAPFEN (AUS)   fritters with whipped cream
INDISCHE REISCREMESUPPE   Indian rice cream soup
INGWER   ginger
INGWERBROT   gingerbread
INGWERCREME   ginger cream sauce
INGWERSAHNE   ginger cream
ITALIENISCHER SALAT   veal, salami, tomatoes,
   anchovies, cucumber in mayonnaise

J

JAGDWURST   smoked pork, beef and bacon sausage
JÄGEREINTOPF   beef stew with onions, mushrooms,
   potatoes
JÄGERSCHNITZEL   veal cutlet with wine, mushroom
   and tomato sauce
JÄGERSCHNITZEL MIT PFIFFERLINGEN   fried veal
   cutlet, sauce of mushrooms, shallots, wine, tomato
JÄGERSPIESS   skewered venison, broiled or sautéed in a
   sauce

JÄGERTOPF   casserole or stew, of meat, mushrooms, tomato sauce, shallots

JAKOBSMUSCHEL   scallop

JOGHURT   yogurt

JOHANNISBEERE   redcurrent

JOHANNISBEERSOSSE   redcurrant jelly sauce

JULIENNESUPPE MIT SAGO   vegetable soup with tapioca

JUNG   young, spring

JUNGE ENTE   duckling

JUNGE ENTE, GEBRATEN, GEDÜNSTET, GEFÜLLT (AUS)
   duckling, roast, stewed, stuffed

JUNGER SCHWEINERÜCKEN   roasted young pig's back, loin or saddle

JUNGES GEMÜSE   young vegetables

JUNGES HUHN   spring chicken

JUNGFERNBRATEN   roast pork with bacon

K

KABELJAU   codfish

KABELJAU GEGRILLER   codfish or haddock, grilled with butter, paprika and grated cheese

KABELJAU KUTTERKABELJAU   cutter, codfish

KABELJAU UNGARISCHER   codfish sauteed in butter, onion, sour cream, paprika

KABINETT   wine of high quality

KAFFEE   coffee

KAFFEE HAG   caffeine-free coffee

KAFFEE KIRSCH (AUS)   cup or small jug of black coffee accompanied by a small glass of Kirsch or cherry brandy

KAFFEE MIT SAHNE   coffee with cream

KAFFEE MIT SCHLAG   coffee with whipped cream

KAFFEE MIT ZUCKER   with sugar

KAFFEE, SCHWARZER   black coffee

KAFFEE VERKEHRT (AUS)   more milk than coffee

KAFFEECREME   coffee cream

KAFFEECREMEROLLE   coffee cream roll

KAFFEECREMETORTE   coffee cream cake
KAFFEEKUCHEN   coffeecake
KAFFEEROULADE (AUS)   coffee cream roll
KAISERGRANAT   Norway lobster, Dublin Bay prawn
KAISERKRABBEN   special shrimps
KAISERMELANGE (AUS)   half coffee, half hot milk, to
   which a fresh egg has been added
KAISERSCHMARREN   sweet dessert omelette served in
   cut up pieces
KAISERSCHMARREN MIT KOMPOTT   sweet dessert
   omelette served in cut up pieces with applesauce or
   stewed fruit
KAISERSCHMARRN   sweet dessert omelette served in
   cut up pieces
KAISERSCHOTEN   small peas
KAKAO   cocoa
KALB   veal
KALB FLEISCHBÄLLCHEN   veal meatballs
KALB FLEISCHKLÖSSCHEN   veal meatballs with onions,
   poached in stock
KALB, GEGRILLTES   grilled veal
KALB NACH BERLINER-ART   veal fried in butter with
   onion rings and apples
KALB NACH JÄGERART   veal fried in butter with
   mushrooms, shallots, wine, tomato paste
KALBFLEISCH, GESCHABTET   ground veal
KALBFLEISCHRAGOUT   pieces of veal in brown sauce
KALBFLEISCHRAHMSUPPE   veal cream soup
KALBFLEISCHSCHNITTE MIT RAHMSAUCE   veal slices
   in gravy with cream
KALBFLEISCHSUPPE   clear soup with veal
KALBFLEISCHVOGEL   veal scallops in anchovy cream
   gravy
KALBS BRUST, GEFÜLLTE   breast of veal, stuffed with
   chicken livers or ham
KALBSBRATEN   veal roast
KALBSBRATWURST   grilled sausage made of veal

KALBSBRIES   veal sweetbread

KALBSBRIES IN WEISSWEIN   calf sweetbreads poached in wine

KALBSBRUST   breast of veal

KALBSBRÜSTCHEN   sweetbreads

KALBSFILLET   veal tenderloin or fillet steak

KALBSFLEISCH   veal meat

KALBSFRIKASSEE   veal fricassee

KALBSFÜSSE   calves' feet

KALBSGESCHNETZELTES   veal slices cooked in brown sauce

KALBSGOULASCH   braised pieces of veal with seasonings

KALBSGULASCH (AUS)   veal goulash

KALBSHAXE   veal hocks or shanks

KALBSHAXE, GEBRATENE   baked or roasted veal shanks or hocks

KALBSHAXE IN GEWÜRZGURKENSOSSE   veal shanks in pickle sauce

KALBSHAXE, KNUSPRIGE   crispy roasted veal shank

KALBSHERZ   broiled or baked veal heart

KALBSHIRN   calves' brains

KALBSHIRN MIT RÜHREI   scrambled eggs with calves' brains

KALBSKÄSE   veal meat loaf with cheese

KALBSKOPF   calves' head, boiled, boned, batter-dipped, and deep-fried

KALBSKOTELETT, GEBACKEN, GEBRATEN, GEGRILLT (AUS)   veal cutlet, fried, roast, grilled

KALBSKOTELETTEN NATURELL   plain veal chops

KALBSLEBER   calves' liver

KALBSLEBER, GEBRATENE   fried, breaded calves' liver

KALBSLEBER MIT SPECK   calf's liver with bacon

KALBSLEBERWURST   veal liverwurst

KALBSLENDCHEN   veal loin

KALBSLUNGE   calf's lungs

KALBSMEDALLIONS   veal leg slices

KALBSMILCH sweetbreads
KALBSNIERENBRATEN veal with kidney
KALBSNIERENSTÜCK loin of veal
KALBSNÜSSCHEN roasted veal sirloin
KALBSRAGOUT MIT GEMÜSE (AUS) veal stew with
   vegetables
KALBSRAHMBRATEN veal with sweet or sour cream
   sauce
KALBSRIPPCHEN veal chop
KALBSROLLBRATEN stuffed rolled veal slices
KALBSRÜCKEN back of veal
KALBSSAFTGOULASCH very liquid veal stew
KALBSSCHLEGEL veal leg
KALBSSCHNITZEL veal cutlet
KALBSSCHNITZEL MIT SARDELLEN veal cutlet in
   sauce with anchovies
KALBSSCHNITZEL NATUR MIT CHAMPIGNONS UND
   RAHMSOSSE cutlet natural, with mushrooms and
   cream sauce
KALBSSCHNITZEL PRINZESS cutlet in mushroom sauce
   with potato croquettes and asparagus
KALBSSCHNITZEL RUSSISCH fried cutlet with
   mushrooms and tomatoes in cream sauce
KALBSSCHNITZEL, WIENER cutlet breaded and fried in
   lard
KALBSSCHULTER shoulder of veal
KALBSSTEAK veal steak
KALBSVOGERL stuffed cutlets, pot-roasted with
   vegetables in wine
KALDAUNEN tripe
KALT cold
KALTE refers to cold dishes
KALTE GERICHTE small cold dishes
KALTE KALBSLENDE cold loin of veal
KALTE SPEISEN cold dishes
KALTE VORSPEISEN cold first courses or appetizers
KALTE WEINSUPPE cold wine soup

KALTES GEFLÜGEL   cold poultry

KALTES HUHN (AUS)   cold chicken

KALTSCHALE   chilled fruit soup with white wine base

KAMMÜSCHEL   scallop

KANDIERTE FRÜCHTE   candied fruit

KANDIERTE ORANGENSCHALEN   candied orange peel

KANGURUHSCHWANZSUPPE   kangaroo tail soup

KANINCHEN   rabbit

KAPAUN   capon

KAPERN   capers

KAPERNSOSSE   caper sauce

KAPUZINER (AUS)   small cup of black coffee with cream,
   producing the color dark brown

KAPUZINER   coffee with whipped cream and grated
   chocolate

KARAMELCREME   caramel custard

KARAMELSAUCE   caramel sauce

KARFIOL   cauliflower

KAROTTEN   carrots

KAROTTENEINTOPF MIT FLEISCHEINLAGE   carrot
   casserole with meat

KAROTTENSUPPE   carrot soup

KARPFEN   carp

KARPFEN, GEGRILLTER   grilled carp

KARPFEN, GESÜLZTER (AUS)   carp in aspic

KARTOFFEL KRONPRINZESSIN   mashed potatoes
   breaded and deep-fried

KARTOFFEL LYONNAISE   sliced potatoes, fried in lard
   with fried onions

KARTOFFELBÄLLCHEN   pan-fried mashed potato balls

KARTOFFELBREI   mashed potatoes

KARTOFFELCHIPS   potato chips

KARTOFFELCROQUETTEN (AUS)   potato croquettes

KARTOFFELFÜLLE   potato stuffing

KARTOFFELGERICHTE   potato dishes

KARTOFFELKLÖSSE   potato dumplings

KARTOFFELKLÖSSE MIT PFLAUMENMUS   potato
   dessert dumplings with prune butter filling
KARTOFFELKNÖDEL   potato dumplings
KARTOFFELKROKETTEN   potato croquettes
KARTOFFELKÜCHLEIN   potato pancakes
KARTOFFELN   potatoes
KARTOFFELN, GERÖSTETE   crisp pan-fried potatoes
KARTOFFELN MIT SPECK   fried potatoes with bits of
   bacon
KARTOFFELPASTETCHEN   potato patties, containing
   onion in pastry tart
KARTOFFELPUFFER MIT APFELMUS   potato pancakes
   with applesauce
KARTOFFELPUFFER, REIBEKUCHEN   potato pancakes
KARTOFFELPÜREE   mashed potatoes
KARTOFFELPÜREE MIT GELBEN RÜBEN   whipped
   potatoes and carrots
KARTOFFELPÜREE MIT SAHNE   mashed potatoes with
   cream
KARTOFFELSALAT   potato salad
KARTOFFELSCHALE   potatoes in their jackets
KARTOFFELSUPPE   potato soup
KARTOFFELTTOMATENAUFLAUF   potato and tomato
   casserole
KÄSE   cheese
KÄSEBROT (AUS)   open cheese sandwich
KÄSEFLÄDLE   pastry flavored with sage
KÄSEKUCHEN   white cheese cheesecake
KÄSEPASTETCHEN   baked cheese accompaniment, with
   eggs, sour cream, grated cheese
KÄSEPLATTE   cheese platter
KÄSESALAT (AUS)   cheese salad
KÄSESOSSE   cheese sauce
KÄSESPÄTZLE   cheese with spätzle
KÄSESTANGEN   cheese sticks made of puff pastry
KÄSETORTE   cheesecake

KASSE   cashier

KASSELER RIPPENSPEER   roasted smoked pork chops
with sauerkraut

KASSELER RIPPESPEER   fried salt pork

KASSELER SAFTRIPPE   pickled smoked pork loin chop

KASSLER RIPPCHEN MIT SAUERKRAUT   smoked pork
chops with sauerkraut

KASTANIE   chestnut

KASTANIENCREME   chestnut cream

KASTANIENPÜREE   chestnut purée

KATENRAUCHSCHINKEN   country-style smoked ham

KATENRAUCHSPECK IN PAPRIKA   paprika covered,
cottage smoked bacon

KATENSCHINKEN   cottage-cured ham

KATENWURST   country-style smoked sausage

KATERFISCH   fish with tomato sauce and pickles

KATSUP   catsup

KATZENJAMMER   cold beef slices in mayonnaise with
cucumbers

KAVIAR   caviar

KEKS   biscuit or cookie

KELLNER   waiter

KERBEL   chervil, an herb in the parsley family

KERBELSUPPE   thick potato soup with meat and
chopped chervil

KESSELFLEISCH   boiled pork served with vegetables

KESSELGOULASCH   goulash of pork meat

KEULE   leg

KIELER SPROTTEN   sprats from kiel

KIMBURGER KOTELETTE   breaded and fried ground
pork and veal cutlet

KIPFEL   crescent-shaped roll

KIRSCHE   cherry

KIRSCHEN ÜBERBACKEN MIT SCHOKOLADENCREME
(AUS)   cherry flambé on chocolate sauce

KIRSCHKALTSCHALE   chilled fruit soup with cherries

KIRSCHKNÖDEL (AUS)   cherry dumplings

KIRSCHKUCHEN (AUS)   cherry cake
KIRSCHPFANNKUCHEN   cherry pancakes
KIRSCHPUDDING   cherry pudding
KIRSCHSOSSE   cherry sauce
KIRSCHSTRUDEL (AUS)   cherry strudel
KIRSCHTORTE   cherry tart
KIRSCHWASSER   cherry brandy
KITZ   kid, young goat
KLABEN   white bread filled with currants and almonds
KLARE SUPPE   clear soup (broth)
KLEIN   little or small
KLEIN FEIN   small tasty dishes
KLEINE GERICHTE   small courses, hot or cold
KLEINGEBÄCK   small fine pastries
KLOPS   meatball
KLOSS   dumpling
KLÖSSCHEN   small meat and dough dumplings
KLOSTERLIKÖR   herb liqueur made in monastery
KLUFTSTEAK   rumpsteak
KNACKWURST   garlic flavored sausage
KNOBLAUCH   garlic
KNOCHEN   bone
KNOCHENSCHINKEN   cured ham on the bone
KNÖDEL   dumplings
KNOPFLI   thick noodle
KNUSPRIG   crisp or crunchy
KOCHEN   boil, cook
KOGNAK   cognac
KOHL   cabbage
KOHLRÄBCHENGEMÜSE   kohlrabi
KOHLRABI IN RAHMSOSSE   kohlrabi with sour cream
KOHLRABI, RÜBE   turnip
KOHLRABIGEMÜSE   kohlrabi
KOHLROULADE   meat stuffed cabbage
KOHLROULADE IN RAHMSOSSE   stuffed cabbage
   leaves in cream sauce
KOHLRÜBEN   rutabagas

KOHLSUPPE   cabbage soup

KOKOSNUSSBONBONS   coconut bonbons

KOKOSNUSSMAKRONEN   coconut macaroons

KOMPOTT   stewed fruit in syrup

KONDITOREI   confectioner's or pastry shop

KONFITÜRE   jam

KÖNIGINPASTETCHEN   pastry shells stuffed with chicken, tongue, mushrooms

KÖNIGINPASTETE GEFÜLLT MIT FEINEM RAGOUT   patty shell filed with diced chicken in a cream sauce with mushrooms, wine, herbs. (Chicken a la King)

KÖNIGINSUPPE   creamed chicken soup with pieces of chicken breast

KÖNIGSBERGER KLOPS   poached meatballs in lemon and caper sauce

KÖNIGSCAMPI   medium prawn

KÖNIGSKRABBEN   king crab

KÖNIGSKUCHEN   loaf cake with raisins, almonds and rum

KONSUL (AUS)   black coffee with a dash of cream

KOPFSALAT   green head lettuce salad

KOPFSÜLZE   pork head-cheese in aspic

KORINTHE   currant

KORNBRANNTWEIN   whiskey distilled from grain

KOTELETT IN ASPIK   smoked pork chop in aspic

KOTELETTE   veal rib chop, pork loin chop

KRABBEN   crabs or shrimp

KRABBEN, BÜSUMER   shrimp from the North Sea coast

KRABBEN IN MAYONNAISE   shrimp in mayonnaise dressing

KRABBENSALAT   shrimp salad with mayonnaise

KRAFTBRÜHE   broth

KRAFTBRÜHE MIT EI   broth with beaten egg

KRAFTBRÜHE MIT FADENNUDELN   broth with string noodles

KRAFTBRÜHE MIT FLÄDLE   broth with thin strips of pancake

KRAFTBRÜHE MIT LEBERKNÖDEL broth with liver dumplings

KRAFTBRÜHE MIT LEBERSPÄTZLE broth with liver dumplings

KRAFTBRÜHE MIT MARK broth with marrow

KRAFTBRÜHE MIT NUDELN broth with noodles

KRAFTSUPPE beef soup

KRAINER spiced pork sausage

KRANZKUCHEN ring-shaped cake

KRAPFEN fritter, jelly donut

KRAUSKOHL kale

KRAUT cabbage

KRÄUTER herbs

KRÄUTERBUTTER herb butter

KRÄUTERMAYONNAISE (AUS) mayonnaise sauce with herbs

KRÄUTEROMELETTE omelette with green herbs

KRÄUTEROMELETTE MIT CHAMPIGNONS omelette with green herbs and mushrooms

KRÄUTERQUARK white cheese seasoned with chopped herbs

KRÄUTERSOSSE herb dressing

KRÄUTERSTEAK steak topped with herb butter

KRÄUTERSUPPE soup with chopped herbs

KRAUTSALAT coleslaw

KRAUTSTIEL white beet, Swiss chard

KRAUTSUPPE cabbage soup

KRAUTWICKEL stuffed cabbage

KREBS freshwater crayfish

KREBSCOCKTAIL (AUS) crayfish cocktail

KREBSSCHWÄNZE crayfish tails

KREBSSCHWANZSALAT crayfish salad

KREBSSUPPE crayfish soup

KREMSCHNITTE Napoleon, custard slice

KREN horseradish

KRENFLEISCH pork stew with vegetables and horseradish

KRESSE cress
KRESSESALAT cress salad
KREVETTEN shrimps
KROKANT nut brittle
KROKETTEN croquettes
KRONSBEEREN cranberry
KRUSTENTIER shellfish
KUCHEN cake
KÜCHENRAGOUT sweetbreads stew with green peas, mussels and a cream sauce
KUCHERL Austrian word for fritters
KUKURUZ corn
KÜMMEL caraway
KÜMMELBRANNTWEIN caraway-flavored spirit
KÜMMELKRAUT cabbage with caraway seeds
KÜMMELSUD caraway-flavored poaching liquid
KÜMMELSUPPE caraway soup
KÜRBIS pumpkin
KÜRBISSUPPE pumpkin soup

L

LABSKAUS boiled potatoes, herring, beets and fried onions
LABSKAUSE one dish meal of corned beef hash, potato and salt herring
LACHS salmon
LACHSBRÖTCHEN smoked salmon sandwiches
LACHSFORELLE salmon trout
LACHSMEDALLIONS fillets of salmon
LAMMBRATEN roast leg of lamb
LAMMFLEISCH lamb
LAMMGERICHT, IRISCHES Irish lamb stew
LAMMGULASCH (AUS) lamb goulash
LAMMKOTELETTE, GEBRATEN, GEGRILLT (AUS) lamb chop, roast, grilled
LAMMKOTELETTE VOM ROST broiled lamb chop

LAMMKOTELETTEN   lamb cutlets
LAMMKRONE   crown roast of lamb
LAMMRÜCKEN   back of lamb
LAMMSCHLEGEL   leg of lamb
LAMMSCHULTER   shoulder of lamb
LÄNDLICH   country-style, or local
LANGUSTE   spiny lobster, crawfish
LANGUSTE IN MAYONNAISE   crayfish with mayonnaise
LANGUSTENSCHWÄNZE   lobster tail
LAUCH   leek
LAUCH GRATIN   leeks with sharp Cheddar cheese
LAUCHCREMESUPPE   leek soup
LAUCHRAHMSOSSE   leeks with sour cream
LAUCHSALAT   leek salad
LAUF (AUS)   coffee mixed with whipped cream and
    served in a tall glass
LAUGENBREZEL   pretzel
LAUGENWECKERL   roll-shaped pretzel
LEBER   liver
LEBER BERLINER ART   calf's liver, fried, served covered
    with fried onions and apples
LEBERKÄSE   cold or hot meat loaf of liver, pork and
    bacon
LEBERKLÖSSE   liver dumplings
LEBERKLÖSSE, FEINE   liver patties made with onion
LEBERKLÖSSUPPE   liver dumpling soup
LEBERKNOCKERLSUPPE   soup with liver, chicken,
    chopped onions, stuffed dumplings
LEBERKNÖDEL   chopped liver dumplings
LEBERKNÖDELSUPPE   clear soup with dumplings of
    minced liver and onions
LEBERPRESSACK   pressed liver meat loaf
LEBERRAGOUT BOMBAY   liver in curry sauce
LEBERSCHEIBEN   sliced liver
LEBERSPÄTZEL   thick round liver noodles
LEBERWURST   liverwurst
LEBKUCHEN   gingerbread

LEBKUCHENHÄUSCHEN   gingerbread house
LECKERBISSEN   small morsel or tidbit
LECKERLI   honey flavored ginger biscuit
LEGIERT   thickened as soup or salad sauces
LEGUMES   vegetables which come in a pod, such as peas
LEICHTER KARTOFFELSALAT   summer potato salad
LEIPZIGER ALLERLEI   mixed vegetable dish
LENDEN   loin
LENDENBRATEN   roast tenderloin
LENDENGOULASCH   braised fillet in thick gravy
LENDENSCHNITTEN   tenderloin slices
LENDENSTEAK   beef tenderloin
LENDENSTEAK ESPAGÑOL   fried with onions, rice,
   stuffed tomatoes, sherry, gravy
LENDENSTEAK MIRABEAU   grilled tenderloin with
   anchovies, olives
LENDENSTEAK NATUR   plain fried steak
LENDENSTEAK VIKTORIA   sautéed steak, chicken
   croquette and fried tomato
LENDENSTEAK WESTMORELAND   braised steak in
   tomato sauce with pickles and capers
LENGFISCHFILET   ling cod fillet
LIKÖR   liqueur or cordial
LIMBURGER KÄSE   semi-soft, strong-smelling whole-
   milk cheese
LIMONADE   lemon drink
LINSEN   lentils
LINSENEINTOPF   lentil pot
LINSENEINTOPF MIT WIENER WÜRSTCHEN   lentil pot
   with sausages
LINSENPÜREESUPPE (AUS)   lentil puree soup
LINSENSUPPE   lentil soup
LINSENSUPPE MIT WÜRSTCHEN   lentil soup with
   frankfurters
LINZER TORTE   hazelnut or almond cake or tart with
   raspberry jam
LÖFFEL   spoon

LÖWENZAHN   dandelion green salad
LUCULLUS EIER   eggs with goose liver, truffle in various
   sauces
LUFTGETROCKNETE METTWÜRST   air dried cold
   cooked sausage
LYONER   like baloney, hot or cold

M

MADEIRASAUCE (AUS)   Madeira sauce
MAGER   lean or thin
MAGERER SPECK   lean bacon
MAHLZEIT   meal
MAIFISCH   shad
MAILÄNDER SCHNITZEL   breaded veal cutlet with
   cheese, butter, fried with mushrooms and tongue
MAILÄNDER STEAK   breaded and butter-fried veal steak
MAINAUER KÄSE   semi-hard, full-cream round cheese
MAINZER RIPPCHEN   pork chop
MAÏS   corn
MAISGËBACK   pastry with cornmeal
MAKKARONI   macaroni
MAKKARONI MIT SCHINKEN   macaroni and ham
MAKRELE   mackerel
MAKRELEN IN ÖL (AUS)   mackerels in oil
MAKRONE   macaroon
MAKRONENTORTE   baked macaroon tart
MALZBIER   low alcohol malt beer
MANDARINE   tangerine
MANDEL   almond
MANDELBOGEN   baked almond rainbows
MANDELCREME   almond cream custard dessert
MANDELCREMETORTE (AUS)   almond cream cake
MANDELFLAMMERI   almond pudding
MANDELHALBMONDE   baked almond half-moons
MANDELKRÄNZCHEN   almond wreaths
MANDELKROKETTEN   croquettes of potatoes and almonds

MANDELMAKRONEN   baked almond macaroons
MANDELSAUCE   almond sauce
MANDELSCHNECKEN   baked snail shaped almond
  pastry
MANDELSPLITTER   almond chips
MANDELTORTE   almond pastry
MANGOLD   white beet
MARASCHINO   wild cherry
MARILLE   apricot
MARILLEN ÜBERBACKEN MIT VANILLEEIS (AUS)
  apricot flambé on vanilla ice
MARINIERT   marinated, pickled
MARK   bone marrow
MARKKLÖSSCHEN   marrow balls
MARKKLÖSSE   beef marrow dumplings
MARKKLOSSUPPE   marrow dumpling soup
MARKSOSSE   bone marrow sauce
MARMELADEPALATSCHINKEN (AUS)   pancakes with
  jam
MARMORKUCHEN   baked marble cake
MARONE   chestnut
MÄRZENBIER   beer with high alcohol
MARZIPAN   almond paste
MARZIPANKRANZ   baked almond paste cookies with
  raisins and icing
MASSKRUG   beer mug holding about 1 quart
MAST   grain fed
MASTENTE   grain-fed fattened duck
MASTGANSBRATEN   grain-fed roasted goose
MASTHÄHNCHEN   grain-fed roasting chicken
MASTHUHN   grain-fed roasting chicken
MASTKALBS   grain-fed calf
MASTOCHSE   grain-fattened steer beef
MASTOCHSENFLEISCH   boiled, fattened beef
MASTOCHSENLENDE   grain-fattened tenderloin or fillet
MASTPOULARDE   fattened roasting chicken
MASTPUTER   fattened turkey

MASTRINDFLEISCHSALAT cold, cooked, grain-fed beef cut in strips and put into a salad with mayonnaise

MATJESHERING young salted herring

MATJESHERING NACH HAUSFRAUEN-ART herring filets with apple slices, onion rings, onion sauce and sour cream

MATJESHERINGSFILET fillets of young herring

MATROSENBROT hard chopped egg and anchovy sandwich

MAULBEERE mulberry

MAULTASCHE ravioli filled with meat and vegetables

MAULTASCHE SCHWÄBISCH ravioli with chopped meat, brains, spinach in a sauce

MAYONNAISENSALAT vegetables, meat, fish in mayonnaise

MAZAGRAN (AUS) cold, black, sweetened coffee served with ice cubes and maraschino or rum in a tall glass

MAZEDONISCHE HÜHNERCROQUETTEN chicken croquettes, gravy and mushrooms

MEER sea

MEERESFRÜCHTE seafood

MEERESFRÜCHTESALAT (AUS) sea food salad

MEERKREBSE IN BIERTEIG GEBACKEN (AUS) deep-fried scampi

MEERRETTICH horseradish

MEHLNOCKERL small dumpling

MEHLPUT stewed pears and dumplings

MEHLSPEISEN flour-based dishes like noodles, dumplings, omelette-pancakes, and sweet desserts

MEHLSUPPE brown flour soup

MELANGE (AUS) half coffee, half hot milk, sweetened with sugar

MELONE melon

MELONE AUF EIS chilled melon

MERINGE meringue

MESSER knife

METTWURST   spiced and smoked pork sausage spread
MIESMUSCHEL   mussel
MILCH   milk
MILCHKAFFEE   half coffee and half hot milk
MILCHMIX   milk shake
MILCHRAHMSTRUDEL (AUS)   white bread, eggs, sugar, milk, raisins and warm vanilla sauce
MILCHREIS   rice in milk
MILZWURST   sausage made of veal spleen
MINERALWASSER   mineral water
MIRABELLE   small yellow plum
MISCHGEMÜSE   mixed vegetables
MISCHPILZE   mixed mushrooms
MIT EIER   with egg
MITTAGESSEN   midday meal, lunch
MITTELMEER   Mediterranean Sea
MITTELRHEIN   fresh and dry wine
MOCCA   coffee
MOCCA GESPRITZT (AUS)   black coffee with a dash of brandy or rum
MOCCA MILCH   small black coffee mixed with milk
MOCCA OBERS (AUS)   small black coffee with cream
MOHN   poppy
MOHNBRÖTCHEN   poppyseed rolls
MOHNSAMEN   poppyseeds
MOHNSTRIEZEL   poppyseed cake
MOHNTORTE (AUS)   poppyseed cake
MOHR IM HEMD (AUS)   moist chocolate cake covered with chocolate sauce
MÖHRE, MOHRRÜBE   carrot
MOHRENKOPF   individual white cakes filled with custard or whipped cream and covered with chocolate
MOHRRÜBENSUPPE   carrot soup
MOKKACREMETORTE   mocha or coffee cream torte
MOKKATORTE   coffee-flavored cake
MOLLE   a pint of beer

MORCHEL   morel mushroom
MORGENRÖTESUPPE   thick soup of meat, tapioca, tomatoes and chicken stock
MOSEL-SAAR-RUWER-WEIN   fresh, delicate wine with a fine fruity flavor
MOSELWEIN   a white wine
MOST   young wine
MÜLLERIN-ART   dredged in flour and fried in butter and oil
MÜNSTERLÄNDER TÖPFCHEN   spicy stew of calf's head
MÜRBTEIG   dessert pastry
MUS   stewed fruit, puree, mash
MUSCHEL   mussel
MUSCHEL RAGOUT-FIN   mussels in a thick cream sauce
MUSCHELN, GEBRATENE (AUS)   roast mussels
MUSCHELN IN SPANISCHER SHERRYWEINSOSSE   Spanish mussels in sherry wine sauce
MUSCHELSALAT   mussel salad
MUSCHELSUPPE   mussel soup
MUSKAT   nutmeg
MUSTEWECKE   bread filled with chopped pork

N

NACH JAHRESZEIT   in season
NACHSPEISEN   desserts
NACHTISCH   desserts
NAHE-WEIN   fragrant, fruity, lively wine
NAPFKUCHEN   yeast cake made with raisins
NASI GORENG   rice with chicken, pork or beef
NATUR   plain
NATURSCHNITZEL   sautéed veal chops
NATURWEIN   unblended, unsweetened wine
NELKE   clove
NEUE KARTOFFELN   new potatoes

NIEDRIG   low
NIERCHEN SAUER   braised kidneys in sweet and sour
   sour-cream sauce
NIEREN   kidneys
NIERENBRATEN   roast loin of veal with kidneys
NIERENSTÜCK   loin
NOCKERL   small dumpling
NORDISCHER RAUCHSALM   northern smoked salmon
NORWEGISCHE EIER   poached eggs in aspic on shrimp
   salad with anchovy
NOUGAT   almond and chocolate paste
NOUGAT EISTORTE   an ice cream cake made with an
   almond and chocolate paste
NOUGATTORTE   nougat torte
NUDEL   noodle
NUDELAUFLAUF   noodle pudding
NUDELSUPPE   noodle soup
NUDELSUPPE MIT HUHN   chicken noodle soup
NUDELSUPPE MIT HÜHNERKLEIN   noodle soup with
   chicken giblets
NUDELTOPF MIT HUHN UND SPARGEL   chicken and
   noodle casserole with asparagus
NÜRNBERGER BRATWURST   small grilled, veal and
   pork sausages
NÜRNBERGER LEBKUCHEN   baked spice cake
NUSS   nut
NUSSAUFLAUF   nut pudding soufflé
NUSSKIPFEL   nut crescent cakes
NUSSKUCHEN   nutcake
NUSSLEBKUCHEN   baked nut spice cake
NUSSSTRUDEL   nut strudel
NUSSTORTE (AUS)   nut cake

O

OBST   fruit
OBSTKNÖDEL (AUS)   fruit dumplings

OBSTKUCHEN   pastry or tart baked with fruit
OBSTPASTETEN   fruit pies
OBSTPUDDING   fruit pudding
OBSTSAFT   fruit juice
OBSTSALAT   fruit salad
OBSTTORTE   mixed fruit tart
OCHS   ox or bull
OCHSENBRATEN   roast beef
OCHSENFLEISCH   beef
OCHSENFLEISCH GEKOCHT   boiled beef
OCHSENLENDE   fillet of beef
OCHSENMARK   beef marrow
OCHSENMAULSALAT   ox-muzzle salad
OCHSENNIERE   beef kidney
OCHSENSCHWANZ   oxtail
OCHSENSCHWANZEINTOPF   oxtail stew with
   vegetables
OCHSENSCHWANZRAGOUT   braised oxtail stew
OCHSENSCHWANZSUPPE   oxtail soup
OCHSENSCHWANZSUPPE, GEBUNDENE MADEIRA
   oxtail soup with Madeira wine
OCHSENSCHWANZSUPPE MIT KLÖSSCHEN   oxtail
   soup with dumplings
OCHSENSCHWANZSUPPE MIT PILZEN   oxtail soup
   with mushrooms
OCHSENZUNGE   ox tongue
OCHSENZUNGE IN MADEIRA   ox tongue in wine sauce
OCHSENZUNGENTASCHEN   cold sliced tongue rolls
   with horseradish sauce inside
ODER   or
OEL   oil
OFFENE TORTE   open pastry tart
OHNE   without
ÖL   oil
OLIVEN   olives
ÖLSARDINEN   sardines in oil
OMELETTE GEFÜLLT   stuffed omelette

OMELETTE MIT EDELCHAMPIGNONS IN RAHM
   omelette with mushrooms in cream sauce
OMELETTE MIT FEINEN KRÄUTERN   omelette with
   chopped parsley, chervil, tarragon and chives
OMELETTE MIT GEFLÜGELLEBER   chicken liver omelette
OMELETTE MIT GEFLÜGELRAGOUT   omelette with
   diced chicken in a cream sauce
OMELETTE MIT KALBFLEISCHRAGOUT   omelette with
   diced veal in cream sauce
OMELETTE MIT KÄSE   with cheese
OMELETTE MIT KONFITÜRE   omelette with preserves
OMELETTE MIT LEBER   omelette with chopped liver
OMELETTE MIT NIEREN   omelette with sautéed kidneys
OMELETTE MIT NUDELN   omelette with noodles and a
   butter and cheese sauce
OMELETTE MIT PILZEN   mushroom omelette
OMELETTE MIT SAUERN NIEREN   omelette with
   sautéed kidneys in sour sauce
OMELETTE MIT SCALLOPS   scallop omelette
OMELETTE MIT SCHINKEN   ham omelette
OMELETTE NACH JÄGER-ART   omelette with chicken
   livers and mushrooms in sauce
OMELETTE NATUR   plain omelette
OMELETTE SOUFFLÉ   beaten egg whites added to yolks
OMELETTE SPARGEL   asparagus omelette
OMELETTE TOMATEN   tomato omelette
ORANGENBISKUIT   orange biscuit made with cognac
   orange jelly and egg whites
ORANGENFILETS   orange sections
ORANGENSAFT   orange juice
ORANGENSOUFFLÉ   orange soufflé
ÖSTERREICHISCH   Austrian style

P

PALATSCHINKEN   pancake filled with jam or cheese,
   served with hot chocolate

PALMENMARK   palm hearts
PAMPELMUSE   grapefruit
PANHAS   mixture of ground meat, buckwheat and gravy
PANIERT   breaded
PANIERT GEBACKEN (AUS)   breaded and fried
PANIERTE EIER   eggs cooked with bread crumbs
PANIERTE KALBSSCHNITZEL   breaded veal cutlets
PANIERTE KOTELETT   breaded pork chop
PAPRIKA SCHNITZEL   veal cutlet floured with paprika,
   fried, with sour cream sauce
PAPRIKAGULASCH   beef goulash in sour cream sauce
   with paprika
PAPRIKAHUHN   chicken paprika with sour cream sauce
PAPRIKAKARTOFFELN   paprika potatoes
PAPRIKARAHMSAUCE   paprika-flavored cream sauce
PAPRIKARAHMSCHNITZEL   veal cutlets with bell
   peppers in sour cream sauce and paprika
PAPRIKASAHNEHUHN   braised chicken in cream sauce
   with paprika
PAPRIKASALAT   sweet bell pepper salad
PAPRIKASCHNITZEL   veal cutlet with bell peppers
PAPRIKASCHOTE   sweet pepper, yellow, red or green
PARADIESAPFEL   tomato
PARFAIT   dessert of ice cream, fruit, or syrup and
   whipped cream
PASTETCHEN   puff pastry patty shells
PASTETE   pastry or pie
PASTETE GEFÜLLT MIT FEINEM RAGOUT   patty shell
   filled with diced veal in mushroom and wine cream
   sauce
PASTETE KAPUZINER-ART   a delicate meat stew served
   in a patty shell
PELLKARTOFFEL   potato boiled in its jacket
PELLKARTOFFELN   potatoes in their jackets
PERGAMENTPAPIER GEBACKEN, IN   baked in
   parchment
PERLGRAUPE   pearl barley

PERLHUHN   Guinea hen
PERLWEIN   white, semi-sparkling wine
PERLZWIEBELN   pearl onions
PETERSILIE   parsley
PETERSILIENBUTTER   parsley butter
PETERSILIENKARTOFFELN   boiled potatoes with
   parsley
PETERSILIENSOSSE   parsley sauce
PETERSILKARTOFFELBÄLLCHEN   parsley potato balls
PFAHLMUSCHEL   mussel
PFÄLZER   spicy sausage
PFANNENGERICHTE   pan-fried dishes
PFANNKUCHEN   pancake
PFANNKUCHEN AUS RONEN KARTOFFELN
   GEBACKENEN   raw potatoes fried in a skillet like a
   pancake
PFANNKUCHEN MIT ANANASSCHEIBEN (AUS)   small
   pancakes with pineapples
PFANNKUCHEN MIT FRÜCHTEN (AUS)   small
   pancakes with fruit
PFANNKUCHEN MIT HASELNUSSCREME (AUS)   small
   pancakes with hazelnut cream
PFANNKUCHEN MIT KÄSE   pancake with cheese
PFANNKUCHEN MIT ORANGEN (AUS)   small pancakes
   with oranges
PFANNKUCHEN MIT SCHOKOLADECREME (AUS)
   small pancakes with chocolate cream
PFANNKUCHEN MIT SPECK   pancake with bacon
PFANNKUCHEN NATUR   plain egg pancake
PFANNKUCHENKRAPFEN   fritters
PFANNKUCHENSUPPE   hot consommé with thin strips
   of pancake added
PFEFFER   pepper
PFEFFERKUCHEN   very spicy gingerbread
PFEFFERMINZTEE   peppermint tea
PFEFFERNUSS   gingerbread nut
PFEFFERNÜSSE   gingerbread cookies shaped like nuts

PFEFFERNÜSSE KÜCHLEIN   spice cookies
PFEFFERNUSSPLÄTZCHEN   spice cookies
PFEFFERPOTTHAST   spicy meat and onion casserole
PFEFFERSCHWEINEBRATEN   spiced or peppered pork
stew
PFEFFERSTEAK   steak fried with ground peppercorns
PFEFFERSTEAK FLAMBIERT   peppercorn fried steak
flamed with brandy
PFIFFERLINGE   wild mushroom like chanterelle
PFIFFERLINGE MIT SPECK   sautéed mushrooms with
bacon
PFIRSICH CARDINAL   poached peach in syrup with ice
cream and pureed strawberry
PFIRSICH MELBA   Peach halves poached in syrup,
served over vanilla ice cream, topped with raspberry
sauce and whipped cream
PFIRSICHE ÜBERBACKEN MIT HASELNUSSPARFAIT
(AUS)   peach flambé with hazelnut ice cream
PFIRSICHKNÖDEL (AUS)   peach dumplings
PFLAUME   plum
PFLAUMENKNÖDEL   white cheese plum dumplings
PFLAUMENKUCHEN   plum cake
PFLÜMLIWASSER   liquor distilled from plums
PHARISÄER (AUS)   cup of strong, sweetened coffee with
a dash of rum and topped with whipped cream
PICCOLO (AUS)   black coffee with or without whipped
cream, served in a small cup
PICHELSTEINER   mixed meat and vegetable casserole
PIKANT   spiced, highly seasoned
PIKANTE HAMMELSCHULTER   braised lamb shoulder
with mustard and red wine sauce
PIKANTE SOSSE   spicy sauce
PIKANTES HERZTÖPFLE   casserole of veal heart in
seasoned brown gravy
PIKANTES REHFILET   venison tenderloin in spiced
brandy sauce
PIKANTES SCHNITZEL   veal cutlet in spicy sauce

PILAFREIS (AUS)   rice pilaf
PILS   beer with strong aroma of hops
PILZAUFLAUF MIT NUDELN   baked mushrooms with
   noodles
PILZE   mushrooms
PILZE GLAS   mushroom entree with white bread, sherry,
   cream sauce
PILZE MIT SPECK   sautéed wild mushroom with bacon
PILZE MIT TOMATEN UND SPECK   mushrooms with
   tomatoes and bacon
PILZSALAT   mushroom salad with oil, vinegar, onions
PINKELWURST   spicy oatmeal and bacon fat sausage
PLATTE   platter or dish
PLATTFISCH   plaice fish like flounder
PLÄTZCHEN   cookie, biscuit or fancy cake
PLATZLI   scallop
POCHIERT   poached
POCHIERTE EIER (AUS)   poached eggs
POCHIERTE EIER AUF TOAST MIT SCHINKEN (AUS)
   poached eggs on toast with ham
PÖKEL   pickled
PÖKELFLEISCH   marinated meat
PÖKELZUNGE   pickled tongue
PÖKELZUNGE IN MADEIRA   served hot in Madeira sauce
POMERANZENBRÖTCHEN   baked orange or lemon rolls
POMERANZENSOSSE   bitter orange wine and brandy
   sauce
POMMES FONDANT   baked mashed potatoes
POMMES FRITES   french fries
PORREE   leek
PORREESUPPE   leek soup
PORTWEIN   port wine
POULARDE   grain-fed roasting chicken
POULET   chicken
POWIDLTASCHERL (AUS)   tartlets filled with plum jam
PRAGER STEAK   fried veal steak, scrambled eggs and
   chopped ham with brown gravy

PRALINE   chocolate with sweet filling
PREISELBEERE   cranberry
PRESSACK   a pork headcheese
PRESSKOPF   headcheese from pork pieces
PRINTE   honey-flavored cookie
PRINZESSBOHNEN   thick string beans
PRINZREGENTENTORTE   layer cake with chocolate
   butter-cream covered with chocolate
PRISE   pinch (of salt)
PUFFBOHNEN   lima beans
PUNSCH   punch
PUNSCHTORTE (AUS)   dense rum-flavored cake covered
   with pink icing
PÜREE   mash
PUTER   turkey

Q

QUARGEL   slightly acid and salty round cheese
QUARK   fresh white cheese, farmer's cheese
QUARKAUFLAUF   white cheese soufflé
QUARKKLÖSSE   sweet dumplings made with white
   cheese
QUITTE   quince
QUITTEN KONFEKT   quince candy

R

RADIESCHEN   radish
RAGOUT DEUTSCH   beef and vegetable stew
RAGOUT-FIN   diced veal, tongue, brains, in a cream
   sauce with mushrooms and wine
RAGOUTFIN IN MUSCHELN   stew of ox tongue,
   sweetbread, mushrooms, anchovies, wine, grated
   cheese, baked in shells
RAHM   cream
RAHMCREME   creamy rum filling

RAHMHACKBRATEN   slices of meat loaf slices in brown gravy

RAHMKARTOFFELN   creamed potatoes

RAHMMARINADE   cream dressing with mustard, sugar, butter, vinegar, heavy whipped cream

RAHMMEERRETTICH   horseradish cream sauce

RAHMSCHNITZEL   veal cutlet fried in lemon juice with sour cream sauce

RAHMSPINAT   creamed spinach

RAHMSTRUDEL   cream strudel

RASTSTÄTTE OR RASTHAUS   restaurants and inns along the Autobahns (freeways)

RATSKELLER   upper-medium- to high-quality restaurants found in the city hall

RÄUBERFLEISCH AM SPIESS   corn-fed pork broiled on a skewer

RÄUCHERAAL   smoked eel

RÄUCHERBIER   smoked beer

RÄUCHERHERING   smoked herring

RÄUCHERLACHS   smoked salmon

RÄUCHERSCHINKEN   smoked ham

RÄUCHERSPECK   smoked bacon

RÄUCHFLEISCH   smoked meat

RAUHREIF   apple and cream dessert

RAVIOLI IN TOMATENTUNKE   square pasta filled with cheese or meat in tomato sauce

REBHUHN   partridge

REBHUHN MIT WEINTRAUBEN   roast partridges with grapes

RECHNUNG   bill, check

REGENBOGENFORELLE   rainbow trout

REGENSBURGER   highly-spiced and smoked sausage

REGENSBURGER IN ESSIG UND ÖL   cold slices of beef and pork sausage, dressed with oil and vinegar

REHKEULE   venison leg

REHSCHNITZEL MIT PILZEN   venison cutlets with mushrooms

REIBEKUCHEN   potato pancake
REICHE AUSWAHL   full assortment
REICHLICH   abundant
REIS   rice
REIS TRAUTMANNSDORFF   fruit rice with rum,
   whipped cream, and stewed fruits
REISAUFLAUF MIT ÄPFELN   rice pudding with apple
REISFLEISCH   veal braised with rice
RIESENSCAMPI   large prawn
REISRAND TOULOUSER ART   stew filled rice ring with
   sweetbreads, kidneys, truffles and mushrooms
REISSCHMARREN   rice pancakes
REISSUPPE   broth with rice
REMOULADEN SOSSE   mayonnaise sauce with mustard,
   anchovies, capers, gherkins, tarragon, chervil
RENKE   fresh water whitefish
RENTIER   reindeer
RENTIERSCHINKEN   ham from reindeer leg
RESTAURATIONSBROT   bread served with cold cuts
RETTICH   radish
RETTICH MIT BROT UND BUTTER   radishes with bread
   and butter
RETTICHSALAT   radish salad
RHABARBER   rhubarb
RHEIN   country's best white wines
RHEINGAU   good dessert wine, fruity taste with
   character and elegance
RHEINHESSEN-WEIN   smooth, mild wine
RHEINLACHS   Rhine salmon
RHEINLÄNDER MARINADE   dressing of sugar,
   Worcestershire, ketchup, olive oil, vinegar, mustard,
   Tabasco, lemon juice
RHEINLANDPFALZ-WEIN   mild, aromatic, round and
   full-bodied, strong wine
RIBISEL   redcurrant
RIEBELE   noodles
RIESENBOCKWURST   spicy sausage like knockwurst

RIESENKRABBEN   large crabs
RIEVKOOCHE   fried potato pancakes
RIND GEPÖKELT   pickled beef tongue
RIND OR RINDER   beef
RINDERBRATEN   beef roast
RINDERBRUST   brisket of beef
RINDERGULASCH   beef goulash
RINDERMARK   beef marrow
RINDERROULADE   filled beef roll
RINDERROULADE BURGUNDER-ART   beef slices
    stuffed with bacon, pickle, anchovies, onions, sautéed in
    gravy
RINDERROULADEN   stewed beef rolls
RINDERSAFTBRATEN   beef pot roast
RINDERSCHMORBRATEN   beef pot roast
RINDERWURST   grilled beef sausage
RINDERZUNGE IN MADEIRA   boiled beef tongue in
    Madeira sauce
RINDFLEISCH   beef
RINDFLEISCH Á LA MODE   beef pot roast
RINDFLEISCH IN MEERRETTICHTUNKE   boiled beef
    with horseradish sauce
RINDFLEISCH IN SCHNITTLAUCHSOSSE   boiled beef
    with chive sauce
RINDFLEISCHSALAT (AUS)   beef salad
RINDFLEISCHSALAT   beef strips with spicy vinegar
    sauce
RINDFLEISCHSUPPE   soup made from boiling beef
RINGE   rings, wreaths like apple rings
RIPPCHEN   smoked rib loin pork chop
RIPPCHEN MIT SAUERKRAUT   spareribs and
    sauerkraut
RIPPE   rib
RIPPENSTÜCK   ribs of beef
RISOLEEKARTOFFELN   butter sautéed boiled potatoes
ROASTBEEF MIT WÜRSTCHEN   roast beef with
    sausages

ROASTBEEFRÖLLCHEN   cold roast beef roll
ROCHEN   skate fish
ROGEN   codfish eggs or roe
ROGGENBROT   rye bread
ROGGENBRÖTCHEN   rye roll
ROH   raw
ROHER SCHINKEN   uncooked ham
ROHKOST   uncooked vegetables, vegetarian food
ROHKOSTPLATTE   salad plate
ROHKOSTSALAT   raw vegetable salad
RÖHRE   oven
ROLLMOPS   herring fillet rolled around chopped onions
   and pickles
RÖMER   caraway rolls
ROSENKOHL   brussels sprout
ROSENKOHL MIT SCHINKEN UND
   TOMATEN   brussels sprouts with ham and tomatoes
ROSENSPITZ   top sirloin veal steak
ROSINEN   raisins
ROSINENBRÖTCHEN   baked raisin rolls
ROSINENKUCHEN   raisin cake
ROSINENSOSSE   raisin sauce
ROSMARIN   rosemary
ROST   grill, broil
ROSTBRATEN   rumpsteak
ROSTBRATEN HELGOLÄNDER ART   fried steak on toast
   with tomato strips and Hollandaise sauce
ROSTBRATEN JÄGER-ART   fried with bacon, vegetables
   and wine in a sauce of pan juices
ROSTBRATEN, SCHWÄBISCHER   braised in vegetables
   and a brown sauce
ROSTBRATEN WIENER   fried in butter and covered with
   fried onions
ROSTBRATEN, ZIGEUNER   braised with bacon and
   onions or fried with cabbage and potatoes
ROSTBRATWÜRSTE   pork sausages
RÖSTI   course-grated fried potatoes

RÖSTKARTOFFEL   roast potato
RÖSTKARTOFFELN   raw potatoes parboiled then
  browned in butter
RÖSTZWIEBELN   crisp fried onions
ROTBARBE   red mullet or red seabass
ROTE BETE   red beets
ROTE GRÜTZE   fruit jelly served with cream
ROTE RÜBE   beetroot
ROTE RÜBE IN BUTTER   red beets in butter
ROTE RÜBEN   red beetroots
ROTER RÜBENSALAT   pickled beet salad
ROTKOHL   red cabbage
ROTKOHL MIT ÄPFELN   red cabbage with apples
ROTKRAUT   red cabbage
ROTWEIN   red wine
ROTWEINSOSSE   red wine sauce
ROTWEISSER PRESSACK   Austrian pressed headcheese
  meat loaf
ROTWURST   blood sausage
ROTZUNGE   lemon sole
ROULADE   thin slices of beef, stuffed, rolled and braised
ROULADEN   braised stuffed slice of meat
ROULADENFÜLLUNG   ground meat stuffing of roulade
RÜBEN   turnips
RÜBENEINTOPF   turnip stew with breast of lamb,
  tomatoes and beef stock
RÜCKEN   saddle, usually mutton
RÜHREIER   scrambled eggs
RÜHREIER MIT CHAMPIGNONS (AUS)   scrambled eggs
  with mushrooms
RÜHREIER MIT HÜHNERLEBER (AUS)   scrambled eggs
  with chicken livers
RÜHREIER MIT SCHINKEN (AUS)   scrambled eggs with
  ham
RÜHREIER MIT SPARGELSPITZEN (AUS)   scrambled
  eggs with asparagus tips
RÜHREIER MIT SPECK   scrambled eggs with bacon

RÜHREIER MIT TRÜFFELN (AUS) scrambled eggs with truffle

RÜHREIER MIT ZUCKERERBSEN (AUS) scrambled eggs with green peas

RÜHREIER NATUR (EIERSPEISE) (AUS) plain scrambled eggs

RUMFORDSUPPE pea soup with barley, potatoes and fried bacon

RUMKUCHEN SCHWÄBISCHER BUND baked rum cake with raisins, almonds, lemon juice, lemon icing, toasted almonds, candied fruit

RUMPSTEAK cut from bottom round beef steak

RUMPSTEAK MIRABEAU fried with anchovies and olives

RUMPSTEAK PROVENCIAL fried with tomatoes, mushrooms, and garlic-flavored tomato sauce

RUMPSTEAK RUSSLAND with mushrooms, pickles, onions in brown sauce or horseradish

RUMSTEACK steak cut from beef bottom round

RUNDSTÜCK WARM hot roast meat open-faced sandwich with gravy

RUSSISCHE EIER stuffed hard-boiled egg halves with mayonnaise

RUSSISCHER GEFLÜGELSALAT chicken salad with hard-boiled eggs covered with mayonnaise

S

SACHERTORTE chocolate layer cake with jam filling

SAFRAN saffron

SAFT juice or gravy

SAFTBRATEN beef pot roast in lots of liquid

SAFTGOULASCH veal stew with lots of gravy

SAFTSCHINKEN boiled juicy ham

SAHNE cream

SAHNEKÄSE cream cheese

SAHNEMEERRETTICHSOSSE horseradish cream sauce

SAITENWURST   variety of frankfurter sausage
SALAMI   any salami type cold sausage
SALAT   salad
SALAT MIMOSA   salad of lettuce with grated egg yolk
SALAT UND BEILAGE   salad and an accompaniment or
   side dish
SALAT VON GERÄUCHERTEM AAL   smoked eel salad
SALATE   salads
SALATPLATTE   assorted salad plate
SALATTELLER   salad plate
SALBEI   sage
SALM   salmon
SALZ   salt
SALZBURGER NOCKERLN   dessert of sweet dumplings,
   poached in milk with hot vanilla sauce
SALZFLEISCH   salted meat
SALZGURKE   pickled cucumber
SALZKARTOFFELN   boiled salted potatoes
SALZKARTOFFELN MIT KÄSE   boiled potatoes with
   cheese
SANDDORN   flavoring from small berry
SANDMUSCHEL   clam
SANDTORTE   pound cake
SARDELLE   anchovy
SARDELLENBUTTER   anchovy butter
SARDELLENRING   rolled anchovy
SARDELLENSOSSE   anchovy sauce
SARDINE   pilchard or very small herring
SAUBOHNE   broad bean
SAUER   sour
SAUERAMPFER   sorrel
SAUERAMPFERSUPPE   sorrel soup
SAUERBRATEN   marinated pot roasted beef with herbs
SAUERBRATEN MIT ROTKOHL   marinated pot roast
   with red cabbage
SAUERFLEISCH   sour spiced pork
SAUERKIRSCHEN   sour cherries

SAUERKRAUTSALAT   sauerkraut, olive oil, apples, onions

SAUERRAHM   sour cream

SAURE KARTOFFELN   sour potatoes

SAURE LEBER   liver in brown gravy

SAURE LEBER UND NIEREN   liver and kidney with a sour vinegar sauce

SAURE NIEREN   spiced kidneys

SAURE SAHNE   sour cream

SAUREGURKE   pickle

SCAMPI   shrimp or prawns

SCAMPI COCKTAIL   prawn appetizer

SCHALENTIER   shellfish

SCHALLOTTEN   shallots, a milder type of onion

SCHALOTTE   shallot

SCHARFER FLEISCHEINTOPF   very spicy casserole of veal or beef in brown gravy

SCHARFES TÖPFCHEN   very spicy casserole of veal or beef

SCHASCHLIK   meat, kidneys, tomatoes, onions, bacon grilled on a skewer then braised in spicy sauce

SCHASCHLIK, KAUKASISCHES   marinated lamb, veal or beef grilled on a skewer with onions, peppers and tomato

SCHAUMROLLE   puff-pastry filled with whipped cream or custard

SCHAUMSPEISE   frozen dessert with whipped cream and mousse

SCHAUMTORTE   meringue torte

SCHAUMWEIN   champagne

SCHEIBE   slice

SCHELLFISCH   haddock

SCHICHTKÄSE   fresh white cheese

SCHICHTTORTE   layer cake

SCHILDKRÖTENSUPPE   turtle soup

SCHILDKRÖTENSUPPE LADY CURZON   turtle soup with curry powder and whipped cream garnish

SCHILL (AUS) pike-perch
SCHILLERLOCKE pastry cone with vanilla cream filling
SCHILLERWEIN rosé wine
SCHINKEN ham
SCHINKEN IN BROTTEIG smoked ham in baked shell
SCHINKEN IN BURGUNDER ham braised in burgundy
SCHINKENBROT open faced ham sandwich
SCHINKENFÜLLUNG chopped ham stuffing
SCHINKENHAXE ham shanks
SCHINKENOMELETTE ham omelette
SCHINKENOMELETTE MIT NUDELN UND KÄSE
  omelette filled with noodles, cheese and ham
SCHINKENPASTETE ham pie containing pork, veal,
  onion, Madeira wine
SCHINKENRÖLLCHEN rolled ham slices with or
  without filling
SCHINKENSALAT (AUS) ham salad
SCHINKENSTREIFEN ham strips
SCHINKENWURST ham pieces in pork baloney filling,
  eaten cold
SCHLACHTPLATTE meat, liver sausage and sauerkraut
  plate
SCHLACHTSCHÜSSEL boiled dish of liver sausage,
  blood sausage, pork belly with sauerkraut, potatoes and
  dumplings
SCHLAGOBERS whipped cream
SCHLAGRAHM whipped cream
SCHLAGSAHNE whipped cream
SCHLEGEL leg
SCHLEIE carp fish
SCHLEIE BLAU carp fish boiled with butter
SCHLEIE MIT SAHNEMEERRETTICH carp with
  creamed horseradish sauce
SCHLEMMERSCHNITTE slice of bread with raw ground
  beef, raw egg, chopped raw onions, capers, anchovies,
  like steak tartar

SCHLESISCHES HIMMELREICH   roast pork or goose
with dumplings
SCHLOSSKARTOFFELN   oval-shaped potatoes fried in
butter
SCHLOTFEGER MIT SAHNE   a long pastry tube with
whipped cream and chocolate
SCHMALZGEBACKENES   deep fat baked goods
SCHMELZKARTOFFELN   egg-shaped potatoes, in a
covered pan
SCHMELZKÄSE   soft and pungent cheese, usually for
spreading on bread
SCHMIERKÄSE   a soft, odorous cheese
SCHMINKBOHNEN   kidney beans
SCHMORBRATEN   pot roast
SCHMORBRATEN IN EIGENEM SAFT   pot roast in a rich
white or brown sauce
SCHMORBRATEN MIT CHAMPIGNONS   pot roast
braised with mushrooms
SCHMORBRATEN MIT KALBSBRIES, NIEREN UND
TRUFFLEN   stew with calf sweetbreads, kidneys,
truffles and mushrooms in brown sauce
SCHMORBRATEN MIT PILZEN   stew with mushrooms
SCHMORFLEISCH   stew meat
SCHMORGURKEN IN SAUREM DILLRAHM   stewed
cucumbers with sour cream and dill
SCHNAPS   brandy
SCHNECKEN   round small pastries
SCHNECKEN IN KRÄUTERBUTTER (AUS)   snails with
herb butter
SCHNECKENRAGOUT PROVINZIAL   snails stewed in
tomato and onion sauce
SCHNECKENSPIESS MIT CHAMPIGNONS, SPECK,
KNOBLAUCH UND BUTTER   snails with mushrooms,
bacon and garlic butter, grilled
SCHNECKENSUPPE MIT RAHMCURRY   snail cream
soup flavored with curry

SCHNEEKARTOFFELN   riced boiled potatoes
SCHNELLBÜFFET   short order cafeteria eateries
SCHNELLGASTSTÄTTE   fast food restaurant
SCHNELLIMBISS   fast snacks, as grilled sausages or hot dogs
SCHNEPFE   snipe or woodcock
SCHNITTBOHNE   sliced French bean
SCHNITTE   slice, cut
SCHNITTEN   slices, cuts
SCHNITTLAUCH   chive
SCHNITTLAUCHSAUCE   chopped chive cream sauce
SCHNITZEL   cutlet
SCHNITZEL, HOLSTEINER   veal cutlets served with fried eggs and anchovies
SCHNITZEL HUBERTUS   butter-fried veal cutlet with wine, shallot and mushroom sauce
SCHNITZEL IN SARDELLENSOSSE   veal cutlet butter-fried in anchovy sauce
SCHNITZEL, JÄGER   veal cutlet with wine, mushroom and tomato sauce
SCHNITZEL, MAILÄNDER   breaded veal cutlet with cheese, butter-fried with mushrooms and tongue
SCHNITZEL NATUR   pan-fried veal cutlet
SCHNITZEL PAPRIKA   veal cutlet floured with paprika, fried, with sour cream sauce
SCHNITZEL, PIKANTES   veal cutlet in spicy sauce
SCHNITZEL ZIGEUNER   veal cutlet sauteed in tomato sauce with pickled tongue, peppers, mushrooms, in a cream gravy with paprika
SCHNITZELEINTOPF   bottom round stew with onion, carrots, potatoes, cream
SCHOKOLADE   chocolate
SCHOKOLADECREMETORTE (AUS)   chocolate cream cake
SCHOKOLADENAUFLAUF   chocolate soufflé
SCHOKOLADENBREZELN   chocolate pretzels
SCHOKOLADENCREME   chocolate cream

SCHOKOLADENCREMETORTE chocolate cream layer cake

SCHOKOLADENEIS chocolate ice cream

SCHOKOLADENFLAMMERI chilled chocolate pudding

SCHOKOLADENHÜTCHEN small chocolate caps

SCHOKOLADENMUSCHELN baked chocolate shells

SCHOKOLADENNUSSTORTE chocolate nut torte

SCHOKOLADENPUDDING steamed chocolate pudding

SCHOKOLADENSAUCE chocolate sauce

SCHOKOLADENSOUFFLÉ (AUS) Viennese chocolate soufflé

SCHOKOLADENSUPPE chocolate soup

SCHOKOLADENTORTE chocolate torte

SCHOKOLADENTRÜFFEL chocolate truffles

SCHOLLE flat fish like flounder or plaice

SCHOPPENWEIN wine from a keg (1/4 liter, 1/2 pint) sold by the glass

SCHOTE pod, husk or shell

SCHOTENSALAT bell pepper salad

SCHOTTISCHE KRAFTBRÜHE Scotch mutton broth

SCHULTER shoulder

SCHUPFNUDEL a heavy noodle

SCHUPFNUDELN potato noodles

SCHWÄBISCHER JÄGERBRATEN roast pork in brown sauce with mushrooms

SCHWÄBISCHES KOTELETT pork cutlet simmered in sour cream sauce with little dumplings

SCHWALBENESTERSUPPE bird's nest soup

SCHWAMM sponge mushroom

SCHWAMMNUDELN spongy soup noodles

SCHWÄNZE tails

SCHWARTENMAGEN headcheese loaf in aspic

SCHWARZ black or dark

SCHWARZ-WEISSER PRESSACK dark and light meat pork headcheese

SCHWARZBROT whole-grained dark bread

SCHWARZBROTSUPPE dark bread soup

SCHWARZE JOHANNISBEERE   black currant
SCHWARZER (AUS)   mocha-black coffee
SCHWARZWÄLDER SCHINKEN   Black Forest smoked ham
SCHWARZWÄLDER KIRSCHTORTE (AUS)   Black Forest
  cherry cake with whipped cream
SCHWEDENBRÖTCHEN   small open-faced sandwiches
SCHWEDENPLATTE   tiny assorted sandwiches
SCHWEDISCHE VORSPEISEN   plate with mixed
  appetizers
SCHWEIN   pork
SCHWEINE LENDCHEN UNGARISCH   pork tenderloin
  browned then braised in paprika sauce
SCHWEINEBAUCH   boiled thick bacon slices
SCHWEINEBRATEN   roast pork
SCHWEINEBRUST   pork breast
SCHWEINEFILET   fillet of pork
SCHWEINEFLEISCH   pork meat
SCHWEINEFLEISCH IN TEIG   pork and other meats in a
  loaf
SCHWEINEFLEISCH MIT SAUERKRAUT   pork and
  sauerkraut
SCHWEINEKOTELETT   pork chop
SCHWEINEKOTELETT MIT PFEFFER   spicy pork stew
SCHWEINEKOTELETT MIT SENF ODER MEERRETTICH
  pork chops with mustard or horseradish
SCHWEINEKOTELETT, MÜNCHNER   fried or braised
  pork chop
SCHWEINEKOTELETT NACH ZIGEUNER-ART   fried
  pork chop with peppers, fried onions, tomatoes, pickle,
  cayenne pepper in a brown sauce
SCHWEINEKOTELETT NATUR   plain fried pork chop
SCHWEINEKOTELETT PANIERT   fried breaded pork chop
SCHWEINEKOTELETT ROST   broiled pork chop or cutlet
SCHWEINEKOTELETT UNGARISCH   fried pork chop
  sprinkled with paprika
SCHWEINEKOTELETTDREIRLEI   breaded pork chops
SCHWEINELEBER   pork liver

SCHWEINELEBER, SAUERE   pork liver fried with onions
   then braised in vinegar and lemon juice
SCHWEINELENDCHEN   pork tenderloin or fillet
SCHWEINENACKEN   pork neck and back
SCHWEINENIEREN   pork kidneys
SCHWEINEPRESSACK   pork meat loaf
SCHWEINERAGOUT   pork ragout or stew
SCHWEINERIPPCHEN   pork spare ribs
SCHWEINERIPPCHEN MIT GEWÜRZGURKENSOSSE
   pork spareribs with pickle sauce
SCHWEINEROLLBRATEN   rolled pork roast
SCHWEINERÜCKEN   pork back
SCHWEINESCHNITZEL   pork cutlet or thin steak
SCHWEINESCHNITZEL, GEBRATENES   fried pork cutlet
SCHWEINESCHNITZEL IN SAHNESOSSE   fried pork
   cutlet in a creamy sauce
SCHWEINESCHNITZEL, PANIERTES   fried breaded
   pork cutlet
SCHWEINESCHULTER   pork shoulder
SCHWEINESTEAK   thin pork steak or cutlet
SCHWEINESTEAK METZGERIN-ART   pork cutlet
   buttered, coated with breadcrumbs and fried
SCHWEINESTEAK MIRABEAU   pork cutlet fried with
   anchovies and green olives
SCHWEINEWAMMERL, GESOTTENES   simmered pork
   belly slices
SCHWEINSFÜSSE   pig's feet
SCHWEINSHAXE   pork shank
SCHWEINSHAXE BÜRGERLICH   roasted pork shank
   with onions and carrots
SCHWEINSHIRN   pork brains
SCHWEINSKARREE   roasted pork squares
SCHWEINSKEULE   beer steamed pork leg
SCHWEINSKOPFSÜLZE   pork headcheese loaf
SCHWEINSKOTELETT à LA WESTMORELAND   fried
   pork chop with peppers, cauliflower, dill pickles, pearl
   onions, carrot, asparagus, string beans

SCHWEINSKOTELETT, KNACKWÜRST UND
KARTOFFELN   pork chops with knockwurst and
potatoes
SCHWEINSLEBERKÄSE   liver, pork, bacon meat loaf
SCHWEINSOHREN   pigs' ears
SCHWEINSROULADEN   pork rolls
SCHWEINSSÜLZE   pork headcheese
SCHWEINSWÜRSTL   grilled pork sausages
SCHWEIZER KÄSE   Swiss cheese
SCHWEIZER REIS   sweet rice dessert
SCHWEIZER SAHNEREIS   cream rice pudding
SCHWEIZER SCHNITZEL CORDON BLEU   pork cutlets
with ham and Swiss cheese between, breaded and fried
SCHWEIZER WURSTSALAT   Swiss baloney salad
SCHWEMMKLÖSSCHEN   flour dumplings
SCHWENKKARTOFFELN   potatoes boiled then fried
SCHWETZINGER SPARGEL   asparagus
SEEBARSCH (AUS)   perch
SEEKRABBE   crab
SEELACHS   codfish called sea salmon
SEEZUNGE   sole fish like plaice or flounder
SEEZUNGE COLBERT   sole breaded and fried in butter,
served with herbal butter and wine sauce
SEEZUNGE GEBACKEN   breaded and deep-fried sole
SEEZUNGE IN BUTTER   sole fillets in butter
SEEZUNGE IN WEISSWEIN   sole in white wine
SEEZUNGE MÜLLERIN   floured and fried sole fillets
SEEZUNGENRÖLLCHEN   rolled sole fillets poached in
white wine served with sauce
SEKT   champagne
SELCHFLEISCH   smoked pork
SELCHKARREE   smoked pork
SELLERIE   celery
SELLERIE MIT ÄPFELN   celery root and apple salad
SELLERIECREMESUPPE   cream of celery soup
SELLERIESALAT   celery root salad

SEMMEL   roll
SEMMELAUFLAUF   almond or poppy seed soufflé
SEMMELBRÖSEL   breadcrumbs
SEMMELKNÖDEL   meat and bread dumplings
SEMMELKNÖDEL AUS EIER   bread dumplings made with eggs
SEMMELKNÖDEL OHNE EI   bread dumplings without egg
SEMOLINA   flour of hard durum wheat
SENF   mustard
SENFBUTTER   mustard flavored butter
SENFGELEE   mustard relish
SENFGURKEN   mustard pickles
SENFSOSSE   mustard sauce
SENFTUNKE   mustard sauce
SERBISCHES REISFLEISCH   veal braised with onions, garlic, tomato puree, with rice
SERBISCHES TÖPFCHEN   beef or veal casserole with paprika
SERVIETTE   napkin
SERVIETTENKNÖDEL   large bread dumpling cooked in a napkin flavored with onion and parsley
S-GEBÄCK   butter cookies shaped as letter S
SHRIMPSALAT   shrimp salad
SIEDFLEISCH   boiled meat
SIRUP   syrup
SOCKELREIS   bed of rice
SODAWASSER   soda water
SOLOKREBS   very large prawns
SONNTAGS GESCHLOSSEN   closed Sundays
SORBET   flavored ice sherbet
SOSSEN   sauces
SPANFERKEL   suckling pig
SPANFERKELKÖPFERL   suckling pig head
SPANFERKELLEBER GERUSTET AM SPIESS   spit roasted liver

SPANFERKELSPIESS   roasted on a spit
SPANISCHE SOSSE   brown sauce with herbs
SPANISCHES OMELETTE   omelette with filling of
   sautéed tomatoes and onions
SPARGEL   asparagus
SPARGELCREMESUPPE   cream of asparagus soup
SPARGELGERICHT ÜBERBACKEN   baked asparagus
   with potatoes, ham, parsley, cheese, nutmeg
SPARGELOMELETTE   asparagus omelette
SPARGELSALAT   asparagus salad
SPARGELSPITZEN   white asparagus tips
SPARGELSUPPE   asparagus soup
SPÄTLESE   full bodied wine
SPÄTZLE   small boiled flour dumplings
SPECK   bacon
SPECKBOHNEN   string beans with bacon
SPECKEIER (AUS)   fried eggs with bacon
SPECKKNÖDEL   dumpling made with bacon
SPECKKRAUT   cabbage with bacon
SPECKKRAUTSALAT   cabbage salad with bacon
SPECKPFANNKUCHEN   flat pancake with pieces of
   chopped bacon
SPECKSAUCE   sauce or gravy flavored with bacon
SPECKSTIPPE   sauce or gravy flavored with bacon
SPEISE   food
SPEISEEISE   ice cream or ices
SPEISEKARTE   menu, bill of fare
SPEKULATIUS   spiced cookie
SPEZIALBIER   strong brewed beer
SPEZIALITÄT   specialty
SPEZIALITÄT DES HAUSES   chef's specialty
SPEZIALITÄT DES TAGES   day's specialty
SPEZIALITÄTEN   specialties (of the house)
SPIEGELEI   frieg egg, usually sunny side up
SPIEGELEIER MIT SCHINKEN   fried eggs with ham
SPIEGELEIER MIT SPECK   fried eggs with bacon

SPIESS   on a skewer
SPINAT   spinach
SPINAT UND SPIEGELEI   spinach with fried eggs, sunny side up
SPINATCREMESUPPE   cream of spinach soup
SPINATPFANNKUCHEN   spinach pancakes
SPITZBUBEN   baked cookie sandwiches with almonds, jelly or jam
SPRINGERLE   aniseed-flavored cookies
SPRITZGEBÄCK   pressed hazelnut cookies
SPROSSENKOHL   brussels sprout
SPROTTEN   sprats, like sardines
SPRUDELWASSER   soda water
STACHELBEERE   gooseberry
STADTWURSTSÜLZE   locally made sausage
STANGENBOHNEN   pole or string beans
STANGENSELLERIE   stalk celery
STANGENSPARGEL   asparagus spears
STARKBIER   strong beer with a high malt content
STAUDENSELLERIE   stalk celery
STECKRÜBE   turnip
STEINBEISSER   sea bass
STEINBUSCHER KÄSE   semi-hard creamy cheese; strong and slightly bitter
STEINBUTT   turbot, similar to halibut
STEINBUTT GEKOCHT   boiled turbot
STEINBUTTSALAT   salad made of cold boiled turbot
STEINGARNELE   prawn
STEINHÄGER   juniper flavored spirit
STEINHUDER RÄUCHERAAL   smoked eel from Steinhuder Lake region
STEINPILZE   wild yellow mushrooms
STELZE   knuckle of pork
STIERENAUGE   fried egg, sunny side up
STINT   smelt, small fish like sardine
STOCK   mashed potatoes

STOCKFISCH   dried codfish

STOLLEN   loaf cake with raisins, almonds, nuts and candied lemon peel

STÖR   sturgeon

STÖR GERÄUCHTERTER   smoked sturgeon

STÖRSTEAK   sturgeon steak

STOTZEN   leg, haunch

STRAMMER MAX   sandwich with minced pork, sausage or ham with fried eggs and onions

STRAUBEN   deep-fried dough curls with cinnamon and sugar

STREICHEN   to spread

STREICHKÄSE   soft cheese spread

STREICHWURST   very soft spreadable liverwurst

STREIFEN   strips

STREUSELKUCHEN   coffee crumb cake with topping made of butter, sugar, flour, cinnamon

STRIEZEL   coffee braid cake

STROHKARTOFFELN   shoestring potatoes

STRUDEL   thin layers of pastry filled with apple slices, nuts, raisins, jam

STUBENKÜKEN   young broiler chicken

STÜCK   piece, slice

STULLE   rye bread sandwiches with various fillings

SUD   poached or boiled in broth or other liquid

SULPERKNOCHEN   pig's ears, tail, with sauerkraut and peas

SÜLZE   jellied, in aspic

SÜLZKOTELETTEN   pork chops in aspic

SUPPE   soup

SUPPE NACH WAHL   soup of your choice

SUPPENEINLAGEN   soup garnishes

SUPPENFLEISCH   boiled beef, soup meat

SUPPENHUHNTOPF   chicken soup casserole

SUPPENMAKRONEN   baked almonds and macaroons added to soups

SUPPENTOPF MIT HUHN (AUS) chicken pot with vegetables

SUPREM MASTHUHN boned chicken breast in sauces

SÜSS sweet

SÜSS-SAURE BRATWURST bratwurst in sweet and sour sauce

SÜSS-SAURE ROTE RÜBEN pickled beets

SÜSSE SAUCEN sweet sauces

SÜSSE WEINE dessert wine

SÜSSER UND SAUERER RAHM sweet and sour sauces

SÜSSIGKEITEN sweet, candy

SÜSSKARTOFFELN sweet potatoes

SÜSSKARTOFFELN, SÜDLICHE mashed with butter, sweet cream and sherry

SÜSSKARTOFFELN, ÜBERBACKENE sweet potatoes baked with brown sugar

SÜSSPEISEN desserts, sweet dishes or dessert of the day

SÜSSWEIN dessert wine

SZEGEDINER GOULASCH lard-browned pork cubes braised in onions, then stewed with sauerkraut

T

TAFEL selection or choice suitable for the table

TAFELPILZE select mushrooms

TAGESDESSERT dessert of the day

TAGESGERICHT day's special

TAGESKARTE daily menu

TAGESSUPPE day's soup

TASCHERL pastry turnover with meat, cheese or jam filling

TASSE cup

TATAR raw spiced minced beef

TATARENBROT open faced sandwich of raw, spiced, minced beef

TAUBE pigeon or dove

TEE   tea
TEE MIT MILCH   tea with milk
TEE MIT ZITRONE   tea with lemon
TEEBLATT   oval flake pastry with sugar sprinkled on top
TEEGEBÄCK   tea cakes or petit fours
TEIGGEMÜSE   macaroni dishes
TEIGWAREN   macaroni, noodles, spaghetti
TELLER   plate, dish
TELLERFLEISCH   boiled pork or boiled beef
TELLERGERICHT   one course meal usually boiled
TELTOWER RÜBCHEN   baby turnips cooked in sugar
TERRINE   large bowl
TEUFELSSALAT   a salad with a spicy, vinegar dressing
THUNFISCH   tunafish
THUNFISCH AURORA   tunafish with a tomato flavored
   sauce
THUNFISCH GRIECHISCH   tunafish slices poached in
   with lemon juice and oil
THYMIAN   thyme
TIEFSEE KREBSFLEISCH   deep sea crayfish meat
TILSITER KÄSE   semi-hard cheese, mildly pungent
TINTENFISCH   cuttlefish, like squid
TIROLER KNÖDEL   dumplings made with bacon fat,
   basil, parsley, cooked in salted water
TOAST   toast
TOASTBROT   toast
TOILETTE   lavatory
TOMATEN   tomatoes
TOMATEN MIT FEINER FLEISCHFÜLLUNG   tomatoes
   stuffed with light meat filling
TOMATENCREMESUPPE   cream of tomato soup
TOMATENKRAFTBRÜHE   consommé flavored with
   tomatoes
TOMATENOMELETTE   tomato omelette
TOMATENSAFT   tomato juice
TOMATENSALAT   tomato salad
TOMATENSCHEIBEN   tomato slices

TOMATENSOSSE tomato sauce
TOMATENSUPPE tomato soup
TOMATENWÜRFEL diced or cubed tomatoes
TOPF pot
TÖPFCHEN beef or veal casserole dish
TOPFEN fresh white cheese
TOPFENKNÖDEL (AUS) white cheese dumplings
TOPFENKUCHEN cake with raisins
TOPFENOBERSTORTE (AUS) white cheese cheesecake
TOPFENSTRUDEL (AUS) baked flaky pastry filled with
vanilla flavored white cheese
TÖRTCHEN small pastry dessert or tart
TORTE layer cake, usually rich
TORTENBODEN baked tart crust layers (spread with
cream)
TOULOUSER GEFLÜGELPASTETE chicken stew with
mushrooms in a patty shell
TOULOUSER SCHMORBRATEN stew with calf
sweetbreads, kidneys, truffles and mushrooms in brown
sauce
TOURNEDOS slices of steak fillet
TOURNEDOS CHATELEINE beef fillet on stuffed
artichoke bottoms in wine sauce with chestnuts and
potatoes
TOURNEDOS ROSSINI beef fillet on toast with goose
liver and wine sauce
TRAPANGSUPPE smoked, fried sea cucumber boiled in
broth
TRAUBEN grapes
TRAUBENSAFT grape juice
TRAUBENZUCKER grape sugar, dextrose
TROCKEN dry
TRÜFFEL flavorful mushroom like plant that grows
underground
TRÜFFELKRAFTBRÜHE consommé with truffles
TRUTHAHN turkey
TRUTHAHN, GEFÜLLTER turkey with stuffing

TRUTHAHN VOM ROST   roast turkey
TRUTHAHNBRATEN   roast turkey
TRUTHAHNKEULE   turkey leg
TRUTHAHNKROKETTEN   turkey croquettes
TRUTHAHNSCHINKEN   turkey leg
TUNKE/STIPPE   sauce or gravy
TÜRKENKORN   corn or maize
TÜRKISCHER KAFFEE (AUS)   finely-ground coffee
   brought to a boil with sugar, served foaming in a small
   cup
TUTTI FRUTTI   mixed fruit

U

ÜBERBACKEN   cooked under broiler
ÜBERBACKENER BLUMENKOHL   baked cauliflower
ÜBERKRUSTET   cooked in very hot oven until browned
   on top
ÜBERZOGEN   coated or basted
UNGARISCH   Hungarian
UNGARISCHE PAPRIKASCHOTEN   stuffed peppers
   with rice and ground beef in tomato sauce
UNGARISCHES GEPÖKELTES FLEISCH   Hungarian
   pickled veal
UNGEZUCKERT   unsweetened
UNSER   our

V

VANILLE   vanilla
VANILLECREME   vanilla cream with whipped cream
VANILLEEISCREME   vanilla ice cream
VANILLEKARAMELLEN   vanilla caramels
VANILLEPUDDING   vanilla pudding
VANILLERAHMEIS   vanilla ice cream
VANILLESOSSE   vanilla cream sauce
VANILLEZUCKER   vanilla confectioners' sugar

VERLORENE EIER   poached eggs
VERLORENE EIER BENEDIKT   toast with slice of ham,
  then poached eggs on top, covered with cream sauce
VIERTEL   about 1/2 pint (of wine)
VOLLBIER   typical beer
VOM BRETT   from a pastry cart
VOM GRILL   dishes from the grill
VOM HAMMEL   mutton main dishes
VOM KALB   veal main dishes
VOM LAMM   lamb main dishes
VOM RIND   beef main dishes
VOM ROST   main dishes, grilled, roasted or broiled
VOM SCHWEIN   pork main dishes
VOM SPIESS   skewered dishes, can be from spit or
  braised
VORSICHT   caution
VORSPEISEN   appetizer

W

WACHOLDERBEERE   juniper berry
WACHOLDERBEEREN RAHM   juniper berry cream
  sauce
WACHSBOHNEN   yellow wax beans
WACHSBOHNENSALAT   wax bean salad
WACHSTUM   grower name on a wine label guarantees
  wines
WACHTEL   quail
WAFFELN   waffles
WAHL   of your choice
WALDERDBEEREN   wild strawberries
WALLER   large catfish
WALNUSS   walnut
WALNUSSTORTE   walnut torte
WALSUPPE   whale soup
WAMMERL   home smoked bacon
WARME GERICHTE   small- to medium-sized hot dishes

WARME SPEISEN   hot main dishes

WARME VORGERICHTE   hot first courses or appetizers

WARME WURSTSPEISEN   cooked sausages

WARMER KARTOFFELSALAT MIT SPECK   hot potato salad with bacon

WASSERMELONE   watermelon

WECKEWERK   pork meat and skin mixed with bread and fried

WECKKLÖSSCHEN   bread dumplings

WEICH   soft, as in soft-boiled egg

WEIN   wine

WEINBERGSCHNECKEN   snails

WEINBERGSCHNECKEN MIT KNÖBLÄUCHBUTTER   snails with garlic butter

WEINBERGSCHNECKEN MIT KRÄUTERBUTTER   snails with herbal butter

WEINBRAND   brandy distilled from wine

WEINGELEE MIT FRÜCHTEN   wine jelly with fruit

WEINKARTE   wine list

WEINKRAUT   sauerkraut cooked in white wine, may have apples

WEINSCHAUMCREME   wine cream

WEINSOSSE   wine sauce

WEINSTUBE   Wine and snack tavern

WEINSUD   sauce made from wine and fish stock

WEINTRAUBE   grape

WEINWEISSKRAUT   white cabbage braised with apples and simmered in wine

WEISSBIER   wheat beer

WEISSBROT   white bread

WEISSBROT MIT KÜMMEL   white bread with caraway seeds

WEISSE BOHNEN   white dried beans

WEISSE RÜBEN   turnips

WEISSE SOSSE   medium white sauce

WEISSE WINDSORSUPPE   cream soup with rice and veal seasonings

WEISSFISH   whiting, a type of fish
WEISSGEBÄCK   a type of pastry
WEISSKÄSE   fresh white cheese
WEISSKOHL   white cabbage
WEISSKOHLEINTOPF MIT SCHWEINSPFÖTCHEN
   cabbage casserole with pig's feet
WEISSKRAUT   white cabbage
WEISSKRAUT MIT SPECK   cooked cabbage with bacon
WEISSWEIN   white wine
WEISSWURST   veal sausage
WEIZEN   wheat
WELLFLEISCH   boiled pork
WELS (AUS)   catfish
WELSCHKORN   corn
WERMUT   vermouth liqueur
WESTFÄLISCH PFEFFERPOTTHAST   beef short ribs
   with spicy sauce
WESTFÄLISCHER SCHINKEN   cured raw Westphalian
   ham
WESTFÄLISCHES BLINDHUHN   beans with fruit and
   vegetables
WIENER   from Vienna
WIENER APFELSOUFFLÉ   Viennese apple soufflé
WIENER BACKHENDL   deep-fat fried and baked chicken
WIENER BACKHUHN   deep-fat fried and baked chicken
WIENER EISKAFFEE (AUS)   tall glass half filled with
   vanilla ice to which cold, strong black coffee is added,
   topped with whipped cream
WIENER ERBSENSUPPE   pea soup
WIENER FASCHINGSKRAPFEN (AUS)   Viennese jam
   filled doughnuts
WIENER GOULASCH   beef stew with onions
WIENER RAHMBEUSCHERL   calf's lung braised in
   cream sauce with anchovies
WIENER RAHMSCHLEGEL   pork leg with cream sauce
WIENER SCHNITZEL   breaded veal cutlet
WIENER WÜRSTCHEN   frankfurter type of sausage

WIENER WÜRSTL spicy sausage, usually boiled
WIENER ZWIEBELROSTBRATEN fried steak with fried
  onions on top
WILDBRET venison, game
WILDBRETBRATEN roast venison
WILDBRETKEULE leg or thigh of venison
WILDBRETMEDALLIONS slices of venison loin or
  tenderloin
WILDBRETPFEFFER jugged venison, fried and braised in
  its marinade, with sour cream
WILDBRETRAGOUT stew of venison and vegetables
WILDBRETRÜCKEN saddle of venison
WILDBRETRÜCKEN BADEN-BADEN baked saddle of
  venison in brown sauce with pears and redcurrant jelly
WILDBRETRÜCKEN IN ROTWEINSOSSE roast saddle
  of venison with red wine sauce
WILDBRETRÜCKEN JÄGERMEISTER roasted saddle of
  venison in shallot, mushroom and wine sauce
WILDENTE wild duck
WILDGEFLÜGEL IN BURGUNDER game birds in
  burgundy
WILDRÜCKENSTEAK venison steak
WILDSCHWEIN wild boar
WILDSCHWEINBRATEN wild boar roasted
WILDSCHWEINKEULE haunch of wild boar
WILDSCHWEINRAGOUT stew of wild boar
WILDSCHWEINRÜCKEN saddle of wild boar
WILDSCHWEINSCHINKEN ham from wild boar
WILDSCHWEINSCHINKEN, GERÄUCHERTER (AUS)
  smoked boar ham
WILDSCHWEINSCHNITZEL wild boar boneless cutlet
WILDSTEAK venison steak
WILDTAUBE wild pigeon
WILSTERMARSCHKÄSE semi-hard cheese, similar to
  Tilsiter
WINDBEUTEL baked cream puff

WINTEREINTOPF winter stew, made with chestnuts, yellow turnips, leeks, sausages
WINTERKOHL winter cabbage
WIRSING savoy cabbage
WITTLING whiting
WOLFSBARSCH bass
WOLLWURST mild white veal sausage
WÜRFEL cubed or diced
WÜRFELKARTOFFELN fried diced potatoes
WURST sausage
WURST IN TEIG sausage cooked in dough
WURSTBROT open sausage sandwich
WURSTBRÖTCHEN sausage in a roll
WÜRSTCHEN sausages
WURSTGERICHTE hot sausage dishes
WURSTPLATTE platter of assorted sausages
WURSTSALAT sausage salad (with vegetables, mayonnaise)
WURSTSPEISEN pork products
WURSTSPEZIALITÄTEN house specialties in hot sausages
WÜRTTEMBERGISCHER WEIN wine that is strikingly fruity, with a distinctive after-taste
WÜRZE spice, seasoning, pickled
WURZEL root vegetable
WURZELSUD pickling brew
WÜRZFLEISCH beef in spiced sour cream sauce
WÜRZIG spiced

Z

ZANDER pike-perch
ZANDER SCHNITTE IN SENFBUTTER fillet of walleyed pike with mustard butter
ZART mildly smoked, tender, delicate, soft
ZERLASSENE BUTTER melted butter

ZIEGE   goat

ZIGEUNER   gypsy (style)

ZIGEUNER ROSTBRATEN   braised ribsteak with bacon, cabbage and potatoes

ZIGEUNERSALAT   paprika salad

ZIGEUNERSCHNITZEL   veal or pork cutlet sautéed in tomato sauce with pickled tongue, peppers, mushrooms, in cream gravy with paprika

ZIGEUNERSPIESS   pork tenderloin broiled on a skewer with vegetables

ZIGEUNERSTEAK   fried beef or veal steak with mushrooms, peppers, onions, pickles, chopped ham in sauce

ZIMT   cinnamon

ZIMT UND ZUCKER   cinnamon sugar

ZIMTKUCHEN   cinnamon coffee cake

ZIMTSTERNE   cinnamon star cookies

ZITRONE   lemon

ZITRONENCREME   lemon cream dessert

ZITRONENPUDDING   lemon pudding

ZITRONENREIS   rice pudding with lemon juice, lemon peel, stewed fruits

ZITRONENSAFT   lemon soda

ZITRONENSOUFFLÉ   soufflé of baked egg white with lemon

ZUBEREITET   ready to serve, pre-prepared, prepared at the table, or made with

ZUCCINI   Italian zucchini squash

ZUCKER   sugar

ZUCKERERBSEN   young green peas

ZUCKERMELONE   sweet melon

ZUNGE   tongue

ZUNGENRAGOUT   tongue ragout or stew

ZUNGENRAGOUT MARENGO   braised tongue in oil, tomatoes, white wine, button mushrooms and onions

ZUNGENSTREIFEN   tongue strips

ZUNGENWURST   ox tongue sausage

ZUTAT   added ingredient

ZWETSCHGEN   plums
ZWETSCHGENKNÖDEL   sweet plum dumplings
ZWETSCHGENWASSER   spirit distilled from plums
ZWETSCHKENSTRUDEL   plum strudel
ZWIEBACK   extra dry toast
ZWIEBEL   onions
ZWIEBELFLEISCH   beef sautéed with onions
ZWIEBELFLEISCH MÜNCHNER-ART   thin beef slices
   sautéed in fried onions
ZWIEBELRINGE   onion rings, usually fried
ZWIEBELROSTBRATEN   fried club steak with fried
   onions
ZWIEBELSOSSE   onion sauce
ZWIEBELSUPPE   onion soup
ZWIEBELSUPPE, FRANZÖSISCHE   French onion soup
ZWIEBELWURST   liver and onion sausage
ZWISCHENRIPPENSTÜCK   ribsteak

SOMETHING WICKED
THIS WAY COMES

"The stuff of nightmares."

—*The New York Times*

"Crazy . . . fascinating . . . spellbinding."

—*Sarasota Herald Tribune*

"Brilliantly original."

—*Book-of-the-Month Club News*

"Nightmarish allegory."

—*Christian Science Monitor*

"A world of dark fancy."

—*Oakland Tribune*

"Sinister, disturbing, masterfully told."

—*San Francisco Chronicle*

WALT DISNEY PRODUCTIONS
PRESENTS

RAY BRADBURY'S
SOMETHING WICKED THIS WAY COMES

A JACK CLAYTON FILM

STARRING
JASON ROBARDS
JONATHAN PRYCE
DIANE LADD
PAM GRIER

PRODUCED BY
PETER VINCENT DOUGLAS

SCREENPLAY BY
RAY BRADBURY
BASED ON HIS NOVEL

DIRECTED BY
JACK CLAYTON

MUSIC COMPOSED BY
JAMES HORNER

RELEASED BY BUENA VISTA
DISTRIBUTION CO., INC.

©1983 WALT DISNEY PRODUCTIONS

SOMETHING WICKED THIS WAY COMES

Ray Bradbury

BANTAM BOOKS
TORONTO · NEW YORK · LONDON · SYDNEY

*This low-priced Bantam Book
has been completely reset in a type face
designed for easy reading, and was printed
from new plates. It contains the complete
text of the original hard-cover edition.*
NOT ONE WORD HAS BEEN OMITTED.

SOMETHING WICKED THIS WAY COMES
*A Bantam Book / published by arrangement with
Simon & Schuster, Inc.*

PRINTING HISTORY
*Simon & Schuster edition published September 1962
2nd printing . . . September 1962
Bantam edition / September 1963
25 printings through June 1983*

*A small portion of this novel has
appeared previously in* MADEMOISELLE.

ISBN 0-553-23620-2

Published simultaneously in the United States and Canada

PRINTED IN THE UNITED STATES OF AMERICA

H   34 33 32 31 30 29 28 27 26 25

With gratitude to
JENNET JOHNSON, who taught
me how to write the short story,
and to SNOW LONGLEY HOUSH,
who taught me poetry
at Los Angeles High School
a long time ago,
and to
JACK GUSS,
who helped with this novel
not so long ago

CONTENTS

Man is in love, and loves what vanishes.

—W. B. YEATS

They sleep not, except they have done mischief;
And their sleep is taken away, unless they cause some to fall.
For they eat the bread of wickedness,
And drink the wine of violence.

—Proverbs 4:16–17

I know not all that may be coming, but be it what
it will, I'll go to it laughing.

—STUBB in *Moby Dick*

First of all, it was October, a rare month for boys. Not that all months aren't rare. But there be bad and good, as the pirates say. Take September, a bad month: school begins. Consider August, a good month: school hasn't begun yet. July, well, July's really fine: there's no chance in the world for school. June, no doubting it, June's best of all, for the school doors spring wide and September's a billion years away.

But you take October, now. School's been on a month and you're riding easier in the reins, jogging along. You got time to think of the garbage you'll dump on old man Prickett's porch, or the hairy-ape costume you'll wear to the YMCA the last night of the month. And if it's around October twentieth and everything smoky-smelling and the sky orange and ash gray at twilight, it seems Halloween will never come in a fall of broomsticks and a soft flap of bedsheets around corners.

But one strange wild dark long year, Halloween came early.

One year Halloween came on October 24, three hours after midnight.

At that time, James Nightshade of 97 Oak Street was thirteen years, eleven months, twenty-three days old. Next door, William Halloway was thirteen years, eleven months and twenty-*four* days old. Both touched toward fourteen; it almost trembled in their hands.

And that was the October week when they grew up overnight, and were never so young any more. . . .

I.   ARRIVALS

CHAPTER ONE

The seller of lightning rods arrived just ahead of the storm. He came along the street of Green Town, Illinois, in the late cloudy October day, sneaking glances over his shoulder. Somewhere not so far back, vast lightnings stomped the earth. Somewhere, a storm like a great beast with terrible teeth could not be denied.

So the salesman jangled and clanged his huge leather kit in which oversized puzzles of ironmongery lay unseen but which his tongue conjured from door to door until he came at last to a lawn which was cut all wrong.

No, not the grass. The salesman lifted his gaze. But two boys, far up the gentle slope, lying *on* the grass. Of a like size and general shape, the boys sat carving twig whistles, talking of olden or future times, content with having left their fingerprints on every movable object in Green Town during summer past and their footprints on every open path between here and the lake and there and the river since school began.

"Howdy, boys!" called the man all dressed in storm-colored clothes. "Folks home?"

The boys shook their heads.

"Got any money, yourselves?"

The boys shook their heads.

"Well—" The salesman walked about three feet, stopped and hunched his shoulders. Suddenly he seemed aware of house windows or the cold sky staring at his neck. He turned slowly, sniffing the air. Wind rattled the empty trees. Sunlight, breaking through a small rift in the clouds, minted a last few oak leaves all gold. But the sun vanished, the coins were spent, the air blew gray; the salesman shook himself from the spell.

The salesman edged slowly up the lawn.

"Boy," he said. "What's your name?"

And the first boy, with hair as blond-white as milk thistle, shut up one eye, tilted his head, and looked at the salesman with a single eye as open, bright and clear as a drop of summer rain.

"Will," he said. "William Halloway."

The storm gentleman turned. "And *you?*"

The second boy did not move, but lay stomach down on the autumn grass, debating as if he might make up a name. His hair was wild, thick, and the glossy color of waxed chestnuts. His eyes, fixed to some distant point within himself, were mint rock-crystal green. At last he put a blade of dry grass in his casual mouth.

"Jim Nightshade," he said.

The storm salesman nodded as if he had known it all along.

"Nightshade. That's quite a name."

"And only fitting," said Will Halloway. "I was born one minute *before* midnight, October thirtieth. Jim was born one minute *after* midnight, which makes it October thirty-first."

"Halloween," said Jim.

By their voices, the boys had told the tale all their lives, proud of their mothers, living house next to house, running for the hospital together, bringing sons into the world seconds apart; one light, one dark. There was a history of mutual celebration behind them. Each year Will lit the candles on a single cake at one minute to midnight. Jim, at one minute after, with the last day of the month begun, blew them out.

So much Will said, excitedly. So much Jim agreed to, silently. So much the salesman, running before the storm, but poised here uncertainly, heard looking from face to face.

"Halloway. Nightshade. No money, you say?"

The man, grieved by his own conscientiousness, rummaged in his leathery bag and seized forth an iron contraption.

"Take this, free! Why? One of those houses will be struck by lightning! Without this rod, bang! Fire and ash, roast pork and cinders! Grab!"

The salesman released the rod. Jim did not move. But Will caught the iron and gasped.

"Boy, it's heavy! And funny-looking. Never seen a lightning rod like this. Look, Jim!"

And Jim, at last, stretched like a cat, and turned his head. His green eyes got big and then very narrow.

The metal thing was hammered and shaped half-crescent, half-cross. Around the rim of the main rod little curlicues and doohingies had been soldered on, later. The entire surface of the rod was finely scratched and etched with strange languages, names that could tie the tongue or break the jaw, numerals that added to incomprehensible sums, pictographs of insect-animals all bristle, chaff, and claw.

"That's Egyptian." Jim pointed his nose at a bug soldered to the iron. "Scarab beetle."

"So it is, boy!"

Jim squinted. "And those there—Phoenician hen tracks."

"Right!"

"Why?" asked Jim.

"Why?" said the man. "Why the Egyptian, Arabic, Abyssinian, Choctaw? Well, what tongue does the wind talk? What nationality is a storm? What country do rains come from? What color is lightning? Where does thunder go when it dies? Boys, you got to be ready in every dialect with every shape and form to hex the St. Elmo's fires, the balls of blue light that prowl the earth like sizzling cats. I got the only lightning rods in the world that hear, feel, know, and sass back any storm, no matter what tongue, voice, or sign. No foreign thunder so loud this rod can't soft-talk it!"

But Will was staring beyond the man now.

"Which," he said. "Which house will it strike?"

"Which? Hold on. Wait." The salesman searched deep in their faces. "Some folks draw lightning, suck it like cats suck babies' breath. Some folks' polarities are negative, some positive. Some glow in the dark. Some snuff out. You now, the two of you . . . I—"

"What makes you so sure lightning will strike anywhere around here?" said Jim suddenly, his eyes bright.

The salesman almost flinched. "Why, I got a nose, an eye, an ear. Both those houses, their timbers! Listen!"

They listened. Maybe their houses leaned under the cool afternoon wind. Maybe not.

"Lightning needs channels, like rivers, to run in. One of those attics is a dry river bottom, itching to let lightning pour through! Tonight!"

"Tonight?" Jim sat up, happily.

"No ordinary storm!" said the salesman. "Tom Fury tells you. Fury, ain't that a fine name for one who sells lightning rods? Did I *take* the name? No! Did the name fire *me* to my occupations? Yes! Grown up, I saw cloudy fires jumping the world, making men hop and hide. Thought: I'll chart hurricanes, map storms, then run ahead shaking my iron cudgels, my miraculous defenders, in my fists! I've shielded and made snug-safe one hundred thousand, count 'em, God-fearing homes. So when I tell you, boys, you're in dire need, listen! Climb that roof, nail this rod high, ground it in the good earth before nightfall!"

"But which house, which!" asked Will.

The salesman reared off, blew his nose in a great kerchief, then walked slowly across the lawn as if approaching a huge time bomb that ticked silently there.

He touched Will's front porch newels, ran his hand over a post, a floorboard, then shut his eyes and leaned against the house to let its bones speak to him.

Then, hesitant, he made his cautious way to Jim's house next door.

Jim stood up to watch.

The salesman put his hand out to touch, to stroke, to quiver his fingertips on the old paint.

"This," he said at last, "is the one."

Jim looked proud.

Without looking back, the salesman said, "Jim Nightshade, this your place?"

"Mine," said Jim.

"I should've known," said the man.

"Hey, what about *me?*" said Will.

The salesman snuffed again at Will's house. "No, no.

Oh, a few sparks'll jump on your rainspouts. But the real show's next door here, at the Nightshades'! Well!"

The salesman hurried back across the lawn to seize his huge leather bag.

"I'm on my way. Storm's coming. Don't wait, Jim boy. Otherwise—bamm! You'll be found, your nickels, dimes and Indian-heads fused by electroplating. Abe Lincolns melted into Miss Columbias, eagles plucked raw on the backs of quarters, all run to quicksilver in your jeans. More! Any boy hit by lightning, lift his lid and there on his eyeball, pretty as the Lord's Prayer on a pin, find the last scene the boy ever saw! A box-Brownie photo, by God, of that fire climbing down the sky to blow you like a penny whistle, suck your soul back up along the bright stair! Git, boy! Hammer it high or you're dead come dawn!"

And jangling his case full of iron rods, the salesman wheeled about and charged down the walk, blinking wildly at the sky, the roof, the trees, at last closing his eyes, moving, sniffing, muttering. "Yes, bad, here it comes, feel it, way off now, but running fast. . . ."

And the man in the storm-dark clothes was gone, his cloud-colored hat pulled down over his eyes, and the trees rustled and the sky seemed very old suddenly and Jim and Will stood testing the wind to see if they could smell electricity, the lightning rod fallen between them.

"Jim," said Will. "Don't stand there. *Your* house, he said. You going to nail up the rod or ain't you?"

"No," smiled Jim. "Why spoil the fun?"

"Fun! You *crazy?* I'll get the ladder! You the hammer, some nails and wire!"

But Jim did not move. Will broke and ran. He came back with the ladder.

"Jim. Think of your mom. You want *her* burnt?"

Will climbed the side of the house, alone, and looked down. Slowly, Jim moved to the ladder below and started up.

Thunder sounded far off in the cloud-shadowed hills.

The air smelled fresh and raw, on top of Jim Nightshade's roof.

Even Jim admitted that.

CHAPTER TWO

There's nothing in the living world like books on water cures, deaths-of-a-thousand-slices, or pouring white-hot lava off castle walls on drolls and mountebanks.

So said Jim Nightshade, that's all he read. If it wasn't how to burgle the First National, it was how to build catapults, or shape black bumbershoots into lurking bat costumes for Cabbage Night.

Jim breathed it out all fine.

And Will, he breathed it in.

With the lightning rod nailed to Jim's roof, Will proud, and Jim ashamed of what he considered mutual cowardice, it was late in the day. Supper over, it was time for their weekly jog to the library.

Like all boys, they never walked anywhere, but named a goal and lit for it, scissors and elbows. Nobody won. Nobody wanted to win. It was in their friendship they just wanted to run forever, shadow and shadow. Their hands slapped library door handles together, their chests broke track tapes together, their tennis shoes beat parallel pony tracks over lawns, trimmed bushes, squirreled trees, no one losing, both winning, thus saving their friendship for other times of loss.

So it was on this night that blew warm, then cool, as they let the wind take them downtown at eight o'clock. They felt the wings on their fingers and elbows flying, then, suddenly plunged in new sweeps of air, the clear autumn river flung them headlong where they must go.

Up steps, three, six, nine, twelve! Slap! Their palms hit the library door.

Jim and Will grinned at each other. It was all so good, these blowing quiet October nights and the library waiting inside now with its green-shaded lamps and papyrus dust.

Jim listened. "What's *that?*"

"What, the wind?"

"Like music . . ." Jim squinted at the horizon.

"Don't hear no music."

Jim shook his head. "Gone. Or it wasn't even there. Come on!"

They opened the door and stepped in.

They stopped.

The library deeps lay waiting for them.

Out in the world, not much happened. But here in the special night, a land bricked with paper and leather, anything might happen, always did. Listen! and you heard ten thousand people screaming so high only dogs feathered their ears. A million folk ran toting cannons, sharpening guillotines; Chinese, four abreast, marched on forever. Invisible, silent, yes, but Jim and Will had the gift of ears and noses as well as the gift of tongues. This was a factory of spices from far countries. Here alien deserts slumbered. Up front was the desk where the nice old lady, Miss Watriss, purple-stamped your books, but down off away were Tibet and Antarctica, the Congo. There went Miss Wills, the other librarian, through Outer Mongolia, calmly toting fragments of Peiping and Yokohama and the Celebes. Way down the third book corridor, an oldish man whispered his broom along in the dark, mounding the fallen spices. . . .

Will stared.

It was always a surprise—that old man, his work, his name.

That's Charles William Halloway, thought Will, not grandfather, not far-wandering, ancient uncle, as some might think, but . . . *my father.*

So, looking back down the corridor, was Dad shocked to see he owned a son who visited this separate 20,000-fathoms-deep world? Dad always seemed stunned when Will rose up before him, as if they had met a lifetime ago and one had grown old while the other stayed young, and this fact stood between. . . .

Far off, the old man smiled.

They approached each other, carefully.

"Is that you, Will? Grown an inch since this morning." Charles Halloway shifted his gaze. "Jim? Eyes darker, cheeks paler; you burn yourself at both ends, Jim?"

"Heck," said Jim.

"No such place as Heck. But hell's right here under 'A' for Alighieri."

"Allegory's beyond me," said Jim.

"How stupid of me," Dad laughed. "I mean Dante. Look at this. Pictures by Mister Doré, showing all the aspects. Hell never looked better. Here's souls sunk to their gills in slime. There's someone upside down, wrong-side out."

"Boy howdy!" Jim eyed the pages two different ways and thumbed on. "Got any dinosaur pictures?"

Dad shook his head. "That's over in the next aisle." He strolled them around and reached out. "Here we are: *Pterodactyl, Kite of Destruction!* Or what about *Drums of Doom: The Saga of the Thunder Lizards!* Pep you up, Jim?"

"I'm pepped!"

Dad winked at Will. Will winked back. They stood now, a boy with corn-colored hair and a man with moon-white hair, a boy with a summer-apple, a man with a winter-apple face. Dad, Dad, thought Will, why, why, he looks . . . like *me* in a smashed mirror!

And suddenly Will remembered nights rising at two in the morning to go to the bathroom and spying across town to see that one single light in the high library window and know Dad had lingered on late murmuring and reading alone under these green jungle lamps. It made Will sad and funny to see that light, to know the old man—he stopped to change the word—his father, was here in all this shadow.

"Will," said the old man who was also a janitor who happened to be his father, "what about you?"

"Huh?" Will shook himself.

"You need a white-hat or a black-hat book?"

"Hats?" said Will.

"Well, Jim—" they perambulated, Dad running his fingers along the book spines—"he wears the black ten-gallon hats and reads books to fit. Middle name's Moriarty, right, Jim? Any day now he'll move up from Fu Manchu to Machiavelli here—medium-size dark fedora.

Or over along to Dr. Faustus—extra large black Stetson. That leaves the white-hat boys to you, Will. Here's Gandhi. Next door is St. Thomas. And on the next level, well . . . Buddha."

"You don't mind," said Will, "I'll settle for *The Mysterious Island*."

"What," asked Jim, scowling, "is all this talk about white and black hats?"

"Why—" Dad handed Jules Verne to Will—"it's just, a long time ago, I had to decide, myself, which color I'd wear."

"So," said Jim, "which *did* you pick?"

Dad looked surprised. Then he laughed, uneasily.

"Since you need to ask, Jim, you make me wonder. Will, tell Mom I'll be home soon. Get out of here, both of you. Miss Watriss!" he called softly to the librarian at the desk. "Dinosaurs and mysterious islands, coming up!"

The door slammed.

Outside, a weather of stars ran clear in an ocean sky.

"Heck." Jim sniffed north, Jim sniffed south. "Where's the storm? That darn salesman promised. I just *got* to watch that lightning fizz down my drainpipes!"

Will let the wind ruffle and refit his clothes, his skin, his hair. Then he said, faintly, "It'll be here. By morning."

"Who says?"

"The huckleberries all down my arms. *They* say."

"Great!"

The wind flew Jim away.

A similar kite, Will swooped to follow.

CHAPTER THREE

Watching the boys vanish away, Charles Halloway suppressed a sudden urge to run with them, make the pack. He knew what the wind was doing to them, where it was taking them, to all the secret places that were never so secret again in life. Somewhere in him, a shadow turned mournfully over. You had to run with a night like this, so the sadness could not hurt.

Look! he thought. Will runs because running is its own excuse. Jim runs because something's up ahead of him.

Yet, strangely, they *do* run together.

What's the answer, he wondered, walking through the library, putting out the lights, putting out the lights, putting out the lights, is it all in the whorls on our thumbs and fingers? Why are some people all grasshopper fiddlings, scrapings, all antennae shivering, one big ganglion eternally knotting, slip-knotting, square-knotting themselves? They stoke a furnace all their lives, sweat their lips, shine their eyes and start it all in the crib. Caesar's lean and hungry friends. They eat the dark, who only stand and breathe.

That's Jim, all bramblehair and itchweed.

And Will? Why, he's the last peach, high on a summer tree. Some boys walk by and you cry, seeing them. They feel good, they look good, they are good. Oh, they're not above peeing off a bridge, or stealing an occasional dime-store pencil sharpener; it's not that. It's just, you know, seeing them pass, that's how they'll be all their life; they'll get hit, hurt, cut, bruised, and always wonder why, why does it happen? how can it happen to *them?*

But Jim, now, he knows it happens, he watches for it happening, he sees it start, he sees it finish, he licks the wound he expected, and never asks why: he *knows.* He *always* knew. Someone knew before him, a long time ago, someone who had wolves for pets and lions for night conversants. Hell, Jim doesn't know with his mind. But his body knows. And while Will's putting a bandage on his latest scratch, Jim's ducking, weaving, bouncing away from the knockout blow which must inevitably come.

So there they go, Jim running slower to stay with Will, Will running faster to stay with Jim, Jim breaking two windows in a haunted house because Will's along, Will breaking one window instead of none, because Jim's watching. God, how we get our fingers in each other's clay. That's friendship, each playing the potter to see what shapes we can make of the other.

Jim, Will, he thought, strangers. Go on. I'll catch up, some day. . . .

The library door gasped open, slammed.

Five minutes later, he turned into the corner saloon for his nightly one-and-only drink, in time to hear a man say:

". . . I read when alcohol was invented, the Italians thought it was the big thing they'd been looking for for centuries. The Elixir of Life! Did you know that?"

"No." The bartender's back was turned.

"Sure," the man went on. "Distilled wine. Ninth, tenth century. Looked like water. But it burnt. I mean, it not only burnt the mouth and stomach, but you could set it on fire. So they thought they'd mixed water and fire. Fire-water, the Elixir Vitae, By God. Maybe they weren't so far wrong thinking it was the Cure-all, the thing that worked miracles. Have a drink!?"

"I don't need it," said Halloway. "But someone inside me does."

"Who?"

The boy I once was, thought Halloway, who runs like the leaves down the sidewalk autumn nights.

But he couldn't say that.

So he drank, eyes shut, listening to hear if that thing inside turned over again, rustling in the deep bons that were stacked for burning but never burned.

CHAPTER FOUR

Will stopped. Will looked at the Friday night town.

It seemed when the first stroke of nine banged from the big courthouse clock all the lights were on and business humming in the shops. But by the time the last stroke of nine shook everyone's fillings in his teeth, the barbers had yanked off the sheets, powdered the customers, trotted them forth; the druggist's fount had stopped fizzing like a nest of snakes, the insect neons everywhere had ceased buzzing, and the vast glittering acreage of the dime store with its ten billion metal, glass and paper oddments waiting to be fished over, suddenly blacked out. Shades slithered, doors boomed, keys rattled their bones in locks, people fled with hordes of torn newspaper mice nibbling their heels.

Bang! they were gone!

"Boy!" yelled Will. "Folks run like they thought the storm was here!"

"It is!" shouted Jim. *"Us!"*

They stomp-pound-thundered over iron grates, steel trapdoors, past a dozen unlit shops, a dozen half-lit, a dozen dying dark. The city was dead as they rounded the United Cigar Store corner to see a wooden Cherokee glide in darkness, by himself.

"Hey!"

Mr. Tetley, the proprietor, peered over the Indian's shoulder.

"Scare you, boys?"

"Naw!"

But Will shivered, feeling cold tidal waves of strange rain moving down the prairie as on a deserted shore. When the lightning nailed the town, he wanted to be layered under sixteen blankets and a pillow.

"Mr. Tetley?" said Will, quietly.

For now there were two wooden Indians upright in ripe tobacco darkness. Mr. Tetley, amidst his jest, had frozen, mouth open, listening.

"Mr. Tetley?"

He heard something far away on the wind, but couldn't say what it was.

The boys backed off.

He did not see them. He did not move. He only listened.

They left him. They ran.

In the fourth empty block from the library, the boys came upon a third wooden Indian.

Mr. Crosetti, in front of his barber shop, his door key in his trembling fingers, did not see them stop.

What had stopped them?

A teardrop.

It moved shining down Mr. Crosetti's left cheek. He breathed heavily.

"Crosetti, you fool! *Something* happens, *nothing* happens, you cry like a baby!"

Mr. Crosetti took a trembling breath, snuffing. "Don't you *smell* it?"

Jim and Will sniffed.

"Licorice!"

"Heck, no. Cotton candy!"

"I haven't smelled that in years," said Mr. Crosetti.

Jim snorted. "It's around."

"Yes, but who notices? When? Now, my nose tells me, breathe! And I'm crying. Why? Because I remember how a long time ago, boys ate that stuff. Why haven't I stopped to think and smell the last thirty years?"

"You're busy, Mr. Crosetti," Will said. "You haven't got time."

"Time, time." Mr. Crosetti wiped his eyes. "Where does that smell come from? There's no place in town sells cotton candy. Only circuses."

"Hey," said Will. "That's right!"

"Well, Crosetti is done crying." The barber blew his nose and turned to lock his shop door. As he did this, Will watched the barber pole whirl its red serpentine up out of nothing, leading his gaze around, rising to vanish into more nothing. On countless noons Will had stood here trying to unravel that ribbon, watch it come, go, end without ending.

Mr. Crosetti put his hand to the light switch under the spinning pole.

"Don't," said Will. Then, murmuring, "Don't turn it off."

Mr. Crosetti looked at the pole, as if freshly aware of its miraculous properties. He nodded, gently, his eyes soft. "Where does it come from, where does it go, eh? Who knows? Not you, not him, not me. Oh, the mysteries, by God. So. We'll leave it on!"

It's good to know, thought Will, it'll be running until

dawn, winding up from nothing, winding away to nothing, while we sleep.

"Good night!"

"Good night."

And they left him behind in a wind that very faintly smelled of licorice and cotton candy.

CHAPTER FIVE

Charles Halloway put his hand to the saloon's double swing doors, hesitant, as if the gray hairs on the back of his hand, like antennae, had felt something beyond slide by in the October night. Perhaps great fires burned somewhere and their furnace blasts warned him not to step forth. Or another Ice Age had loomed across the land, its freezing bulk might already have laid waste a billion people in the hour. Perhaps Time itself was draining off down an immense glass, with powdered darkness falling after to bury all.

Or maybe it was only that man in a dark suit, seen through the saloon window, across the street. Great paper rolls under one arm, a brush and bucket in his free hand, the man was whistling a tune, very far away.

It was a tune from another season, one that never ceased making Charles Halloway sad when he heard it. The song was incongruous for October, but immensely moving, overwhelming, no matter what day or what month it was sung:

> I heard the bells on Christmas Day
> Their old, familiar carols play,
>   And wild and sweet
>   Their words repeat
> Of peace on earth, good will to men!

Charles Halloway shivered. Suddenly there was the

old sense of terrified elation, of wanting to laugh and cry
together when he saw the innocents of the earth wandering the snowy streets the day before Christmas among
all the tired men and women whose faces were dirty with
guilt, unwashed of sin, and smashed like small windows
by life that hit without warning, ran, hid, came back and
hit again.

> Then pealed the bells more loud and deep:
> "God is not dead, nor doth He sleep!
>> The Wrong shall fail,
>> The Right prevail,
> With peace on earth, good will to men!"

The whistling died.

Charles Halloway stepped out. Far up ahead, the man
who had whistled the tune was motioning his arms by a
telegraph pole, silently working. Now he vanished into the
open door of a shop.

Charles Halloway, not knowing why, crossed the street
to watch the man pasting up one of the posters inside the
unrented and empty store.

Now the man stepped out the door with his brush, his
paste bucket, his rolled papers. His eyes, a fierce and lustful shine, fixed on Charles Halloway. Smiling, he gestured an open hand.

Halloway stared.

The palm of that hand was covered with fine black
silken hair. It looked like—

The hand clenched, tight. It waved. The man swept
around the corner. Charles Halloway, stunned, flushed
with sudden summer heat, swayed, then turned to gaze
into the empty shop.

Two sawhorses stood parallel to each other under a
single spotlight.

Placed over these two sawhorses like a funeral of
snow and crystal was a block of ice six feet long. It
shone dimly with its own effulgence, and its color was
light green-blue. It was a great cool gem resting there in
the dark.

On a little white placard at one side near the window the following calligraphic message could be read by lamplight:

Cooger & Dark's Pandemonium Shadow Show—
Fantoccini, Marionette Circus, and Your
Plain Meadow Carnival. Arriving
Immediately! Here on Display, one of
our many attractions:

THE MOST BEAUTIFUL WOMAN IN THE WORLD!

Halloway's eyes leaped to the poster on the inside of the window.

THE MOST BEAUTIFUL WOMAN IN THE WORLD!

And back to the cold long block of ice.

It was such a block of ice as he remembered from traveling magician's shows when he was a boy, when the local ice company contributed a chunk of winter in which, for 12 hours on end, frost maidens lay embedded, on display while people watched and comedies toppled down the raw white screen and coming attractions came and went and at last the pale ladies slid forth all rimed, chipped free by perspiring sorcerers to be led off smiling into the dark behind the curtains.

THE MOST BEAUTIFUL WOMAN IN THE WORLD!

And yet this vast chunk of wintry glass held nothing but frozen river water.

No. Not quite empty.

Halloway felt his heart pound one special time.

Within the huge winter gem was there not a special vacuum? a voluptuous hollow, a prolonged emptiness which undulated from tip to toe of the ice? and wasn't this vacuum, this emptiness waiting to be filled with summer flesh, was it not shaped somewhat like a . . . woman?

Yes.

The ice. And the lovely hollows, the horizontal flow of emptiness within the ice. The lovely nothingness. The exquisite flow of an invisible mermaid daring the ice to capture it.

The ice was cold.

The emptiness within the ice was warm.

He wanted to go away from here.

But Charles Halloway stood in the strange night for a long time looking in at the empty shop and the two saw-horses and the cold waiting arctic coffin set there like a vast Star of India in the dark. . . .

CHAPTER SIX

Jim Nightshade stopped at the corner of Hickory and Main, breathing easily, his eyes fixed tenderly on the leafy darkness of Hickory Street.

"Will . . . ?"

"No!" Will stopped, surprised at his own violence.

"It's just there. The fifth house. Just *one* minute, Will," Jim pleaded, softly.

"Minute . . . ?" Will glanced down the street.

Which was the street of the Theater.

Until this summer it had been an ordinary street where they stole peaches, plums and apricots, each in its day. But late in August, while they were monkey-climbing for the sourest apples, the "thing" happened which changed the houses, the taste of the fruit, and the very air within the gossiping trees.

"Will! It's waiting. Maybe something's *happening!*" hissed Jim.

Maybe something is. Will swallowed hard, and felt Jim's hand pinch his arm.

For it was no longer the street of the apples or plums or apricots, it was the one house with a window at the side and this window, Jim said, was a stage, with a curtain—the shade, that is—up. And in that room, on that strange stage, were the actors, who spoke mysteries, mouthed wild things, laughed, sighed, murmured so much; so *much* of it was whispers Will did not understand.

"Just one last time, Will."

"You know it won't be last!"

Jim's face was flushed, his cheeks blazing, his eyes green-glass fire. He thought of that night, them picking the apples, Jim suddenly crying softly, "Oh, there!"

And Will, hanging to the limbs of the tree, tight-pressed, terribly excited, staring in at the Theater, that peculiar stage where people, all unknowing, flourished shirts above their heads, let fall clothes to the rug, stood raw and animal-crazy, naked, like shivering horses, hands out to touch each other.

What're they *doing!* thought Will. Why are they laughing? What's wrong with them, what's *wrong!?*

He wished the light would go out.

But he hung tight to the suddenly slippery tree and watched the bright window Theater, heard the laughing, and numb at last let go, slid, fell, lay dazed, then stood in dark gazing up at Jim, who still clung to his high limb. Jim's face, hearth-flushed, cheeks fire-fuzzed, lips parted, stared in. "Jim, Jim, come down!" But Jim did not hear. "Jim!" And when Jim looked down at last he saw Will as a stranger below with some silly request to give off living and come down to earth. So Will ran off, alone, thinking too much, thinking nothing at all, not knowing what to think.

"Will, please . . ."

Will looked at Jim now, with the library books in his hands.

"We been to the library. Ain't that enough?"

Jim shook his head. "Carry these for me."

He handed Will his books and trotted softly off under the hissing whispering trees. Three houses down he called back: "Will? Know what you *are?* A darn old dimwit Episcopal Baptist!"

Then Jim was gone.

Will seized the books tight to his chest. They were wet from his hands.

Don't look back! he thought.

I won't! I won't!

And looking only toward home, he walked that way. Quickly.

CHAPTER SEVEN

Halfway home, Will felt a shadow breathing hard behind him.

"Theater closed?" said Will, not looking back.

Jim walked in silence beside him for a long while and then said, "Nobody home."

"Swell!"

Jim spat. "Darn Baptist preacher, you!"

And around the corner a tumbleweed slithered, a great cotton ball of pale paper which bounced, then clung shivering to Jim's legs.

Will grabbed the paper, laughing, pulled it off, let it fly! He stopped laughing.

The boys, watching the pale throwaway rattle and flit through the trees, were suddenly cold.

"Wait a minute . . ." said Jim, slowly.

All of a sudden they were yelling, running, leaping. "Don't tear it! Careful!"

The paper fluttered like a snare drum in their hands.

"COMING, OCTOBER TWENTY-FOURTH!"

Their lips moved, shadowing the words set in rococo type.

"Cooger and Dark's . . ."

"Carnival!"

"October twenty-fourth! That's tomorrow!"

"It can't be," said Will. "All carnivals stop after Labor Day—"

"Who cares? A thousand and one wonders! See! MEPHISTOPHELE, THE LAVA DRINKER! MR. ELECTRICO! THE MONSTER MONTGOLFIER?"

"Balloon," said Will. "A Montgolfier is a balloon."

"MADEMOISELLE TAROT!" read Jim. "THE DANGLING MAN. THE DEMON GUILLOTINE! THE ILLUSTRATED MAN! Hey!"

"That's just an old guy with tattoos."

"No." Jim breathed warm on the paper. "He's *illustrated*. Special. See! Covered with monsters! A menagerie!" Jim's eyes jumped. "SEE! THE SKELETON! Ain't that fine, Will? Not Thin Man, no, but SKELETON! SEE! THE DUST WITCH! What's a Dust Witch, Will?"

"Dirty old Gypsy—"

"No." Jim squinted off, seeing things. "A Gypsy that was born in the Dust, raised in the Dust, and some day winds up *back* in the Dust. Here's more: EGYPTIAN MIRROR MAZE! SEE YOURSELF TEN THOUSAND TIMES! SAINT ANTHONY'S TEMPLE OF TEMPTATION!"

"THE MOST BEAUTIFUL—" read Will.

"—WOMAN IN THE WORLD," finished Jim.

They looked at each other.

"*Can* a carnival have the Most Beautiful Woman on Earth in its side show, Will?"

"You ever *seen* carnival ladies, Jim?"

"Grizzly bears. But how come this handbill claims—"

"Oh, shut up!"

"You mad at me, Will?"

"No, it's just—get it!"

The wind had torn the paper from their hands.

The handbill blew over the trees and away in an idiot caper, gone.

"It's not true, anyway," Will gasped. "Carnivals don't come this late in the year. Silly darn-sounding thing. Who'd *go* to it?"

"Me." Jim stood quiet in the dark.

Me, thought Will, seeing the guillotine flash, the Egyptian mirrors unfold accordions of light, and the sulphur-skinned devil-man sipping lava, like gunpowder tea.

"That music . . ." Jim murmured. "Calliope. Must be coming *tonight*!"

"Carnivals come at sunrise."

"Yeah, but what about the licorice and cotton candy we smelled, close?"

And Will thought of the smells and the sounds flowing

on the river of wind from beyond the darkening houses, Mr. Tetley listening by his wooden Indian friend, Mr. Crosetti with the single tear shining down his cheek, and the barber pole sliding its red tongue up and around forever out of nowhere and away to eternity.

Will's teeth chattered.

"Let's go home."

"We *are* home!" cried Jim, surprised.

For, not knowing it, they had reached their separate houses and now moved up separate walks.

On his porch, Jim leaned over and called softly.

"Will. You're not mad?"

"Heck, no."

"We won't go by that street, that house, the Theater, again for a month. A *year!* I swear."

"Sure, Jim, sure."

They stood with their hands on the doorknobs of their houses, and Will looked up at Jim's roof where the lightning rod glittered against the cold stars.

The storm was coming. The storm *wasn't* coming.

No matter which, he was glad Jim had that grand contraption up there.

"Night!"

"Night."

Their separate doors slammed.

CHAPTER EIGHT

Will opened the door and shut it again. Quietly, this time.

"That's better," said his mother's voice.

Framed through the hall door Will saw the only theater he cared for now, the familiar stage where sat his father (home already! he and Jim *must* have run the long way round!) holding a book but reading the empty spaces. In a chair by the fire mother knitted and hummed like a tea-kettle.

He wanted to be near and not near them, he saw

them close, he saw them far. Suddenly they were aw-
fully small in too large a room in too big a town and
much too huge a world. In this unlocked place they
seemed at the mercy of anything that might break in
from the night.

Including me, Will thought. Including me.

Suddenly he loved them more for their smallness than
he ever had when they seemed tall.

His mother's fingers twitched, her mouth counted, the
happiest woman he had ever seen. He remembered a
greenhouse on a winter day, pushing aside thick jungle
leaves to find a creamy pink hothouse rose poised alone
in the wilderness. That was mother, smelling like fresh
milk, happy, to herself, in this room.

Happy? But how and why? Here, a few feet off, was
the janitor, the library man, the stranger, his uniform
gone, but his face still the face of a man happier at night
alone in the deep marble vaults, whispering his broom in
the drafty corridors.

Will watched, wondering why this woman was so
happy and this man so sad.

His father stared deep in the fire, one hand relaxed.
Half cupped in that hand lay a crumpled paper ball.

Will blinked.

He remembered the wind blowing the pale handbill
skittering in the trees. Now the same color paper lay
crushed, its rococo type hidden, in his father's fingers.

"Hey!"

Will stepped into the parlor.

Immediately Mom opened a smile that was like lighting a second fire.

Dad, stricken, looked dismayed, as if caught in a criminal act.

Will wanted to say, "Hey, what'd you think of the
handbill . . . ?"

But Dad was cramming the handbill deep in the chair
upholstery.

And mother was leafing the library books.

"Oh, these are fine, Willy!"

So Will just stood with Cooger and Dark on his tongue
and said:

"Boy, the wind really *flew* us home. Streets full of *paper* blowing."

Dad did not flinch at this.

"Anything new, Dad?"

Dad's hand still lay tucked in the side of the chair. He lifted a gray, slightly worried, very tired gaze to his son:

"Stone lion blew off the library steps. Prowling the town now, looking for Christians. Won't find any. Got the only one in captivity here, and she's a good cook."

"Bosh," said Mom.

Walking upstairs, Will heard what he half expected to hear.

A soft fluming sigh as something fresh was tossed on the fire. In his mind, he saw Dad standing at the hearth looking down as the paper crinkled to ash:

". . . COOGER . . . DARK . . . CARNIVAL . . . WITCH . . . WONDERS . . ."

He wanted to go back down and stand with Dad, hands out, to be warmed by the fire.

Instead he went slowly up to shut the door of his room.

Some nights, abed, Will put his ear to the wall to listen, and if his folks talked things that were right, he stayed, and if not right he turned away. If it was about time and passing years or himself or town or just the general inconclusive way God ran the world, he listened warmly, comfortably, secretly, for it was usually Dad talking. He could not often speak with Dad anywhere in the world, inside or out, but this was different. There was a thing in Dad's voice, up, over, down, easy as a hand winging soft in the air like a white bird describing flight patterns, made the ear want to follow and the mind's eye to see.

And the odd thing in Dad's voice was the sound truth makes being said. The sound of truth, in a wild roving land of city or plain country lies, will spell any boy. Many nights Will drowsed this way, his senses like stopped clocks long before that half-singing voice was

still. Dad's voice was a midnight school, teaching deep
fathom hours, and the subject was life.

So it was this night, Will's eyes shut, head leaned to the
cool plaster. At first Dad's voice, a Congo drum, boomed
softly, horizons away. Mother's voice, she used her
water-bright soprano in the Baptist choir, did not sing, yet
sang back replies. Will imagined Dad sprawled talking to
the empty ceiling:

". . . Will . . . makes me feel so *old* . . . a man
should play baseball with his son. . . ."

"Not necessary," said the woman's voice, kindly.
"You're a good man."

"—in a bad season. Hell, I was forty when he was
born! And *you.* Who's your *daughter?* people say. God,
when you lie down your thoughts turn to mush. Hell!"

Will heard the shift of weight as Dad sat up in the
dark. A match was being struck, a pipe was being
smoked. The wind rattled the windows.

". . . man with posters under his arm . . ."

". . . carnival . . ." said his mother's voice, ". . . *this*
late in the year??"

Will wanted to turn away, but couldn't.

". . . most beautiful . . . woman . . . in the world,"
Dad's voice murmured.

Mother laughed softly. "You know I'm not."

No! thought Will, that's from the handbill! Why doesn't
Dad *tell!!?*

Because, Will answered himself. Something's going on.
Oh, something *is* going on!

Will saw that paper frolicked in the trees, its words
THE MOST BEAUTIFUL WOMAN, and fever prickled his
cheeks. He thought: Jim, the street of the Theater, the
naked people in the stage of that Theater window, crazy
as Chinese opera, darn odd crazy as old Chinese opera,
judo, jujitsu, Indian puzzles, and now his father's voice,
dreaming off, sad, sadder, saddest, much too much to
understand. And suddenly he was scared because Dad
wouldn't talk about the handbill he had secretly burned.
Will gazed out the window. There! Like a milkweed
plume! White paper danced in the air.

"No," he whispered, "no carnival's coming *this* late. It can't!" He hid under the covers, switched on his flashlight, opened a book. The first picture he saw was a pre-historic reptile trap-drumming a night sky a million years lost.

Heck, he thought, in the rush I got Jim's book, he's got one of mine.

But it was a pretty fine reptile.

And flying toward sleep, he thought he heard his father, restless, below. The front door shut. His father was going back to work late, for no reason, with brooms, or books, downtown, away . . . away. . . .

And mother asleep, content, not knowing he had gone.

CHAPTER NINE

No one else in the world had a name came so well off the tongue.

"Jim Nightshade. That's me."

Jim stood tall and now lay long in bed, strung together by marsh-grass, his bones easy in his flesh, his flesh easy on his bones. The library books lay unopened by his relaxed right hand.

Waiting, his eyes were dark as twilight, with shadows under the eyes from the time, his mother said, he had almost died when he was three and still remembered. His hair was dark autumn chestnut and the veins in his temples and brow and in his neck and ticking in his wrists and on the backs of his slender hands, all these were dark blue. He was marbled with dark, was Jim Nightshade, a boy who talked less and smiled less as the years increased.

The trouble with Jim was he looked at the world and could not look away. And when you never look away all your life, by the time you are thirteen you have done *twenty* years taking in the laundry of the world.

Will Halloway, it was in him young to always look just beyond, over or to one side. So at thirteen he had saved up only six years of staring.

Jim knew every centimeter of his shadow, could have cut it out of tar paper, furled it, and run it up a flagpole—his banner.

Will, he was occasionally surprised to see his shadow following him somewhere, but that was that.

"Jim? You awake?"

"Hi, Mom."

A door opened and now shut. He felt her weight on the bed.

"Why, Jim, your hands are ice. You shouldn't have the window so high. Mind your health."

"Sure."

"Don't say 'sure' that way. You don't know until you've had three children and lost all but one."

"Never going to have any," said Jim.

"You just say that."

"I *know* it. I know everything."

She waited a moment. "What do you know?"

"No use making more people. People die."

His voice was very calm and quiet and almost sad.

"That's everything."

"Almost everything. *You're* here, Jim. If you weren't, I'd given up long ago."

"Mom." A long silence. "Can you remember Dad's face? Do I look like him?"

"The day you go away is the day he leaves forever."

"Who's going away?"

"Why, just lying there, Jim, you run so fast. I never saw anyone move so much, just sleeping. Promise me, Jim. Wherever you go and come back, bring lots of kids. Let them run wild. Let me spoil them, some day."

"I'm never going to own anything can hurt me."

"You going to collect rocks, Jim? No, some day, you've got to be hurt."

"No, I don't."

He looked at her. Her face had been hit a long time ago. The bruises had never gone from around her eyes.

"You'll live and get hurt," she said, in the dark. "But

when it's time, tell me. Say goodbye. Otherwise, I might not let you go. Wouldn't that be terrible, to just grab ahold?"

She rose up suddenly and went to put the window down.

"Why do boys want their windows open wide?"

"Warm blood."

"Warm blood." She stood alone. "That's the story of all our sorrows. And don't ask why."

The door shut.

Jim, alone, raised the window, and leaned into the absolutely clear night.

Storm, he thought, you *there?*

Yes.

Feel . . . away to the west . . . a real humdinger, rushing along!

The shadow of the lightning rod lay on the drive below.

He sucked in cold air, gave out a vast exhilaration of heat.

Why, he thought, why don't I climb up, knock that lightning rod loose, throw it away?

And then see what happens?

Yes.

And *then* see what happens!

CHAPTER TEN

Just after midnight.

Shuffling footsteps.

Along the empty street came the lightning-rod salesman, his leather valise swung almost empty in his baseball-mitt hand, his face at ease. He turned a corner and stopped.

Paper-soft white moths tapped at an empty store window, looking in.

And in the window, like a great coffin boat of star-colored glass, beached on two sawhorses lay a chunk of

Alaska Snow Company ice chopped to a size great enough to flash in a giant's ring.

And sealed in this ice was the most beautiful woman in the world.

The lightning-rod salesman's smile faded.

In the dreaming coldness of ice like someone fallen and slept in snow avalanches a thousand years, forever young, was this woman.

She was as fair as this morning and fresh as tomorrow's flowers and lovely as any maid when a man shuts up his eyes and traps her, in cameo perfection, on the shell of his eyelids.

The lightning-rod salesman remembered to breathe.

Once, long ago, traveling among the marbles of Rome and Florence, he had seen women like this, kept in stone instead of ice. Once, wandering in the Louvre, he had found women like this, washed in summer color and kept in paint. Once, as a boy, sneaking the cool grottos behind a motion picture theater screen, on his way to a free seat, he had glanced up and there towering and flooding the haunted dark seen a woman's face as he had never seen it since, of such size and beauty built of milk-bone and moon-flesh as to freeze him there alone behind the stage, shadowed by the motion of her lips, the bird-wing flicker of her eyes, the snow-pale-death-shimmering illumination from her cheeks.

So from other years there jumped forth images which flowed and found new substance here within the ice.

What color was her hair? It was blond to whiteness and might take any color, once set free of cold.

How tall was she?

The prism of the ice might well multiply her size or diminish her as you moved this way or that before the empty store, the window, the night-soft rap-tapping ever-fingering, gently probing moths.

Not important.

Far above all—the lightning-rod salesman shivered—he knew the most extraordinary thing.

If by some miracle her eyelids should open within that sapphire and she should look at him, he knew what color her eyes would be.

He knew what color her eyes would be.

If one were to enter this lonely night shop—

If one were to put forth one's hand, the warmth of that hand would . . . what?

Melt the ice.

The lightning-rod salesman stood there for a long moment, his eyes quickened shut.

He let his breath out.

It was warm as summer on his teeth.

His hand touched the shop door. It swung open. Cold arctic air blew out around him. He stepped in.

The door shut.

The white snowflake moths tapped at the window.

CHAPTER ELEVEN

Midnight then and the town clocks chiming on toward one and two and then three in the deep morning and the peals of the great clocks shaking dust off old toys in high attics and shedding silver off old mirrors in yet higher attics and stirring up dreams about clocks in all the beds where children slept.

Will heard it.

Muffled away in the prairie lands, the chuffing of an engine, the slow-following dragon-glide of a train.

Will sat up in bed.

Across the way, like a mirror image, Jim sat up, too.

A calliope began to play oh so softly, grieving to itself, a million miles away.

In one single motion, Will leaned from his window, as did Jim. Without a word they gazed over the trembling surf of trees.

Their rooms were high, as boys' rooms should be. From these gaunt windows they could rifle-fire their gaze artillery distances past library, city hall, depot, cow barns, farmlands to empty prairie!

There, on the world's rim, the lovely snail-gleam of the

railway tracks ran, flinging wild gesticulations of lemon
or cherry-colored semaphore to the stars.

There, on the precipice of earth, a small steam feather
uprose like the first of a storm cloud yet to come.

The train itself appeared, link by link, engine, coal-
car, and numerous and numbered all-asleep-and-slumber-
ing-dreamfilled cars that followed the firefly-sparked
churn, chant, drowsy autumn hearthfire roar. Hellfires
flushed the stunned hills. Even at this remote view, one
imagined men with buffalo-haunched arms shoveling black
meteor falls of coal into the open boilers of the engine.

The engine!

Both boys vanished, came back to lift binoculars.

"The engine!"

"Civil War! No other stack like that since 1900!"

"The rest of the train, *all* of it's old!"

"The flags! The cages! It's the carnival!"

They listened. At first Will thought he heard the air
whistling fast in his nostrils. But no—it was the train,
and the calliope sighing, weeping, on that train.

"Sounds like church music!"

"Hell. Why would a carnival play church music?"

"Don't say hell," hissed Will.

"Hell." Jim ferociously leaned out. "I've saved up all
day. Everyone's asleep so—hell!"

The music drifted by their windows. Goose pimples rose
big as boils on Will's arms.

"That *is* church music. Changed."

"For cri-yi, I'm froze, let's go watch them set up!"

"At three A.M.?"

"At three A.M.!"

Jim vanished.

For a moment, Will watched Jim dance around over
there, shirt uplifted, pants going on, while off in night
country, panting, churning was this funeral train all black
plumed cars, licorice-colored cages, and a sooty calliope
clamoring, banging three different hymns mixed and lost,
maybe not there at all.

"Here goes nothing!"

Jim slid down the drainpipe on his house, toward the
sleeping lawns.

"Jim! Wait!"

Will thrashed into his clothes.

"Jim, don't go *alone!*"

And followed after.

CHAPTER TWELVE

Sometimes you see a kite so high, so wise it almost knows the wind. It travels, then chooses to land in one spot and no other and no matter how you yank, run this way or that, it will simply break its cord, seek its resting place and bring you, blood-mouthed, running.

"Jim! Wait for me!"

So now Jim was the kite, the wild twine cut, and whatever wisdom was his taking him away from Will who could only run, earthbound, after one so high and dark silent and suddenly strange.

"Jim, here I come!"

And running, Will thought, Boy, it's the same old thing. I talk. Jim runs. I tilt stones, Jim grabs the cold junk under the stones and—lickety-split! I climb hills. Jim yells off church steeples. I got a bank account. Jim's got the hair on his head, the yell in his mouth, the shirt on his back and the tennis shoes on his feet. How come I think *he's* richer? Because, Will thought, I sit on a rock in the sun and old Jim, he prickles his arm-hairs by moonlight and dances with hoptoads. I tend cows. Jim tames Gila monsters. Fool! I yell at Jim. Coward! he yells back. And here we—*go!*

And they ran from town, across fields and both froze under a rail bridge with the moon ready beyond the hills and the meadows trembling with a fur of dew.

WHAM!

The carnival train thundered the bridge. The calliope wailed.

"There's no one playing it!" Jim stared up.

"Jim, no jokes!"

"Mother's honor, look!"

Going away, away, the calliope pipes shimmered with star explosions, but no one sat at the high keyboard. The wind, sluicing ice-water air in the pipes, made the music.

The boys ran. The train curved away, gonging its undersea funeral bell, sunk, rusted, green-mossed, tolling, tolling. Then the engine whistle blew a great steam whiff and Will broke out in pearls of ice.

Way late at night Will had heard—how often?—train whistles jetting steam along the rim of sleep, forlorn, alone and far, no matter how near they came. Sometimes he woke to find tears on his cheek, asked why, lay back, listened and thought, Yes! *they* make me cry, going east, going west, the trains so far gone in country deeps they drown in tides of sleep that escape the towns.

Those trains and their grieving sounds were lost forever between stations, not remembering where they had been, not guessing where they might go, exhaling their last pale breaths over the horizon, gone. So it was with all trains, ever.

Yet *this* train's whistle!

The wails of a lifetime were gathered in it from other nights in other slumbering years; the howl of moon-dreamed dogs, the seep of river-cold winds through January porch screens which stopped the blood, a thousand fire sirens weeping, or worse! the outgone shreds of breath, the protests of a billion people dead or dying, not wanting to be dead, their groans, their sighs, burst over the earth!

Tears jumped to Will's eyes. He lurched. He knelt. He pretended to lace one shoe.

But then he saw Jim's hands clap *his* ears, his eyes wet, too. The whistle screamed. Jim screamed against the scream. The whistle shrieked. Will shrieked against the shriek.

Then the billion voices ceased, instantly, as if the train had plunged in a fire storm off the earth.

The train skimmed on softly, slithering, black pennants fluttering, black confetti lost on its own sick-sweet candy wind, down the hill, with the boys pursuing, the air so cold they ate ice cream with each breath.

They climbed a last rise to look down.

"Boy," whispered Jim.

The train had pulled off into Rolfe's moon meadow, so-called because town couples came out to see the moon rise here over a land so wide, so long, it was like an inland sea, filled with grass in spring, or hay in late summer or snow in winter, it was fine walking here along its crisp shore with the moon coming up to tremble in its tides.

Well, the carnival train was crouched there now in the autumn grass on the old rail spur near the woods, and the boys crept and lay down under a bush, waiting.

"It's so quiet," whispered Will.

The train just stood in the middle of the dry autumn field, no one in the locomotive, no one in the tender, no one in any of the cars behind, all black under the moon, and just the small sounds of its metal cooling, ticking on the rails.

"Ssst," said Jim. "I *feel* them *moving* in there."

Will felt the cat fuzz on his body bramble up by the thousands.

"You think they *mind* us watching?"

"Maybe," said Jim, happily.

"Then why the noisy calliope?"

"When I figure that," Jim smiled, "I'll tell you. Look!"

Whisper.

As if exhaling itself straight down from the sky, a vast moss-green balloon touched at the moon.

It hovered two hundred yards above and away, quietly riding the wind.

"The basket under the balloon, someone *in* it!"

But then a tall man stepped down from the train caboose platform like a captain assaying the tidal weathers of this inland sea. All dark suit, shadow-faced, he waded to the center of the meadow, his shirt as black as the gloved hands he now stretched to the sky.

He gestured, once.

And the train came to life.

At first a head lifted in one window, then an arm, then

another head like a puppet in a marionette theater. Suddenly two men in black were carrying a dark tent pole out across the hissing grass.

It was the silence that made Will pull back, even as Jim leaned forward, eyes moon-bright.

A carnival should be all growls, roars like timberlands stacked, bundled, rolled and crashed, great explosions of lion dust, men ablaze with working anger, pop bottles jangling, horse buckles shivering, engines and elephants in full stampede through rains of sweat while zebras neighed and trembled like cage trapped in cage.

But this was like old movies, the silent theater haunted with black-and-white ghosts, silvery mouths opening to let moonlight smoke out, gestures made in silence so hushed you could hear the wind fizz the hair on your cheeks.

More shadows rustled from the train, passing the animal cages where darkness prowled with unlit eyes and the calliope stood mute save for the faintest idiot tune the breeze piped wandering up the flues.

The ringmaster stood in the middle of the land. The balloon like a vast moldy green cheese stood fixed to the sky. Then—darkness came.

The last thing Will saw was the balloon swooping down, as clouds covered the moon.

In the night he felt the men rush to unseen tasks. He sensed the balloon, like a great fat spider, fiddling with the lines and poles, rearing a tapestry in the sky.

The clouds arose. The balloon sifted up.

In the meadow stood the skeleton main poles and wires of the main tent, waiting for its canvas skin.

More clouds poured over the white moon. Shadowed, Will shivered. He heard Jim crawling forward, seized his ankle, felt him stiffen.

"Wait!" said Will. "They're bringing out the canvas!"

"No," said Jim. "Oh, no . . ."

For somehow instead, they both knew, the wires highflung on the poles were catching swift clouds, ripping them free from the wind in streamers which, stitched and sewn by some great monster shadow, made canvas and more canvas as the tent took shape. At last there was the clear-water sound of vast flags blowing.

The motion stopped. The darkness within darkness was still.

Will lay, eyes shut, hearing the beat of great oil-black wings as if a huge, ancient bird had drummed down to live, to breathe, to survive in the night meadow.

The clouds blew away.

The balloon was gone.

The men were gone.

The tents rippled like black rain on their poles.

Suddenly it seemed a long way to town.

Instinctively, Will glanced behind himself.

Nothing but grass and whispers.

Slowly he looked back at the silent, dark, seemingly empty tents.

"I don't like it," he said.

Jim could not tear his eyes away.

"Yeah," he whispered. "Yeah."

Will stood up. Jim lay on the earth.

"Jim!" said Will.

Jim jerked his head as if slapped. He was on his knees, he swayed up. His body turned, but his eyes were fastened to those black flags, the great side-show signs swarming with unguessed wings, horns, and demon smiles.

A bird screamed.

Jim jumped. Jim gasped.

Cloud shadows panicked them over the hills to the edge of town.

From there, the two boys ran alone.

CHAPTER THIRTEEN

The air was cold blowing in through the wide-open library window.

Charles Halloway had stood there for a long time.

Now, he quickened.

Along the street below fled two shadows, two boys above them matching shadow stride for stride. They softly printed the night air with treads.

"Jim!" cried the old man. "Will!"

But not aloud.

The boys went away toward home.

Charles Halloway looked out into the country.

Wandering alone in the library, letting his broom tell him things no one else could hear, he had heard the whistle and the disjointed calliope hymns.

"Three," he now said, half-aloud. "Three in the morning . . ."

In the meadow, the tents, the carnival waited. Waited for someone, anyone to wade along the grassy surf. The great tents filled like bellows. They softly issued forth exhalations of air that smelled like ancient yellow beasts.

But only the moon looked in at the hollow dark, the deep caverns. Outside, night beasts hung in midgallop on a carousel. Beyond lay fathoms of Mirror Maze which housed a multifold series of empty vanities one wave on another, still, serene, silvered with age, white with time. Any shadow, at the entrance, might stir reverberations the color of fright, unravel deep-buried moons.

If a man stood here would he see himself unfolded away a billion times to eternity? Would a billion images look back, each face and the face after and the face after that old, older, oldest? Would he find himself lost in a fine dust away off deep down there, not fifty but sixty, not sixty but seventy, not seventy but eighty, ninety, ninety-nine years old?

The maze did not ask.

The maze did not tell.

It simply stood and waited like a great arctic floe.

"Three o'clock . . ."

Charles Halloway was cold. His skin was suddenly a lizard's skin. His stomach filled with blood turned to rust. His mouth tasted of night damps.

Yet he could not turn from the library window.

Far off, something glittered in the meadow.

It was moonlight, flashing on a great glass.

Perhaps the light said something, perhaps it spoke in code.

I'll *go* there, thought Charles Halloway, I *won't* go there.

I *like* it, he thought, I *don't* like it.

A moment later the library door slammed.

Going home, he passed the empty store window.

Inside stood two abandoned sawhorses.

Between lay a pool of water. In the water floated a few shards of ice. In the ice were a few long strands of hair.

Charles Halloway saw but chose not to see. He turned and was gone. The street was soon as empty as the hardware-store window.

Far away, in the meadow, shadows flickered in the Mirror Maze, as if parts of someone's life, yet unborn, were trapped there, waiting to be lived.

So the maze waited, its cold gaze ready, for so much as a bird to come look, see, and fly away shrieking.

But no bird came.

CHAPTER FOURTEEN

"Three," a voice said.

Will listened, cold but warming, glad to be in with a roof above, floor below, wall and door between too much exposure, too much freedom, too much night.

"Three . . ."

Dad's voice, home now, moving down the hall, speaking to itself.

"Three . . ."

Why, thought Will, that's when the train came. Had Dad seen, heard, followed?

No, he *mustn't!* Will hunched himself. Why not? He trembled. What did he fear?

The carnival rushing in like a black stampede of storm waves on the shore out beyond? Of him and Jim and Dad knowing, of the town asleep, not knowing, was *that* it?

Yes. Will buried himself, deep. Yes . . .

"Three . . ."

Three in the morning, thought Charles Halloway, seated on the edge of his bed. Why did the train come at that hour?

For, he thought, it's a special hour. Women never wake then, do they? They sleep the sleep of babes and children. But men in middle age? They know that hour well. Oh God, midnight's not bad, you wake and go back to sleep, one or two's not bad, you toss but sleep again. Five or six in the morning, there's hope, for dawn's just under the horizon. But three, now, Christ, three A.M.! Doctors say the body's at low tide then. The soul is out. The blood moves slow. You're the nearest to dead you'll ever be save dying. Sleep is a patch of death, but three in the morn, full wide-eyed staring, is living death! You dream with your eyes open. God, if you had strength to rouse up, you'd slaughter your half-dreams with buckshot! But no, you lie pinned to a deep well-bottom that's burned dry. The moon rolls by to look at you down there, with its idiot face. It's a long way back to sunset, a far way on to dawn, so you summon all the fool things of your life, the stupid lovely things done with people known so very well who are now so very dead— And wasn't it true, had he read it somewhere, more people in hospitals die at 3 A.M. than at any other time . . . ?

Stop! he cried silently.

"Charlie?" his wife said in her sleep.

Slowly, he took off the other shoe.

His wife smiled in her sleep.

Why?

She's immortal. She has a son.

Your son, too!

But what father ever really believes it? He carries no burden, he feels no pain. What man, like woman, lies down in darkness and gets up with child? The gentle, smiling ones own the good secret. Oh, what strange wonderful clocks women are. They nest in Time. They make the flesh that holds fast and binds eternity. They live inside the gift, know power, accept, and need not mention it. Why speak of Time when you *are* Time, and shape the universal moments, as they pass, into warmth and action? How men envy and often hate these warm clocks, these wives, who know they will live forever. So what do we do? We men turn terribly mean, because we can't hold to the world or ourselves or anything. We are blind to continuity, all breaks down, falls, melts, stops, rots, or runs away. So, since we cannot shape Time, where does that leave men? Sleepless. Staring.

Three A.M. That's our reward. Three in the morn. The soul's midnight. The tide goes out, the soul ebbs. And a train arrives at an hour of despair. . . . *Why?*

"Charlie . . . ?"

His wife's hand moved to his.

"You . . . *all right* . . .Charlie?"

She drowsed.

He did not answer.

He could not tell her how he was.

CHAPTER FIFTEEN

The sun rose yellow as a lemon.

The sky was round and blue.

The birds looped clear water songs in the air.

Will and Jim leaned from their windows.

Nothing had changed.

Except the look in Jim's eyes.

"Last night . . ." said Will. "Did or didn't it happen?"

They both gazed toward the far meadows.

The air was sweet as syrup. They could find no shadows, anywhere, even under trees.

"Six minutes!" cried Jim.

"Five!"

Four minutes later, corn flakes lurching in their stomachs, they frisked the leaves to a fine red dust going out of town.

With a wild flutter of breath, they raised their eyes from the earth they had been treading.

And the carnival was there.

"Hey . . ."

For the tents were lemon like the sun, brass like wheat fields a few weeks ago. Flags and banners bright as bluebirds snapped above lion-colored canvas. From booths painted cotton-candy colors, fine Saturday smells of bacon and eggs, hot dogs and pancakes swam the wind. Everywhere ran boys. Everywhere, sleepy fathers followed.

"It's just a plain old carnival," said Will.

"Like heck," said Jim. "We weren't blind last night. Come on!"

They marched one hundred yards straight on and deep into the midway. And the deeper they went, the more obvious it became they would find no night men cat-treading balloon shadow while strange tents plumed like thunder clouds. Instead, close up, the carnival was mildewed rope, moth-eaten canvas, rain-worn, sun-bleached tinsel. The side show paintings, hung like sad albatrosses on their poles, flapped and let fall flakes of ancient paint, shivering and at the same time revealing the unwondrous wonders of a thin man, fat man, needle-head, tattooed man, hula dancer. . . .

They prowled on but found no mysterious midnight spheres of evil gas tied by mysterious Oriental knots to daggers plunged in dark earth, no maniac ticket takers bent on terrible revenges. The calliope by the ticket booth neither screamed deaths nor hummed idiot songs to itself. The train? Pulled off on a spur in the warming grass, it was old, yes, and welded tight with rust, but it looked like a titanic magnet that had collected to itself, from locomotive boneyards across three continents, drive shafts, flywheels, smoke stacks, and hand-me-down second-rate nightmares. It did not cut a black and mortuary silhouette. It asked permission but to lie dead in autumn strewings, so much tired steam and iron gunpowder blowing away.

"Jim! Will!"

Here came Miss Foley, their seventh-grade schoolteacher, along the midway, all smiles.

"Boys," she said, "what's wrong? You look as if you lost something."

"Well," said Will, "last night, did you hear that calliope—"

"Calliope? No—"

"Then why're you out here so early, Miss Foley?" asked Jim.

"I love carnivals," said Miss Foley, a little woman lost somewhere in her gray fifties, beaming around. "I'll buy hot dogs and you eat while I look for my fool nephew. You *seen* him?"

"Nephew?"

"Robert. Staying with me a few weeks. Father's dead, mother's sick in Wisconsin. I took him in. He ran out here early today. Said he'd meet me. But you know boys! My, you look glum." She shoved food at them. "Eat! Cheer up! Rides'll open in ten minutes. Meantime, I think I'll spy through that Mirror Maze and—"

"No," said Will.

"No what?" asked Miss Foley.

"No Mirror Maze." Will swallowed. He stared at fathoms of reflections. You could never strike bottom there. It was like winter standing tall, waiting to kill you with a glance. "Miss Foley," he said at last, and wondered to hear his mouth say it, "don't go in there."

"Why not?"

Jim peered, fascinated, into Will's face. "Yeah, tell us. Why not?"

"People get lost," said Will, lamely.

"All the more reason. Robert might be wandering, loose, and not find his way out if I don't grab his ear—"

"Never can tell—" Will could not take his eyes off the millions of miles of blind glass—"what might be swimming around in there. . . ."

"Swimming!" Miss Foley laughed. "What a lovely mind you have, Willy. Well, yes, but I'm an old fish. So . . ."

"Miss Foley!"

Miss Foley waved, poised, took a step, and vanished into the mirror ocean. They watched as she settled, wandered, sank deep, deep, and was finally dissolved, gray among silver.

Jim grabbed Will. "What was all *that?*"

"Gosh, Jim, it's the mirrors! They're the only things I don't like. I mean, they're the only things *like* last night."

"Boy, boy, you been out in the sun," snorted Jim. "That maze there is . . ." His voice trailed off. He sniffed the cold air blowing out as from an ice house between the tall reflections.

"Jim? You were saying?"

But Jim said nothing. After a long time he clapped his hand to the back of his neck. "It really *does!*" he cried, in soft amaze.

"What does?"

"Hair! I read it all my life. In scary stories, it stands on end! Mine's doing it—now!"

"Gosh, Jim. So's mine!"

They stood entranced with the delicious cold bumps on their necks and the suddenly stiffened small hairs quilled up over their scalps.

There was a flourish of light and shadow.

Bumping out through the Mirror Maze they saw two, four, a dozen Miss Foleys.

They didn't know which one was real, so they waved to all of them.

But none of the Miss Foleys saw or waved back. Blind, she walked. Blind, she tacked her nails to cold glass.

"Miss Foley!"

Her eyes, flexed wide as from blasts of photographic powder, were skinned white like a statue's. Deep under the glass, she spoke. She murmured. She whimpered. Now she cried. Now she shouted. Now she yelled. She knocked glass with her head, her elbows, tilted drunken as a light-blind moth, raised her hands in claws. "Oh God! Help!" she wailed. "Help, oh God!"

Jim and Will saw their own faces, pale, their own eyes, wide, in the mirrors as they plunged.

"Miss Foley, here!" Jim cracked his brow.

"*This* way!" But Will found only cold glass.

A hand flew from empty space. An old woman's hand, sinking for the last time. It seized anything to save itself. The anything was Will. She pulled him under.

"Will!"

"Jim! Jim!"

And Jim held him and he held her and pulled her free of the silently rushing mirrors coming in coming in from the desolate seas.

They stepped into sunlight.

Miss Foley, one hand to her bruised cheek, bleated, muttered, then laughed quickly, then gasped, and wiped her eyes.

"Thank you, Will, Jim, oh thank you, I'd of drowned! I mean . . . oh, Will you were *right!* My God, did you *see* her, she's lost, drowned in there, poor girl, oh the poor lost sweet . . . save her, oh, we must *save* her!"

"Miss Foley, boy, you're hurting." Will firmly removed her fists from clenching the flesh of his arm. "There's no one in there."

"I saw her! Please! Look! Save her!"

Will jumped to the maze entrance and stopped. The ticket taker gave him an idle glance of contempt. Will backed away to Miss Foley.

"I swear, no one went in ahead or after you, ma'am. It's my fault, I joked about the water, you must've got mixed up, lost, and scared. . . ."

But if she heard, she went on biting the back of her hand, her voice the voice of someone come out of the sea after no air, a long dread time deep, no hope of life and now set free.

"Gone? She's at the bottom! Poor girl. I knew her. 'I *know* you!' I said when I first saw her a minute ago. I waved, she waved. 'Hello!' I ran!—bang! I fell. *She* fell. A dozen, a thousand of her fell. 'Wait!' I said. Oh, she looked so fine, so lovely, so young. But it scared me. 'What're you doing *here?*' I said. 'Why,' I think she said, '*I'm* real. You're *not!*' she laughed, way under water. She ran off in the maze. We *must* find her! before—"

Miss Foley, Will's arm around her, took a last trembling breath and grew strangely quiet.

Jim was staring deep into those cold mirrors, looking for sharks that could not be seen.

"Miss Foley," he said, "what did *she* look like?"

Miss Foley's voice was pale but calm.

"The fact is . . . she looked like myself, many, many years ago.

"I'll go home now," she said.

"Miss Foley, we'll—"

"No. Stay. I'm just fine. Have fun, boys. Enjoy."

And she walked slowly away, alone, down the midway. Somewhere a vast animal made water. Ammonia made the wind turn ancient as it passed.

"I'm leaving!" said Will.

"Will," said Jim. "We're staying until sundown, boy, dark sundown, and figure it *all*. You chicken?"

"No," murmured Will. "But . . . anybody want to dive back in that maze?"

Jim gazed fiercely deep into the bottomless sea, where now only the pure light glanced back at itself, held up emptiness upon emptiness beyond emptiness before their eyes.

"Nobody." Jim let his heart beat twice. ". . . I guess."

CHAPTER SIXTEEN

A bad thing happened at sunset.

Jim vanished.

Through noon and after noon, they had screamed up half the rides, knocked over dirty milk-bottles, smashed kewpie-doll winning plates, smelling, listening, looking their way through the autumn crowd trampling the leafy sawdust.

And then quite suddenly Jim was gone.

And Will, not asking anyone but himself, absolutely silent certain-sure, walked steadily through the late crowd as the sky was turning plum colored until he came to the maze and paid his dime and stepped up inside and called softly just one time:

". . . Jim . . . ?"

And Jim was there, half in, half out of the cold glass

tides like someone abandoned on a seashore when a close friend has gone far out, and there is wonder if he will ever come back. Jim stood as if he had not moved so much as an eyelash in five minutes, staring, his mouth half-open, waiting for the next wave to come in and show him more.

"Jim! Get outa there!"

"Will . . ." Jim sighed faintly. "Let me be."

"Like heck!" With one leap, Will grabbed Jim's belt and hauled. Shuffling backward, Jim did not seem to know he was being dragged from the maze, for he kept protesting in awe at some unseen wonder: "Oh, Will, oh, Willy, Will, oh, Willy . . ."

"Jim, you nut, I'm taking you home!"

"What? What? What?"

They were in the cold air. The sky was darker than plums now, with a few clouds burning late sun-fire above. The sun-fire flamed on Jim's feverish cheeks, his open lips, his wide and terribly rich green shining eyes.

"Jim, what'd you see in there? The same as Miss Foley?"

"What, what?"

"I'm gonna bust your nose! Come on!" He hustled, pulled, shoved, half carried this fever, this elation, this unstruggling friend.

"Can't tell you, Will, wouldn't believe, can't tell you, in there, oh, in there, in there . . ."

"Shut up!" Will socked his arm. "Scare heck outa me, just like *she* scared us. Bugs! It's almost suppertime. Folks'll think we're dead and buried!"

They were striding now, slashing the autumn grass with their shoes, beyond the tents in the hay-smelling, leaf-mold fields, Will glaring at town, Jim staring back at the high now-darkening banners as the last of the sun hid under the earth.

"Will, we got to come back. Tonight—"

"Okay, come back alone."

Jim stopped.

"You wouldn't let me come alone. You're always going to be around, aren't you, Will? To protect me?"

"Look who needs protection." Will laughed and then

did not laugh again, for Jim was looking at him, the last wild light dying in his mouth and caught in the thin hollows of his nostrils and in his suddenly deep-set eyes.

"You'll always be with me, huh, Will?"

Jim simply breathed warm upon him and his blood stirred with the old, the familiar answers: yes, yes, you know it, yes, yes.

And turning together, they stumbled over a clanking dark mound of leather bag.

CHAPTER SEVENTEEN

They stood for a long moment over the huge leather bag.

Almost secretively, Will kicked it. It made a sound of iron indigestion.

"Why," said Will, "that belongs to the lightning-rod salesman!"

Jim slipped his hand through the leather mouth and hefted forth a metal shaft clustered with chimeras, Chinese dragons all fang, eyeball and moss-green armor, all cross and crescent; every symbol around the world that made men safe, or seemed to, clung here, greaving the boys' hands with odd weight and meaning.

"Storm never came. But he *went*."

"Where? And why did he leave his bag?"

They both looked to the carnival where dusk colored the canvas billows. Shadows ran coolly out to engulf them. People in cars honked home in tired commotions. Boys on skeleton bikes whistled dogs after. Soon night would own the midway, while shadows rode the ferris wheel up to cloud the stars.

"People," said Jim, "don't leave their whole life lying around. This is everything that old man owned. Something important—" Jim breathed soft fire—"made him forget. So he just walked off and left this here."

"What? What's so important you forget *everything?*"

"Why—" Jim examined his friend, curiously, twilight

in his face—"no one can tell you. You find out yourself. Mysteries and mysteries. Storm salesman. Storm salesman's bag. If we don't look now, we might never know."

"Jim, in ten minutes—"

"Sure! Midway'll be dark. Everyone home for dinner. Just us alone. But won't it feel great? Just *us!* And here we go, back in!"

Passing the Mirror Maze, they saw two armies—a billion Jims, a billion Wills—collide, melt, vanish. And like those armies, so vanished the real army of people.

The boys stood alone among the encampments of dusk thinking of all the boys in town sitting down to warm food in bright rooms.

CHAPTER EIGHTEEN

The red-lettered sign said: OUT OF ORDER! KEEP OFF!

"Sign's been up all day. I don't believe signs," said Jim.

They peered in at the merry-go-round which lay under a dry rattle and roar of wind-tumbled oak trees. Its horses, goats, antelopes, zebras, speared through their spines with brass javelins, hung contorted as in a death rictus, asking mercy with their fright-colored eyes, seeking revenge with their panic-colored teeth.

"Don't look broke to me."

Jim ambled across the clanking chain, leaped to a turntable surface vast as the moon, among the frantic but forever spelled beasts.

"Jim!"

"Will, this is the only ride we haven't *looked* at. So . . ."

Jim swayed. The lunatic carousel world stirred atilt with his lean bulk. He strolled through brass forests amidst animal rousts. He swung astride a plum-dusk stallion.

"Ho, boy, *git!*"

A man rose from machinery darkness.

"Jim!"

Reaching out from the shadows among the calliope tubes and moon-skinned drums the man hoisted Jim yelling out on the air.

"Help, Will, help!"

Will leaped through the animals.

The man smiled easily, welcomed him handily, swung him high beside Jim. They stared down at bright flame-red hair, bright flame-blue eyes, and rippling biceps.

"Out of order," said the man. "Can't you read?"

"Put them down," said a gentle voice.

Hung high, Jim and Will glanced over at a second man standing tall beyond the chains.

"Down," he said again.

And they were carried through the brass forest of wild but uncomplaining brutes and set in the dust.

"We were—" said Will.

"Curious?" This second man was tall as a lamp post. His pale face, lunar pockmarks denting it, cast light on those who stood below. His vest was the color of fresh blood. His eyebrows, his hair, his suit were licorice black, and the sun-yellow gem which stared from the tie pin thrust in his cravat was the same unblinking shade and bright crystal as his eyes. But in this instant, swiftly, and with utter clearness, it was the suit which fascinated Will. For it seemed woven of boar-bramble, clock-spring hair, bristle, and a sort of ever-trembling, ever-glistening dark hemp. The suit caught light and stirred like a bed of black tweed-thorns, interminably itching, covering the man's long body with motion so it seemed he should excruciate, cry out, and tear the clothes free. Yet here he stood, moon-calm, inhabiting his itch-weed suit and watching Jim's mouth with his yellow eyes. He never looked once at Will.

"The name is Dark."

He flourished a white calling card. It turned blue.

Whisper. Red.

Whisk. A green man dangled from a tree stamped on the card.

Flit. Shh.

"Dark. And my friend with the red hair there is Mr. Cooger. Of Cooger and Dark's . . ."

Flip-flick-shhh.

Names appeared, disappeared on the white square:

". . . Combined Shadow Shows . . ."

Tick-wash.

A mushroom-witch stirred moldering herb pots.

". . . and cross-continental Pandemonium Theater Company . . ."

He handed the card to Jim. It now read:

> *Our specialty: to examine, oil,*
> *polish, and repair Death-Watch*
> *Beetles.*

Calmly, Jim read it. Calmly, Jim put a fist into his copious and richly treasured pockets, rummaged, and held out his hand.

On his palm lay a dead brown insect.

"Here," Jim said. "Fix *this.*"

Mr. Dark exploded his laugh. "Superb! I will!" He extended his hand. His shirt sleeve pulled up.

Bright purple, black, green and lightning-blue eels, worms, and Latin scrolls slid to view on his wrist.

"Boy!" cried Will. "You must be the Tattooed Man!"

"No." Jim studied the stranger. "The Illustrated Man. There's a difference."

Mr. Dark nodded, pleased. "What's your name, boy?"

Don't tell him! thought Will, and stopped. Why not? he wondered, why?

Jim's lips hardly twitched.

"Simon," he said.

He smiled to show it was a lie.

Mr. Dark smiled to show he knew it.

"Want to see more, 'Simon'?"

Jim would not give him the satisfaction of a nod.

Slowly, with great mouth-working pleasure, Mr. Dark pushed his sleeve high to his elbow.

Jim stared. The arm was like a cobra weaving, bobbing, swaying to strike. Mr. Dark clenched his fist, wriggled his fingers. The muscles danced.

Will wanted to run around and see, but could only watch, thinking Jim, oh, Jim!

For there stood Jim and there was this tall man, each examining the other as if he were a reflection in a shop window late at night. The tall man's brambled suit, shadowed out now to color Jim's cheeks and storm over his wide and drinking eyes with a look of rain instead of the sharp cat-green they always were. Jim stood like a runner who has come a long way, fever in his mouth, hands open to receive any gift. And right now it was a gift of pictures twitched in pantomime, as Mr. Dark made his illustrations jerk cold-skinned over his warm-pulsed wrist as the stars came out above and Jim stared and Will could not see and a long way off the last of the town people went away toward town in their warm cars, and Jim said, faintly, "Gosh . . ." and Mr. Dark rolled down his sleeve.

"Show's over. Suppertime. Carnival's shut up until seven. Everyone out. Come back, 'Simon,' and ride the merry-go-round, when it's fixed. Take this card. Free ride."

Jim stared at the hidden wrist and put the card in his pocket.

"So long!"

Jim ran. Will ran.

Jim whirled, glanced back, leaped, and for the second time in the hour, vanished.

Will looked up into the tree where Jim squirmed on a limb, hidden. He looked back. Mr. Dark and Mr. Cooger were turned away, busy with the merry-go-round.

"Quick, Will!"

"Jim . . . ?"

"They'll *see* you. Jump!"

Will jumped. Jim hauled him up. The great tree shook. A wind roared by in the sky. Jim helped him cling, gasping, among the branches.

"Jim, we don't belong here!"

"Shut up! Look!" whispered Jim.

Somewhere in the carousel machinery there were taps and brass knockings, a faint squeal and whistle of calliope steam.

"What was on his arm, Jim?"

"A picture."

"Yeah, but what kind?"

"It was—" Jim shut his eyes. "It was—a picture of a
. . . snake . . . that's it . . . snake." But when he
opened his eyes, he would not look at Will.

"Okay, if you don't want to tell me."

"I told you, Will, a snake. I'll get him to show it to you,
later, you want that?"

No, thought Will, I don't want that.

He looked down at the billion footprints left in the
sawdust on the empty midway and suddenly it was a lot
closer to midnight than to noon.

"I'm going home. . . ."

"Sure, Will, go on. Mirror mazes, old teacher-ladies,
lost lightning-rod bags, lightning-rod salesmen disappear,
snake pictures dancing, unbroken merry-go-rounds, and
you want to go home!? Sure, old friend Will, so long."

"I . . ." Will started down the tree, and froze.

"All clear?" cried a voice below.

"Clear!" someone shouted at the far end of the midway.

Mr. Dark moved, not fifty feet away, to a red control box near the merry-go-round ticket booth. He glared
in all directions. He glared into the tree.

Will hugged, Jim hugged the limb, tightened into smallness.

"Start up!"

With a pop, a bang, a jangle of reins, a lift and down-
fall, a rise and descent of brass, the carousel moved.

But, thought Will, it's broke, out of order!

He flicked a glance at Jim, who pointed wildly down.
The merry-go-round was running, yes, but . . .

It was running *backward*.

The small calliope inside the carousel machinery rattle-
snapped its nervous-stallion shivering drums, clashed its
harvest-moon cymbals, toothed its castanets, and throat-
ily choked and sobbed its reeds, whistles, and baroque
flutes.

The music, Will thought, it's backwards, *too!*

Mr. Dark jerked about, glanced up, as if he had heard

Will's thought. A wind shook the trees in black tumults. Mr. Dark shrugged and looked away.

The carousel wheeled faster, shrieking, plunging, going roundabout-back!

Now Mr. Cooger, with his flaming red hair and fire-blue eyes, was pacing the midway, making a last check. He stood under their tree. Will could have let spit down on him. Then the calliope gave a particularly violent cry of foul murder which made dogs howl in far countries, and Mr. Cooger, spinning, ran and leaped on the back-whirling universe of animals who, tail first, head last, pursued an endless circling night toward unfound and never to be discovered destinations. Hand-slapping brass poles, he flung himself into a seat where with his bristly red hair, pink face, and incredible sharp blue eyes he sat silent, going back around, back around, the music squealing swift back with him like insucked breath.

The music, thought Will, what is it? And how do I know it's backside first? He hugged the limb, tried to catch the tune, then hum it forward in his head. But the brass bells, the drums, hammered his chest, revved his heart so he felt his pulse reverse, his blood turn back in perverse thrusts through all his flesh, so he was nearly shaken free to fall, so all he did was clutch, hang pale, and drink the sight of the backward-turning machine and Mr. Dark, alert at the controls, on the sidelines.

It was Jim who first noticed the new thing happening, for he kicked Will, once, Will looked over, and Jim nodded frantically at the man in the machine as he came around the next time.

Mr. Cooger's face was melting like pink wax.

His hands were becoming doll's hands.

His bones sank away beneath his clothes; his clothes then shrank down to fit his dwindling frame.

His face flickered going, and each time around he melted more.

Will saw Jim's head shift, circling.

The carousel wheeled, a great back-drifting lunar dream, the horses thrusting, the music in-gasped after, while Mr. Cooger, as simple as shadows, as simple as light, as simple as time, got younger. And younger. And younger.

Each time he wheeled to view he sat alone with his bones, which shaped like warm candles burning away to tender years. He gazed serenely at the fiery constellations, the children-inhabited trees, which went away from him as he removed himself from them and his nose diminished and his sweet wax ears reshaped themselves to small pink roses.

Now no longer forty where he had begun his back-spiraled journey, Mr. Cooger was nineteen.

Around went the reverse parade of horse, pole, music, man become young man, young man fast rendered down to boy. . . .

Mr. Cooger was seventeen, sixteen. . . .

Another and another time around under the sky and trees and Will whispering, Jim counting the times around, around, while the night air warmed to summer heat by friction of sun-metal brass, the passionate backturned flight of beasts, wore the wax doll down and down and washed him clean with still stranger musics until all ceased, all died away to stillness, the calliope shut up its brassworks, the ironmongery machines hissed off, and with a last faint whine like desert sands blown back up Arabian hourglasses, the carousel rocked on seaweed waters and stood still.

The figure seated in the carved white wooden sleigh chair was very small.

Mr. Cooger was twelve years old.

No. Will's mouth shaped the word. No. Jim's did the same.

The small shape stepped down from the silent world, its face in shadow, but its hands, newborn wrinkled pink, held out in raw carnival lamplight.

The strange man-boy shot his gaze up, down, smelling fright somewhere, terror and awe in the vicinity. Will balled himself tight and shut his eyes. He felt the terrible gaze shoot through the leaves like blown needle-darts, pass on. Then, rabbit-running, the small shape lit off down the empty midway.

Jim was first to stir the leaves aside.

Mr. Dark was gone, too, in the evening hush.

It seemed to take Jim forever to fall down to earth. Will fell after and they both stood, clamorous with alarms, shaken by concussions of silent pantomime, blasted by events all the more numbing because they ran off into night and unknown. And it was Jim who spoke from their mutual confusion and trembling as each held to the other's arm, seeing the small shadow rush, luring them across the meadow.

"Oh, Will, I wish we could go home, I wish we could eat. But it's too late, we saw! We got to see more! *Don't* we?"

"Lord," said Will, miserably. "I guess we do."

And they ran together, following they didn't know what on out and away to who could possibly guess where.

CHAPTER NINETEEN

Out on the highway the last faint water colors of the sun were gone beyond the hills and whatever they were chasing was so far ahead as to be only a swift fleck now shown in lamplight now set free, running, into dark.

"Twenty-eight!" gasped Jim. "Twenty-eight times!"

"The merry-go-round, sure!" Will jerked his head. "Twenty-eight times I counted, it went around back!"

Up ahead, the small shape stopped and looked back.

Jim and Will ducked in by a tree and let it move on.

"It," thought Will. Why do I think "it"? He's a boy, he's a man . . . no . . . *it* is something that has changed, that's what *it* is.

They reached and passed the city limits, and swiftly jogging, Will said, "Jim, there must've been *two* people on that ride, Mr. Cooger *and* this boy and—"

"No. I never took my eyes off him!"

They ran by the barber shop. Will saw but did not see a sign in the window. He read but did not read. He remembered, he forgot. He plunged on.

"Hey! He's turned on Culpepper Street! Quick!"

They rounded a corner.

"He's gone!"

The street lay long and empty in the lamplight.

Leaves blew on the hopscotch-chalked sidewalks.

"Will, Miss Foley lives on this street."

"Sure, fourth house, but—"

Jim strolled, casually whistling, hands in pockets, Will with him. At Miss Foley's house, they glanced up.

In one of the softly lit front windows, someone stood looking out.

A boy, no more and no less than twelve years old.

"Will!" cried Jim, softly. "That boy—"

"Her nephew . . . ?"

"Nephew, heck! Keep your head away. Maybe he can read lips. Walk slow. To the corner and back. You see his face? The eyes, Will! That's one part of people don't change, young, old, six or sixty! Boy's face, sure, but the eyes were the eyes of Mr. Cooger!"

"No!"

"Yes!"

They both stopped to enjoy the swift pound of each other's heart.

"Keep moving." They moved. Jim held Will's arm tight, leading him. "You did see Mr. Cooger's eyes, huh? When he held us up fit to crack our heads together? You did see the boy, just off the ride? He looked right up near me, hid in the tree, and boy! it was like opening the door of a furnace! I'll never forget those eyes! And there they are now, in the window. Turn around. Now, let's walk back easy and nice and slow. . . . We got to warn Miss Foley what's hiding in her house, don't we?"

"Jim, look, you don't give a darn about Miss Foley or what's in her house!"

Jim said nothing. Walking arm in arm with Will he just looked over at his friend and blinked once, let the lids come down over his shiny green eyes and go up.

And again Will had the feeling about Jim that he had always had about an old almost forgotten dog. Some time every year that dog, good for many months, just ran on out into the world and didn't come back for days and finally did limp back all burred and scrawny and odorous of swamps and dumps; he had rolled in the dirty mangers and foul dropping places of the world, simply to turn home with a funny little smile pinned to his muzzle. Dad had named the dog Plato, the wilderness philosopher, for you saw by his eyes there was nothing he didn't know. Returned, the dog would live in innocence again, tread patterns of grace, for months, then vanish, and the whole thing start over. Now, walking here he thought he heard Jim whimper under his breath. He could feel the bristles stiffen all over Jim. He felt Jim's ears flatten, saw him sniff the new dark. Jim smelled smells that no one knew, heard ticks from clocks that told another time. Even his tongue was strange now, moving along his lower, and now his upper lip as they stopped in front of Miss Foley's house again.

The front window was empty.

"Going to walk up and ring the bell," said Jim.

"What, meet him face to face?!"

"My aunt's eyebrows, Will. We got to check, don't we? Shake his paw, stare him in his good eye or some such, and if it *is* him—"

"We don't warn Miss Foley right in front of him, *do* we?"

"We'll phone her, later, dumb. Up we go!"

Will sighed and let himself be walked up the steps wanting but not wanting to know if the boy in this house had Mr. Cooger hid but showing like a firefly between his eyelashes.

Jim rang the bell.

"What if *he* answers?" Will demanded. "Boy, I'm so scared I could sprinkle dust. Jim, why aren't you scared, why?"

Jim examined both of his untrembled hands. "I'll be darned," he gasped. "You're right! I'm *not!*"

The door swung wide.

Miss Foley beamed out at them.

"Jim! Will! How nice."

"Miss Foley," blurted Will. "You *okay?*"

Jim glared at him. Miss Foley laughed.

"Why shouldn't I be?"

Will flushed. "All those darn carnival mirrors—"

"Nonsense, I've forgotten all about it. Well, boys, are you coming in?"

She held the door wide.

Will shuffled a foot and stopped.

Beyond Miss Foley, a beaded curtain hung like a dark blue thunder shower across the parlor entry.

Where the colored rain touched the floor, a pair of dusty small shoes poked out. Just beyond the downpour the evil boy loitered.

Evil? Will blinked. Why evil? Because. "Because" was reason enough. A boy, yes, and evil.

"Robert?" Miss Foley turned, calling through the dark blue always-falling beads of rain. She took Will's hand and gently pulled him inside. "Come meet two of my students."

The rain poured aside. A fresh candy-pink hand broke through, all by itself, as if testing the weather in the hall.

Good grief, thought Will, he'll look me in the eye! see the merry-go-round and himself on it moving back, back. I *know* it's printed on my eyeball like I been struck by lightning!

"Miss Foley!" said Will.

Now a pink face stuck out through the dim frozen necklaces of storm.

"We got to tell you a terrible thing."

Jim struck Will's elbow, hard, to shut him.

Now the body came out through the dark watery flow of beads. The rain shushed behind the small boy.

Miss Foley leaned toward him, expectant. Jim gripped his elbow, fiercely. He stammered, flushed, then spat it out:

"Mr. Crosetti!"

Quite suddenly, clearly, he saw the sign in the barber's window. The sign seen but not seen as they ran by:

CLOSED ON ACCOUNT OF ILLNESS.

"Mr. Crosetti!" he repeated, and added, swiftly, "He's . . . dead!"

"What . . . the barber?"

"The barber?" echoed Jim.

"See this haircut?" Will turned, trembling, his hand to his head. "He did it. And we just walked by there and the sign was up and people told us—"

"What a shame." Miss Foley was reaching out to fetch the strange boy forward. "I'm so sorry. Boys, this is Robert, my nephew from Wisconsin."

Jim stuck out his hand. Robert the Nephew examined it, curiously. "What are you *looking* at?" he asked.

"You look familiar," said Jim.

Jim! Will yelled to himself.

"Like an uncle of mine," said Jim, all sweet and calm.

The nephew flicked his eyes to Will, who looked only at the floor, afraid the boy would see his eyeballs whirl with the remembered carousel. Crazily, he wanted to hum the backward music.

Now, he thought, face him!

He looked up straight at the boy.

And it was wild and crazy and the floor sank away beneath for there was the pink shiny Halloween mask of a small pretty boy's face, but almost as if holes were cut where the eyes of Mr. Cooger shone out, old, old, eyes as bright as sharp blue stars and the light from those stars taking a million years to get here. And through the little nostrils cut in the shiny wax mask, Mr. Cooger's breath went in steam came out ice. And the Valentine candy tongue moved small behind those trim white candy-kernel teeth.

Mr. Cooger, somewhere behind the eye slits, went *blink-click* with his insect-Kodak pupils. The lenses exploded like suns, then burnt chilly and serene again.

He swiveled his glance to Jim. *Blink-click*. He had Jim flexed, focussed, shot, developed, dried, filed away in dark. *Blink-click*.

Yet this was only a boy standing in a hall with two other boys and a woman. . . .

And all the while Jim gazed steadily back, feathers unruffled, taking his own pictures of Robert.

"Have you boys had supper?" asked Miss Foley. "We're just sitting down—"

"We got to go!"

Everyone looked at Will as if amazed he didn't want to stick here forever.

"Jim—" he stammered. "Your mom's home alone—"

"Oh, sure," Jim said, reluctantly.

"I know what." The nephew paused for their attention. When their faces turned, Mr. Cooger inside the nephew went silently *blink-click, blink-click,* listening through the toy ears, watching through the toy-charm eyes, whetting the doll's mouth with a Pekingese tongue. "Join us later for dessert, huh?"

"Dessert?"

"I'm taking Aunt Willa to the carnival." The boy stroked Miss Foley's arm until she laughed nervously.

"Carnival?" cried Will, and lowered his voice. "Miss Foley, you said—"

"I said I was foolish and scared myself," said Miss Foley. "It's Saturday night, the best night for tent shows and showing my nephew the sights."

"Join us?" asked Robert, holding Miss Foley's hand. "Later?"

"Great!" said Jim.

"Jim," said Will. "We been out all day. Your mom's sick."

"I forgot." Jim flashed him a look filled with purest snake poison.

Flick. The nephew made an X-ray of both, showing them, no doubt, as cold bones trembling in warm flesh. He stuck out his hand.

"Tomorrow, then. Meet you by the side shows."

"Swell!" Jim grabbed the small hand.

"So long!" Will jumped out the door, then turned with a last agonized appeal to the teacher.

"Miss Foley . . . ?"

"Yes, Will?"

Don't go with that boy, he thought. Don't go near the shows. Stay home, oh, please! But then he said:

"Mr. Crosetti's dead."

She nodded, touched, waiting for his tears. And while she waited, he dragged Jim outside and the door swung shut on Miss Foley and the pink small face with the lenses in it going *blink-click,* snapshotting two incoherent boys, and them fumbling down the steps in October dark, while the merry-go-round started again in Will's head, rushing while the leaves in the trees above cracked and fried with wind. Aside, Will spluttered, "Jim, you shook hands with him! Mr. Cooger! You're not going to *meet* him!?"

"It's Mr. Cooger, all right. Boy, those eyes. If I met him tonight, we'd solve the whole shooting match. What's eating you, Will?"

"Eating *me!*" At the bottom of the steps now, they tussled in fierce and frantic whispers, glancing up at the empty windows where, now and again, a shadow passed. Will stopped. The music turned in his head. Stunned, he squinched his eyes. "Jim, the music that the calliope played when Mr. Cooger got younger—"

"Yeah?"

"It was the 'Funeral March'! Played *backwards!*"

"*Which* 'Funeral March'?"

"Which! Jim, Chopin only wrote one tune! *The* 'Funeral March'!"

"But why played backward?"

"Mr. Cooger was marching *away* from the grave, not toward it, wasn't he, getting younger, smaller, instead of older and dropping dead?"

"Willy, you're terrific!"

"Sure, but—" Will stiffened. "He's there. The window, again. Wave at him. So long! Now, walk and whistle something. *Not* Chopin, for gosh sakes—"

Jim waved. Will waved. Both whistled, "Oh, Susanna." The shadow gestured small in the high window.

The boys hurried off down the street.

CHAPTER TWENTY

Two suppers were waiting in two houses.

One parent yelled at Jim, two parents yelled at Will.

Both were sent hungry upstairs.

It started at seven o'clock. It was done by seven-three.

Doors slammed. Locks clacked.

Clocks ticked.

Will stood by the door. The telephone was locked away outside. And even if he called, Miss Foley wouldn't answer. By now she'd be gone beyond town . . . good grief! Anyway, what could he say? Miss Foley, that nephew's no nephew? That boy's no boy? Wouldn't she laugh? She would. For the nephew was a nephew, the boy was a boy, or seemed such.

He turned to the window. Jim, across the way, stood facing the same dilemma, in his room. Both struggled. It was too early to raise the windows and stage-whisper to each other. Parents below were busy growing crystal-radio peach fuzz in their ears, alert.

The boys threw themselves on their separate beds in their separate houses, probed mattresses for chocolate chunks put away against the lean years, and ate moodily.

Clocks ticked.

Nine. Nine-thirty. Ten.

The knob rattled, softly, as Dad unlocked the door.

Dad! thought Will. Come in! We got to talk!

But Dad chewed his breath in the hall. Only his confusion, his always puzzled, half-bewildered face could be felt beyond the door.

He won't come in, thought Will. Walk around, talk around, back off from a thing, yes. But come sit, listen? When had he, when *would* he, ever?

"Will . . . ?"

Will quickened.

"Will . . ." said Dad, ". . . be careful."

"Careful?" cried mother, coming along the hall. "Is *that* all you're going to say?"

"What else?" Dad was going downstairs now. "He jumps, I creep. How can you get two people together like that? He's too young, I'm too old. God, sometimes I wish we'd never . . ."

The door shut. Dad was walking away on the sidewalk.

Will wanted to fling up the window and call. Suddenly, Dad was so lost in the night. Not me, don't worry about me, Dad, he thought, you, Dad, stay in! It's not safe! Don't go!

But he didn't shout. And when he softly raised the window at last, the street was empty, and he knew it would be just a matter of time before that light went on in the library across town. When rivers flooded, when fire fell from the sky, what a fine place the library was, the many rooms, the books. With luck, no one found you. How could they!—when you were off to Tanganyika in '98, Cairo in 1812, Florence in 1492!?

"... careful ..."

What did Dad mean? Did he smell the panic, had he heard the music, had he prowled near the tents? No. Not Dad ever.

Will tossed a marble over at Jim's window.

Tap. Silence.

He imagined Jim seated alone in the dark, his breath like phosphorus on the air, ticking away to himself.

Tap. Silence.

This wasn't like Jim. Always before, the window slid up, Jim's head popped out, ripe with yells, secret hissings, giggles, riots and rebel charges.

"Jim, I know you're there!"

Tap.

Silence.

Dad's out in the town. Miss Foley's with you-know-who! he thought. Good gosh, Jim, we got to do something! Tonight!

He threw a last small marble.

... tap ...

It fell to the hushed grass below.

Jim did not come to the window.

Tonight, thought Will. He bit his knuckles. He lay back cold straight stiff on his bed.

CHAPTER TWENTY-ONE

In the alley behind the house was a huge old-fashioned pine-plank boardwalk. It had been there ever since Will remembered, since civilization unthinkingly poured forth the dull hard unresisting cement sidewalks. His grandfather, a man of strong sentiment and wild impulse, who let nothing go without a roar, had flexed his muscles in favor of this vanishing landmark, and with a dozen handymen had toted a good forty feet of the walk into the alley where it had lain like the skeleton of some indefinable monster through the years, baked by sun, lushly rotted by rains.

The town clock struck ten.

Lying abed, Will realized he had been thinking about Grandfather's vast gift from another time. He was waiting to hear the boardwalk speak. In what language? Well . . .

Boys have never been known to go straight up to houses to ring bells to summon forth friends. They prefer to chunk dirt at clapboards, hurl acorns down roof shingles, or leave mysterious notes flapping from kites stranded on attic window sills.

So it was with Jim and Will.

Late nights, if there were gravestones to be leapfrogged or dead cats to be hurled down sour people's chimneys, one or the other of the boys would prowl out under the moon and xylophone-dance on that old hollow-echoing musical boardwalk.

Over the years, they had *tuned* the walk, prying up an *A* board and nailing it here, lifting up an *F* board and pounding it back down there until the walk was as near onto being melodious as weather and two entrepreneurs could fashion it.

By the tune treaded out, you could tell the night's venture. If Will heard Jim tromping hard on seven or eight notes of "Way Down Upon the Swanee River," he scrambled out knowing it was moon-trail time on the creek leading to the river caves. If Jim heard Will out leaping about like a scalded airedale on the timbers and the tune remotely suggested "Marching Through Georgia," it meant plums, peaches, or apples were ripe enough to get sick on out beyond town.

So this night Will held his breath waiting for some tune to call him forth.

What kind of tune would Jim play to represent the carnival, Miss Foley, Mr. Cooger, and/or the evil nephew?

Ten-fifteen. Ten-thirty.

No music.

Will did not like Jim sitting in his room thinking *what?* Of the Mirror Maze? What *had* he seen there? And, seeing, what did he plan?

Will stirred, restively.

Especially he did not like to think of Jim with no father between him and the tent shows and all that lay dark in the meadows. And a mother who wanted him around so very much, he just *had* to get away, get out, breathe free night air, know free night waters running toward bigger freer seas.

Jim! he thought. Let's have the music!

And at ten-thirty-five, it came.

He heard, or thought he heard, Jim out in the starlight leaping way up and coming flat down like a spring tomcat on the vast xylophone. And the tune! Was or wasn't it like the funeral dirge played backwards by the old carousel calliope?!!

Will started to raise his window to be sure. But suddenly, Jim's window slid quietly up.

He hadn't been down on the boards! It was just Will's wild wish that made the tune! Will started to whisper, but stopped.

For Jim, without a word, scuttled down the drainpipe.

Jim! Will thought.

Jim, on the lawn, stiffened as if hearing his name.

You're not going without me, Jim?

Jim glanced swiftly up.

If he saw Will, he made no sign.

Jim, Will thought, we're still pals, smell things nobody

else smells, hear things no one else hears, got the same blood, run the same way. Now, this first time ever, you're sneaking out! Ditching me!

But the driveway was empty.

A salamander flicking the hedge, there went Jim.

Will was out the window, down the trellis, and over the hedge, before he thought: *I'm* alone. If I lose Jim, it's the first ever I'll be out alone at night, too. And where am I going? Wherever Jim goes.

Lord, let me keep up!

Jim skimmed like a dark owl after a mouse. Will loped like a weaponless hunter after the owl. They sailed their shadows over October lawns.

And when they stopped . . .

There was Miss Foley's house.

CHAPTER TWENTY-TWO

Jim glanced back.

Will became a bush behind a bush, a shadow among shadows, with two starlight rounds of glass, his eyes, holding the image of Jim calling up in a whisper toward the second-floor windows.

"Hey there . . . hey . . ."

Good grief, thought Will, he wants to be slit and stuffed with broken Mirror Maze glass.

"Hey!" called Jim, softly. "You . . . !"

A shadow uprose on a dim-lit shade, above. A small shadow. The nephew had brought Miss Foley home, they were in their separate rooms or— Oh Lord, thought Will, I *hope* she's safe home. Maybe, like the lightning-rod salesman, she—

"Hey . . . !"

Jim gazed up with that funny warm look of breathless anticipation he often had nights in summer at the shadow-show window Theater in that house a few streets over. Looking up with love, with devotion, like a cat Jim waited for some special dark mouse to run forth.

Crouched, now slowly he seemed to grow taller, as if his bones were pulled by the thing in the window above, which now suddenly vanished.

Will ground his teeth.

He felt the shadow sift down through the house like a cold breath. He could wait no longer. He leaped forth.

"Jim!"

He seized Jim's arm.

"Will, what *you* doing here?!"

"Jim, don't talk to *him!* Get out of here. My gosh, he'll chew and spit out your bones!"

Jim writhed himself free.

"Will, go home! You'll spoil everything!"

"He scares me, Jim, what you *want* from him!? This afternoon . . . in the maze, did you *see* something!!?"

". . . Yes . . ."

"For gosh sakes, *what!*"

Will grabbed Jim's shirt front, felt his heart bang under the chest bones. "Jim—"

"Let go." Jim was terribly quiet. "If he knows you're here, he won't come out. Willy, if you don't let go, I'll remember when—"

"When *what!*"

"When I'm older, darn it, *older!*"

Jim spat.

As if he was struck by lightning, Will jumped back.

He looked at his empty hands and put one up to wipe the spittle off his cheek.

"Oh, Jim," he mourned.

And he heard the merry-go-round motioning, gliding on black night waters around, around, and Jim on a black stallion riding off and about, circling in tree-shadow and he wanted to cry out, Look! the merry-go-round! you want it to go forward, don't you, Jim? forward instead of back! and you on it, around once and you're fifteen, circling and you're sixteen, three times more and nine-teen! music! and you're twenty and off, standing tall! not Jim any more, still thirteen, almost fourteen on the empty midway, with me small, me young, me scared!

Will hauled off and hit Jim, hard, on the nose.

Then he jumped Jim, wrapped him tight, and toppled

him rolling down, yelling, in the bushes. He slapped Jim's mouth, stuffed it, mashed it full of fingers to snap and bite at, suffocating the angry grunts and yells.

The front door opened.

Will crushed the air out of Jim, lay heavy on him, fisting his mouth tight.

Something stood on the porch. A tiny shadow scanned the town, searching for but not finding Jim.

But it was just the boy Robert, the friendly nephew, come almost casually forth, hands in pockets, whistling under his breath, to breathe the night air as boys do, curious for adventures that they themselves must make, that rarely happen by. Threshed tight, mortally locked and bound to Jim, staring up, Will was all the more shaken to see the normal boy, the airy glance, the unassuming poise, the small, the easy self in which no man at all was revealed by street light.

At any moment, Robert, in full cry, might leap to play with them, tangle legs, lock arms, bark-snap like pups in May, the whole thing end with them strewn in laughing tears on the lawn, the terror spent, the fear melted off in dew, a dream of nothings quickly gone as such dreams go when the eye snaps wide. For there indeed stood the nephew, his face round fresh, and cream-smooth as a peach.

And he was smiling down at the two boys he now saw locked limb in limb on the grass.

Then, swiftly, he darted in. He must have run upstairs, scrabbled about, and hurtled down again, for suddenly as the two boys outthrashed, outgripped, outraged each other, there was a rain of tinkling, rattling glitter on the lawn.

The nephew leaped the porch rail and landed panther-soft, imbedded in his shadow, on the grass. His hands were delicious with stars. These he liberally sprinkled. They thudded, slithered, winked at Jim's side. Both boys lay stricken by the rain of gold and diamond fire that pelted them.

"Help, police!" cried Robert.

Will was so shocked he let go Jim.

Jim was so shocked he let go Will.

Both reached at the same time for the cold strewn ice.

"Good grief, a bracelet!"

"A ring! A necklace!"

Robert kicked. Two trash cans at the curb fell thundering.

A bedroom light, above, flicked on.

"Police!" Robert threw one last spray of glitter at their feet, shut up his fresh-peach smile like locking an explosion away in a box, and shot away down the street.

"Wait!" Jim jumped. "We won't hurt you!"

Will tripped him, Jim fell.

The window upstairs opened. Miss Foley leaned out. Jim, on his knees, held a woman's wrist watch. Will blinked at a necklace in his hands.

"Who's there!" she cried. "Jim? Will? What's *that* you got?!"

But Jim was running. Will stopped only long enough to see the window empty itself with a wail as Miss Foley pulled in to see her room. When he heard her full scream, he knew she had discovered the burglary.

Running, Will knew he was doing just what the nephew wanted. He should turn back, pick up the jewels, tell Miss Foley what happened. But he must save Jim!

Far back, he heard Miss Foley's new cries turn on more lights! Will Halloway! Jim Nightshade! Night runners! Thieves! That's us, thought Will, oh my Lord! That's us! No one'll believe *anything* we say from now on! Not about carnivals, not about carousels, not about mirrors or evil nephews, not about nothing!

And so they ran, three animals in starlight. A black otter. A tomcat. A rabbit.

Me, thought Will, I'm the rabbit.

And he was white, and much afraid.

CHAPTER TWENTY-THREE

They hit the carnival grounds at a good twenty miles an hour, give or take a mile, the nephew in the lead, Jim close behind, and Will further back, gasping, shotgun blasts of fatigue in his feet, his head, his heart.

The nephew, running scared, looked back, not smiling.

Fooled him, thought Will, he figured I wouldn't follow, figured I'll call the police, get stuck, not be believed, or run hide. Now he's scared I'll beat the tar out of him, and wants to jump on that ride and run around getting older and bigger than me. Oh, Jim, Jim, we got to stop him, keep him young, tear his skin off!

But he knew from Jim's running there'd be no help from Jim. Jim wasn't running after nephews. He was running toward free rides.

The nephew vanished around a tent far ahead. Jim followed. By the time Will reached the midway, the merry-go-round was popping to life. In the pulse, the din, the squeal-around of music the small fresh-faced nephew rode the great platform in a swirl of midnight dust.

Jim, ten feet back, watched the horses leap, his eyes striking fire from the high-jumped stallion's eyes.

The merry-go-round was going *forward!*

Jim *leaned* at it.

"Jim!" cried Will.

The nephew swept from sight borne around by the machine. Drifted back again he stretched out pink fingers urging softly: ". . . Jim . . . ?"

Jim twitched one foot forward.

"No!" Will plunged.

He knocked, seized, held Jim; they toppled; they fell in a heap.

The nephew, surprised, whisked on in darkness, one year older. One year older, thought Will, on the earth, one year taller, bigger, meaner!

"Oh God, Jim, quick!" He jumped up, ran to the control box, the complex mysteries of brass switch and porcelain covering and sizzling wires. He struck the switch. But Jim, behind, babbling, tore at Will's hands.

"Will, you'll spoil it! No!"

Jim knocked the switch full back.

Will spun and slapped his face. Each clenched the

other's elbows, rocked, flailed. They fell against the control box.

Will saw the evil boy, a year older still, glide around into night. Five or six more times around and he'd be bigger than the two of them!

"Jim, he'll kill us!"

"Not me, no!"

Will felt a sting of electricity. He yelled, pulled back, hit the switch handle. The control box spat. Lightning jumped to the sky. Jim and Will, flung by the blast, lay watching the merry-go-round run wild.

The evil boy whistled by, clenched to a brass tree. He cursed. He spat. He wrestled with wind, with centrifuge. He was trying to clutch his way through the horses, the poles, to the outer rim of the carousel. His face came, went, came, went. He clawed. He brayed. The control box erupted blue showers. The carousel jumped and bucked. The nephew slipped. He fell. A black stallion's steel hoof kicked him. Blood printed his brow.

Jim hissed, rolled, thrashed, Will riding him hard, pressing him to grass, trading yell for yell, both fright-pale, heart ramming heart. Electric bolts from the switch flushed up in white stars a gush of fireworks. The carousel spun thirty, spun forty—"Will, let me up!"—spun fifty times. The calliope howled, boiled steam, ran ancient dry, then played nothing, its keys gibbering as only chitterings boiled up through the vents. Lightning unraveled itself over the sweated outflung boys, delivered flame to the silent horse stampede to light their way around, around with the figure lying on the platform no longer a boy but a man no longer a man but more than a man and even more and even more, much more than that, around, around.

"He's, he's, oh he's, oh look, Will, he's—" gasped Jim, and began to sob, because it was the only thing to do, locked down, nailed tight. "Oh God, Will, get up! We *got* to make it run backward!"

Lights flashed on in the tents.

But no one came out.

Why not? Will thought crazily. The explosions? The

electric storm? Do the freaks think the whole world's jumping through the midway? Where's Mr. Dark? In town? Up to no good? What, where, why?

He thought he heard the agonized figure sprawled on the carousel platform drum his heart superfast, then slow, fast, slow, very fast, very slow, incredibly fast, then as slow as the moon going down the sky on a white night in winter.

Someone, something, on the carousel wailed faintly.

Thank God it's dark, thought Will. Thank God, I can't see. There goes someone. Here comes something. There, whatever it is, goes again. There . . . there . . .

A bleak shadow on the shuddering machine tried to stagger up, but it was late, late, later still, very late, latest of all, oh, very late. The shadow crumbled. The carousel, like the earth spinning, whipped away air, sunlight, sense and sensibility, leaving only dark, cold, and age.

In a final vomit, the switch box blew itself completely apart.

All the carnival lights blinked out.

The carousel slowed itself through the cold night wind.

Will let Jim go.

How many times, thought Will, did it go around? Sixty, eighty . . . ninety . . . ?

How many times? said Jim's face, all nightmare, watching the dead carousel shiver and halt in the dead grass, a stopped world now which nothing, not their hearts, hands or heads, could send back anywhere.

They walked slowly to the merry-go-round, their shoes whispering.

The shadowy figure lay on the near side, on the plank floor, its face turned away.

One hand hung off the platform.

It did not belong to a boy.

It seemed a huge wax hand shriveled by fire.

The man's hair was long, spidery, white. It blew like milkweed in the breathing dark.

They bent to see the face.

The eyes were mummified shut. The nose was collapsed upon gristle. The mouth was a ruined white flower, the petals twisted into a thin wax sheath over the clenched teeth through which faint bubblings sighed. The man was small inside his clothes, small as a child, but tall, strung out, and old, so old, very old, not ninety, not one hundred, no, not one hundred ten, but one hundred twenty or one hundred thirty impossible years old.

Will touched.

The man was cold as an albino frog.

He smelled of moon swamps and old Egyptian bandages. He was something found in museums, wrapped in nicotine linens, sealed in glass.

But he was alive, puling like a babe, and shriveling unto death, fast, very fast, before their eyes.

Will was sick over the side of the carousel.

Then, falling against each other, Jim and Will sledge-hammered the insane leaves, the unbelievable grass, the insubstantial earth with their numbed shoes, fleeing off down the midway. . . .

CHAPTER TWENTY-FOUR

Moths ticked off the high tin-shaded arc light which swung abandoned above the crossroads. Below, in a deserted gas station in the midst of country wilderness there was another ticking. In a coffin-sized phone booth speaking to people lost somewhere across night hills, two white-faced boys were crammed, holding to each other at every flit of bat, each sliding of cloud across the stars.

Will hung up the phone. The police and an ambulance were coming.

At first he and Jim had shout-whispered-wheezed at each other, pumping along, stumbling: they should go home, sleep, forget—no! they should take a freight train west!—no! for Mr. Cooger, if he survived what they'd done to him, that old man, that old old old man, would follow them over the world until he found and tore them apart! Arguing, shivering, they ended up in a phone booth, and now saw the police car bouncing along the road, its siren moaning, with the ambulance behind. All the men looked out at the two boys whose teeth chattered in the moth-flicked light.

Three minutes later they all advanced down the dark midway, Jim leading the way, talking, gibbering.

"He's alive. He's *got* to be alive. We didn't mean to do it! We're sorry!" He stared at the black tents. "You hear? We're sorry!"

"Take it easy, boy," said one of the policemen. "Go on."

The two policemen in midnight blue, the two internes like ghosts, the two boys, made the last turn past the ferris wheel and reached the merry-go-round.

Jim groaned.

The horses trampled the night air, in midplunge. Starlight glittered on the brass poles. That was all.

"He's *gone*. . . ."

"He was here, we swear!" said Jim. "One hundred fifty, two hundred years old, and *dying* of it!"

"Jim," said Will.

The four men stirred uneasily.

"They must've taken him in a tent." Will started off. A policeman took his elbow.

"Did you say one hundred fifty years old?" he asked Jim. "Why not *three* hundred?"

"Maybe he was! Oh God." Jim turned, yelling. "Mr. Cooger! We brought *help!*"

Lights blinked on in the Freak Tent. The huge banners out front rumbled and lashed as arc lights flushed over them. The police glanced up. MR. SKELETON, THE DUST WITCH, THE CRUSHER, VESUVIO THE LAVA SIPPER! danced soft, big, painted each on its separate flag.

Jim paused by the rustling freak show entry.

"Mr. Cooger?" he pleaded. "You . . . *there?*"

The tent flaps mouthed out a warm lion air.

"What?" asked a policeman.

Jim read the moving flaps.

"They said 'Yes.' They said, 'Come in.' "

Jim stepped through. The others followed.

Inside they squinted through crisscrossed tent pole

shadows to the high freak platforms and all the world-wandered aliens, crippled of face, of bone, of mind, waiting there.

At a rickety card table nearby four men sat playing orange, lime-green, sun-yellow cards printed with moon beasts and winged sun-symboled men. Here the akimbo Skeleton one might play like a piccolo; here the Blimp who could be punctured every night, pumped up at dawn; here the midget known as The Wart who could be mailed parcel post dirt-cheap; and next to him an even littler accident of cell and time, a Dwarf so small and perched in such a way you could not see his face behind the cards clenched before him in arthritic and tremulous oak-gnarled fingers

The Dwarf! Will started. Something about those hands! Familiar, familiar. Where? Who? What? But his eyes snapped on.

There stood Monsieur Guillotine, black tights, black long stockings, black hood over head, arms crossed over his chest, stiff straight by his chopping machine, the blade high in the tent sky, a hungry knife all flashes and meteor shine, much desiring to cleave space. Below, in the head cradle, a dummy sprawled waiting quick doom.

There stood the Crusher, all ropes and tendons, all steel and iron, all bone-monger, jaw-cruncher, horseshoe-taffy-puller.

And there the Lava Sipper, Vesuvio of the chafed tongue, of the scalded teeth, who spun scores of fireballs up, hissing in a ferris of flame which streaked shadows along the tent roof.

Nearby, in booths, another thirty freaks watched the fires fly until the Lava Sipper glanced, saw intruders, and let his universe fall. The suns drowned in a water tub.

Steam billowed. All froze in a tableau.

An insect stopped buzzing.

Will glanced swiftly.

There, on the biggest stage, a tattoo needle poised like a blowgun dart in his rose-crusted hand, stood Mr. Dark, the Illustrated Man.

His picture crowds flooded raw upon his flesh. Stripped bare to the navel, he had been stinging himself, adding a picture to his left palm with this dragonfly contraption. Now with the insect droned dead in his hand, he wheeled. But Will, staring beyond him, cried:

"There is he! There's Mr. Cooger!"

The police, the internes, quickened.

Behind Mr. Dark sat the Electric Chair.

In this chair sat a ruined man, last seen strewn wheezing in a collapse of bones and albino wax on the broken carousel. Now he was erected, propped, strapped in this device full of lightning power.

"That's him! He was . . . *dying.*"

The Blimp *ascended* to his feet.

The Skeleton spun about, tall.

The Wart flea-hopped to the sawdust.

The Dwarf let fall his cards and flirted his now mad, now idiot eyes ahead, around, over.

I *know* him, thought Will. Oh, God, what they've *done* to him!

The lightning-rod salesman!

That's who it was. Squeezed tight, smashed small, convulsed by some terrible nature into a clenched fist of humanity . . .

The seller of lightning rods.

But now two things happened with beautiful promptitude.

Monsieur Guillotine cleared his throat.

And the blade, above, in the canvas sky, like a homing hawk scythed down. Whisper-whisk-slither-thunder-rush —wham!

The dummy head, chop-cut, fell.

And falling, looked like Will's own head, own face, destroyed.

He wanted, he did not want, to run lift the head, turn it to see if it held his own profile. But how could you ever dare do that? Never, never in a billion years, could one empty that wicker basket.

The second thing happened.

A mechanic, working at the back of an upright glass-fronted coffin booth, released a trip wire. This made a last cog click within the machinery under the sign, MLLE TAROT, THE DUST WITCH. The wax woman's figure

within the glass box nodded her head and fixed the boys
with her pointing nose as the boys passed, leading the
men. Her cold wax hand brushed the Dust of Destiny
on a ledge within the coffin. Her eyes did not see; they
were sewn shut with laced black-widow web, dark
threads. A waxworks fright, good and proper, she was,
and the policemen beamed, viewing her, and strolled on,
and beamed at Monsieur Guillotine for his act, too, and
moving, the police were relaxing now, and seemed not
to mind being called late on a jolly venture into a rehearsing world of acrobats and seedy magicians.

"Gentlemen!" Mr. Dark and his mob of illustrations
surged forward on the pine platform, a jungle beneath
each arm, an Egyptian viper scrolled on each bicep.
"Welcome! You're just in time! We're rehearsing all our
new acts!" Mr. Dark waved, and strange monsters gaped
their fangs from his chest, a Cyclops with a navel for a
squinted moron eye twitched on his stomach as he strode.

Lord, thought Will, is he bringing that crowd with
him or is the crowd pulling him along by his skin?

From all the creaked platforms, from the muffled sawdust, Will felt the freaks wheel and fix their eyes, enchanted, as were internes and police, by this illustrated
throng of humanity that in one agglomerative move domi-
nated and filled the immediate air and tent sky with silent
shoutings for attention.

Now part of the wasp-needle tattooed population
spoke. It was Mr. Dark's mouth over and above this
calligraphic explosion, this railroad accident of monsters
in tumult upon his sweating skin. Mr. Dark chanted forth
the organ tones from his chest. His personal electric blue-
green populations trembled, even as the real freaks on
the sawdust tent floor trembled, even as, hearing in their
most secret marrow, Jim and Will trembled and felt
more freak than the freaks themselves.

"Gentlemen! Boys! We've just perfected the new act!
You'll be the first to see!" cried Mr. Dark.

The first policeman, his hand casually nestled to his
pistol holster, squinted up at that vast corral of beasts
and beings. "This boy said—"

"Said?!" The Illustrated Man barked a laugh. The freaks leaped in a frolic of shock, then calmed as the carnival owner continued with great ease, patting and soothing his own illustrations, which somehow patted and soothed the freaks. "Said? But what did he *see?* Boys always scare themselves at side shows, eh? Run like rabbits when the freaks pop out. But tonight, especially tonight!"

The policemen glanced beyond to the Erector-set-papier-mâché relic constricted in the Electric Chair.

"Who's he?"

"Him?" Will saw fire lick up through Mr. Dark's smoke-clouded eyes, saw him just as quickly snuff it out. "The new act. Mr. Electrico."

"No! Look at the old man! Look!" Will yelled. The police turned to appraise his demon cry.

"Don't you see!" said Will. "He's dead! Only thing holds him up is the straps!"

The internes gazed up at the great flake of winter flung into and held by the black chair.

Oh gosh, thought Will, we thought it would all be simple. The old man, Mr. Cooger, dying, so we bring doctors to save him, so he forgives us, maybe, maybe the carnival doesn't hurt us, lets us go. But now this, what's next? He's dead! It's too late! Everyone hates us!

And Will stood among the others feeling the cold air waft down from the unearthed mummy, from the cold mouth and cold eyes locked up in frozen eyelids. Inside the frozen nostrils not a white hair stirred. Mr. Cooger's ribs under his collapsed shirt were stone-rigid and his teeth under his clay lips were dry-ice cold. Put him out at noon and fog would steam off him.

The internes glanced at each other. They nodded.

The policemen, at this, took one step forward.

"Gentlemen!"

Mr. Dark scuttled a tarantula hand up an electric brass switchboard.

"One hundred thousand volts will now burn Mr. Electrico's body!"

"No, don't let him!" Will cried.

The policemen took another step. The internes opened their mouths to speak. Mr. Dark flicked a swift demanding glance at Jim. Jim cried:

"No! It's all right!"

"Jim!"

"Will, yes, it's okay!"

"Stand back!" The spider clutched the switch handle. "This man is in a trance! As part of our new act, I have hypnotized him! He could suffer injury if you shocked him from his spell!"

The internes shut their mouths. The police stopped moving.

"One hundred thousand volts! Yet he will come forth alive, whole in sound mind and body!"

"No!"

A policeman grabbed Will.

The Illustrated Man and all the men and beasts asprawl in frenzies on him now snatched and banged the switch.

The tent lights snuffed out.

Policemen, internes, boys jumped up their flesh in cobbles and boils.

But now in the swift midnight shuttering, the Electric Chair was a hearth and on it the old man blazed like a blue autumn tree.

The police flinched back, the internes leaned ahead, as did the freaks, blue fire in their eyes.

The Illustrated Man, hand glued to switch, looked upon the old old old man.

The old man was flintrock dead, yes, but electricity alive sheathed over him. It swarmed on his cold shell ears, it flickered in his deep-as-an-abandoned-stone-well nostrils. It crept blue eels of power on his praying-mantis fingers and his grasshopper knees.

The Illustrated Man's lips thrust wide, perhaps he yelled, but no one heard against the immense fry, blast, the slam and sizzle of power which prowled in around over under about man and prisoning chair. Come alive! cried the hum! Come alive! cried the storming color and light. Come alive! yelled Mr. Dark's mouth, which no one heard but Jim, reading lips, read thunderous loud in his mind, and Will the same, Come alive! willing the old man to live, start up, tick, hum, work juice, summon spit, ungum spirit, melt wax soul. . . .

"He's dead!" But no one heard Will, either, no matter how he pushed against the lightning clamor.

Alive! Mr. Dark's lips licked and savored. Alive. Come alive. He racheted the switch to the last notch. Live, live! Somewhere, dynamos protested, skirled, shrilled, moaned a bestial energy. The light turned bottle-green. Dead, dead, thought Will. But live alive! cried machines, cried flame and fire, cried mouths of crowds of livid beasts on illustrated flesh.

So the old man's hair stood up in prickling fumes. Sparks, bled from his fingernails, dripped seething spatters on pine planks. Green simmerings wove shuttles through dead eyelids.

The Illustrated Man bent violently above the old old dead dead thing, his prides of beasts drowned deep in sweat, his right hand thrust in hammering demand upon the air: Live, live.

And the old man came alive.

Will yelled himself hoarse.

And no one heard.

For now, very slowly, as if roused by thunder, as if the electric fire were new dawn, one dead eyelid peeled itself slowly open.

The freaks gaped.

A long way off in the storm, Jim was yelling, too, for Will had his elbow tight and felt the yell pouring out through the bones, as the old man's lips fell apart and frightful sizzles zigzagged between lips and threaded teeth.

The Illustrated Man cut the power to a whine. Then, turning, he fell to his knees, and put out his hand.

Away off up there on the platform, there was the faintest stir as of an autumn leaf beneath the old man's shirt.

The freaks exhaled.

The old old man sighed.

Yes, Will thought, they're breathing for him, helping him, making him to live.

Inhale, exhale, inhale, exhale—yet it looked like an act. What could he say, or do?

". . . lungs so . . . so . . . so . . ." someone whispered.

The Dust Witch, back in her glass box?

Inhale. The freaks breathed. Exhale. Their shoulders slumped.

The old old man's lips trembled.

". . . heart beat . . . one . . . two . . . so . . . so . . ."

The Witch again? Will feared to look.

A vein ticked a small watch in the old man's throat.

Very slowly now that right eye of the old man opened full wide, fixed, stared like a broken camera. It was like looking through a hole in space, with no bottom forever. He grew warmer.

The boys, below, grew colder.

Now the old and terribly-wise-with-nightmare eye was so wide and so deep and so alive all to itself in that smashed porcelain face that there at the bottom of the eye somewhere the evil nephew peered along and out at the freaks, internes, police, and . . .

Will.

Will saw himself, saw Jim, two little pictures posed in reflection on that single eye. If the old man blinked, the two images would be *crushed* by his lid!

The Illustrated Man, on his knees, turned at last and gentled all with his smile.

"Gentlemen, boys, here *indeed* is the man who lives with lightning!"

The second policeman laughed; this motion shook his hand off his holster.

Will shuffled to the right.

The old spittle-eye followed, sucking at him with its emptiness.

Will squirmed left.

As did the phlegm that was the old man's gaze, while his chill lips peeled wide to shape, reshape an echoed gasp, a flutter. From deep below the old man bounced his voice ricocheting off the dank stone walls of his body until it fell out his mouth:

". . . welcome . . . mmmmmm . . ."

The word fell back in.

"well . . . cummm . . . mmmm . . ."

The policemen nudged each other with identical smiles.

"No!" cried Will, suddenly. "That's no act! He was dead! He'd die again if you cut the power—!"

Will slapped his own hand to his mouth.

Oh Lord, he thought, what am I doing? I want him alive, so he'll forgive us, let us be! But, oh Lord, even more I want him dead, I want them all dead, they scare me so much I got hairballs big as cats in my stomach!

"I'm sorry. . . ." he whispered.

"Don't be!" cried Mr. Dark.

The freaks made a commotion of blinks and glares. What next from the statue in the cold sizzling chair? The old old man's one eye gummed itself. The mouth collapsed, a bubble of yellow mud in a sulphur bath.

The Illustrated Man banged the switch a notch, grinning wildly at no one. He thrust a steel sword in the old man's empty glove-like hand.

A drench of electricity prickled from the sere music-box tines of the ancient stubbled cheeks. That deep eye showed swift as a bullet hole. Hungry for Will, it found and ate of his image. The lips steamed:

"I . . . sssaw . . . the . . . boysssssss . . . ssssneak into . . . thee . . . tent . . . tttttt. . . ."

The desiccated bellows refilled, then pin-punctured the swamp air out in faint wails:

". . . We . . . rehearsing . . . sssso I thought . . . play . . . thissss trick . . . pretend to be . . . dead."

Again the pause to drink oxygen like ale, electricity like wine.

". . . let myself fall . . . like . . . I . . . wasssss . . . dying. . . . The . . . boyssssssss . . . ssscreaming . . . ran!"

The old man husked out syllable on syllable.

"Ha." Pause. "Ha." Pause. "Ha."

Electricity hemstitched the whistling lips.

The Illustrated Man coughed gently. "This act, it *tires* Mr. Electrico. . . ."

"Oh, sure." One of the policemen started. "Sorry." He touched his cap. "Fine show."

"Fine," said one of the internes.

Will glanced swiftly to see the interne's mouth, what it looked like saying this, but Jim stood in the way.

"Boys! A dozen free passes!" Mr. Dark held them out. "Here!"

Jim and Will didn't move.

"Well?" said one policeman.

Sheepishly, Will reached up for the flame-colored tickets, but stopped as Mr. Dark said, "Your names?"

The officers winked at each other.

"Tell him, boys."

Silence. The freaks watched.

"Simon," said Jim. "Simon Smith."

Mr. Dark's hand, holding the tickets, constricted.

"Oliver," said Will. "Oliver Brown."

The Illustrated Man sucked in a mighty breath. The freaks *inhaled!* The vast ingasped sigh might have, seemed to, stir Mr. Electrico. His sword twitched. Its tip leaped to spark-sting Will's shoulder, then sizzle over in blue-green explosions at Jim. Lightning shot Jim's shoulder.

The policemen laughed.

The old old man's one wide eye blazed.

"I dub thee . . . asses and foolssssss . . . I dub . . . thee . . . Mr. Sickly . . . and . . . Mr. Pale . . . !"

Mr. Electrico finished. The sword tapped them.

"A . . . sssshort . . . sad life . . . for you both!"

Then his mouth slit shut, his raw eye glued over. Containing his cellar breath, he let the simple sparks swarm his blood like dark champagne.

"The tickets," murmured Mr. Dark. "Free rides. Free rides. Come any time. Come back. Come back."

Jim grabbed, Will grabbed the tickets.

They jumped, they bolted from the tent.

The police, smiling and waving all around, followed at their leisure.

The internes, not smiling, like ghosts in their white suits, came after.

They found the boys huddled in the back of the police car.

They looked as though they wanted to go home.

II. PURSUITS

CHAPTER TWENTY-FIVE

She could feel the mirrors waiting for her in each room much the same as you felt, without opening your eyes, that the first snow of winter has just fallen outside your window.

Miss Foley had first noticed, some years ago, that her house was crowded with bright shadows of herself. Best, then, to ignore the cold sheets of December ice in the hall, above the bureaus, in the bath. Best skate the thin ice, lightly. Paused, the weight of your attention might crack the shell. Plunged through the crust, you might drown in depths so cold, so remote, that all the Past lay carved in tombstone marbles there. Ice water would syringe your veins. Transfixed at the mirror sill, you would stand forever, unable to lift your gaze from the proofs of Time.

Yet tonight, with the echo of the running feet of the three boys dying away, she kept feeling snow fall in the mirrors of her house. She wanted to thrust through the frames to test their weather. But she was afraid that doing this might cause all the mirrors to somehow assemble in billionfold multiplications of self, an army of women marching away to become girls and girls marching to become infinitely small children. So many people, crammed in one house, would provoke suffocation.

So what must she do about mirrors, Will Halloway, Jim Nightshade, and . . . the nephew?

Strange. Why not say *my* nephew?

Because, she thought, from the first when he came in the door, he didn't belong, his proof was not proof, she kept waiting for . . . what?

Tonight. The carnival. Music, the nephew said, that *must* be heard, rides that *must* be ridden. Stay away from the maze where winter slept. Swim around with the carousel where summer, sweet as clover, honey-grass, and wild mint, kept its lovely time.

She looked out at the night lawn from which she had not yet retrieved the scattered jewels. Somehow she guessed this was a way the nephew had of getting rid of the two boys who might stop her using this ticket she took from the mantel:

CAROUSEL. ADMIT ONE.

She had waited for the nephew to come back. With time passing, she must act on her own. Something must be done not to hurt, no, but slow down interference from such as Jim and Will. No one must stand between her and nephew, her and carousel, her and lovely gliding ride-around summer.

The nephew had said as much, by saying nothing, by just holding her hands, and breathing baked-apple-pie scent from his small pink mouth upon her face.

She lifted the telephone.

Across town she saw the light in the stone library building, as all the town had seen it, over the years. She dialed. A quiet voice answered. She said:

"Library? Mr. Halloway? This is Miss Foley. Will's teacher. In ten minutes, please, meet me in the police station. . . . Mr. Halloway?"

A pause.

"Are you still *there* . . . ?"

CHAPTER TWENTY-SIX

"I'd have sworn," said one interne. "When we first got there . . . that old man was dead."

The ambulance and the police car had pulled up at the same moment at the crossroads, going back into town. One of the internes had called over. Now one of the policemen called back:

"You're joking!"

The internes sat in their ambulance. They shrugged. "Yeah. Sure. Joking."

They drove on ahead, their faces as quiet and white as their uniforms.

The police followed, with Jim and Will huddled in back, trying to say more, but the police started talking and laughing, retelling everything that happened to one another, so Will and Jim wound up lying, giving wrong names again, saying they lived around the corner from the police station.

They let the police drop them at two dark houses near the station and they ran up on those porches and grabbed the doorknobs and waited for the prowl car to swing off around the corner into the station, and then they came down and followed and stood looking at the yellow lights of the station all sun-colored at midnight and Will glanced over and saw the whole evening come and go in Jim's face and Jim watching the police station windows as if at any moment darkness might fill every room and put the lights out forever.

On my way back into town, thought Will, I threw away my tickets. But—look . . .

Jim still has his, in his hand.

Will trembled.

What did Jim think, want, plan, now that dead men lived and only lived through the fire of white-hot electric chair machines? Did he still very much love carnivals? Will searched. Faint echoes, yes, they came, they went in Jim's eyes, for Jim, after all, was Jim, even standing here with the calm light of Justice falling on his cheekbones.

"The Chief of Police," Will said. "He'd listen to us—"

"Yeah," said Jim. "He'd wake just long enough to send for the butterfly net. Hell, William, hell, even *I* don't believe what's happened the last twenty-four hours."

"But we got to find someone higher up, keep trying, now we know what the score is."

"Okay, what's the score? What's the carnival done is so bad? Scared a woman with a mirror maze? So, she scared herself, the police'd say. Burgled a house? Okay, where's the burglar? Hiding inside an old man's skin? Who'd believe that? Who'd believe an old old man was ever a boy twelve? What else is the score? Did a lightning-rod salesman disappear? Sure, and left his bag. But he could've left town—"

"That dwarf in the side show—"

"I saw him, you saw him, looks kinda like the lightning-rod man, sure, but again, can you prove he was ever big? No, just like you can't prove Cooger was ever small, so that leaves us right here, Will, on the sidewalk, no proof except what we saw, and us just kids, the carnival's word against ours, and the police had a fine time anyway there. Oh gosh, it's a mess. If only, if only there was *still* some way to apologize to Mr. Cooger—"

"Apologize?" Will yelled. "To a man-eating crocodile? Jehoshaphat! You still don't see we can't do business with those ulmers and goffs!"

"Ulmers? Goffs?" Jim gazed upon him thoughtfully, for that was how the boys talked of the creatures who dragged and swayed and slumped through their dreams. In the bad dreams of William, the "ulmers" moaned and gibbered and had no faces. In the equally bad dreams of Jim, the "goffs," his peculiar name for them, grew like monster meringue-paste mushrooms, which fed on rats which fed on spiders which fed, in turn, because they were large enough, on cats.

"Ulmers! Goffs!" said Will. "You need a ten-ton safe to fall on you? Look what happened to two folks already, Mr. Electrico, and that terrible crazy dwarf! All kinds of things can go wrong with people on that darn machine. We know, we seen it. Maybe they squashed the lightning-rod man down that way on purpose, or maybe something went wrong. Fact is, he wound up in a wine press anyway, got run over by a steam-roller carousel and's so crazy now he doesn't even *know* us! Ain't that enough to scare the Jesus out of you, Jim? Why, maybe even Mr. Crosetti—"

"Mr. Crosetti's on vacation."

"Maybe yes, maybe no. There's his shop. There's the sign: CLOSED ON ACCOUNT OF ILLNESS. What *kind* of illness, Jim? He eat too much candy out at the show? He get seasick on everybody's favorite ride?"

"Cut it, Will."

"No, sir, I won't cut it. Sure, sure, the merry-go-round sounds keen. You think *I* like being thirteen all the time? Not me! But for cri-yi, Jim, face it, you don't *really* want to be twenty!"

"What *else* we talked about all summer?"

"Talk, sure. But throwing yourself head first in that taffy machine and getting your bones pulled long, Jim, you wouldn't know what to do with your bones then!"

"I'd know," said Jim, in the night. "I'd know."

"Sure. You'd just go away and leave me here, Jim."

"Why," protested the other, "I wouldn't leave you, Will. We'd be together."

"Together? You two feet taller and going around feeling your leg-and-arm-bones? You looking down at me, Jim, and what'd we talk about, me with my pockets full of kite-string and marbles and frog-eyes, and you with clean nice and empty pockets and making fun, is that what we'd talk, and you able to run faster and ditch me—"

"I'd never ditch you, Will—"

"Ditch me in a minute. Well, go on, Jim, just go on leave me because I got my pocket knife and there's nothing wrong with me sitting under a tree playing mumblety-peg while you get yourself plain crazy with the heat of all those horses racing around, but thank God they're not racing any more—"

"And it's your fault!" cried Jim. He stopped.

Will stiffened and made fists. "You mean I should've let young mean-and-terrible get old mean-and-terrible enough to chew our heads off? Just let him ride around and hock his spit in our eye? and maybe you with him, waving good-bye, going around again, waving so long! and all I got to do is wave back, Jim, that what you mean?"

"Sh," said Jim. "Like you say, it's too late. The carousel's broke—"

"And when it's fixed, they ride old horrible Cooger back, make him young enough so he can speak and remember our names, and then they come like cannibals after us, or just me, if you want to get in good with them and go tell them my name and where I live—"

"I wouldn't do that, Will." Jim touched him.

"Oh, Jim, Jim, you *do* see, don't you? Everything in its time, like the preacher said only last month, everything one by one, not two by two, will you remember?"

"Everything," said Jim, "in its time . . ."

And then they heard voices from the police station. In one of the rooms to the right of the entrance, a woman was talking now, and men were talking.

Will nodded to Jim and they ran quietly over to pick their way through bushes and look into the room.

There sat Miss Foley. There sat Will's father.

"I don't understand," said Miss Foley. "To think Will and Jim would break in my house, steal, run off—"

"You saw their faces?" asked Mr. Halloway.

"When I screamed, they looked back under the light."

She's not mentioning the nephew, thought Will. And she won't, of course.

You see, Jim, he wanted to shout, it was a trap! The nephew *waited* for us to come prowling. He wanted to get us in so much trouble, no matter what we said to anybody, police, parents, that nobody'd listen to us about carnivals, late hours, merry-go-rounds, because our word'd be no good!

"I don't want to prosecute," said Miss Foley. "But if they are innocent, where are the boys?"

"Here!" someone cried.

"Will!" said Jim.

Too late.

For Will had jumped high and was scrambling through the window.

"Here," he said, simply, as he touched the floor.

CHAPTER TWENTY-SEVEN

They walked home quietly on the moon-colored sidewalks, Mr. Halloway between the boys. When they reached home, Will's father sighed.

"Jim, I don't see any reason to tear your mother to bits at this hour. If you promise to tell her this whole thing at breakfast, I'll let you off. Can you get in without waking her up?"

"Sure. Look what we got."

"We?"

Jim nodded and took them over to fumble among the clusters of thick moss and leaves on the side of the house until they found the iron rungs they had secretly nailed and placed to make a hidden ladder up to Jim's room. Mr. Halloway laughed, once, almost with pain, and a strange wild sadness shook his head.

"How long has this gone on? No, don't tell. I did it, too, your age." He looked up the ivy toward Jim's window. "Fun being out late, free as all hell." He caught himself. "You don't stay out too long—?"

"This week was the very first time after midnight."

Dad pondered a moment. "Having permission would spoil everything, I suppose? It's sneaking out to the lake, the graveyard, the rail tracks, the peach orchards summer nights that counts. . . ."

"Gosh, Mr. Halloway, did you once—"

"Yes. But don't let the women know I told you. Up." He motioned. "And don't come out again *any* night for the next month."

"Yes, sir!"

Jim swung monkeywise to the stars, flashed through his window, shut it, drew the shade.

Dad looked up at the hidden rungs coming down out of the starlight to the running-free world of sidewalks that invited the one-thousand-yard dash, and the high hurdles of the dark bushes, and the pole-vault cemetery trellises and walls. . . .

"You know what I hate most of all, Will? Not being able to run any more, like you."

"Yes, sir," said his son.

"Let's have it clear now," said Dad. "Tomorrow, go apologize to Miss Foley again. Check her lawn. We may have missed some of the—stolen property—with matches and flashlights. Then go to the Police Chief to report.

You're lucky you turned yourself in. You're lucky Miss Foley won't press charges."

"Yes, sir."

They walked back to the side of their own house. Dad raked his hand in the ivy.

"Our place, too?"

His hand found a rung Will had nailed away among the leaves.

"Our place, too."

He took out his tobacco pouch, filled his pipe as they stood by the ivy, the hidden rungs leading up to warm beds, safe rooms, then lit his pipe and said, "I know you. You're not *acting* guilty. You didn't steal anything."

"No."

"Then why did you say you did, to the police?"

"Because Miss Foley—who knows why?—*wants* us guilty. If she says we are, we are. You saw how surprised she was to see us come in through the window? She never figured we'd confess. Well, we did. We got enough enemies without the law on us, too. I figured if we made a clean breast, they'd go easy. They did. At the same time, boy, Miss Foley's won, too, because now we're criminals. Nobody'll believe what we say."

"I'll believe."

"Will you?" Will searched the shadows on his father's face, saw whiteness of skin, eyeball, and hair.

"Dad, the other night, at three o'clock in the morning—"

"Three in the morning—"

He saw Dad flinch as from a cold wind, as if he smelled and knew the whole thing and simply could not move, reach out, touch and pat Will.

And he knew he could not say it. Tomorrow, yes, some other day, yes, for perhaps with the sun coming up, the tents would be gone, the freaks off over the world, leaving them alone, knowing they were scared enough not to push it, say anything, just keep their mouths shut. Maybe it would all blow over, maybe . . . maybe. . . .

"Yes, Will?" said his father, with difficulty, the pipe in his hand going dead. "Go on."

No, thought Will, let Jim and me be cannibalized, but

no one else. Anyone that knows gets hurt. So no one else must know. Aloud he said:

"In a couple days, Dad, I'll tell you everything. I swear. Mom's honor."

"Mom's honor," said Dad, at last, "is good enough for me."

CHAPTER TWENTY-EIGHT

The night was sweet with the dust of autumn leaves that smelled as if the fine sands of ancient Egypt were drifting to dunes beyond the town. How come, thought Will, at a time like this, I can even think of four thousand years of dust of ancient people sliding around the world, and me sad because no one notices except me and Dad here maybe, and even us not telling each other.

It was indeed a time between, one second their thoughts all brambled airedale, the next all silken slumbering cat. It was a time to go to bed, yet still they lingered reluctant as boys to give over and wander in wide circles to pillow and night thoughts. It was a time to say much but not all. It was a time after first discoveries but not last ones. It was wanting to know everything and wanting to know nothing. It was the new sweetness of men starting to talk as they must talk. It was the possible bitterness of revelation.

So while they should have gone upstairs, they could not depart this moment that promised others on not so distant nights when man and boy-becoming-man might almost sing. So Will at last said, carefully:

"Dad? Am I a good person?"

"I think so. I *know* so, yes."

"Will—will that help when things get really rough?"

"It'll help."

"Will it save me if I need saving? I mean, if I'm around bad people and there's no one else good around for miles, what then?"

"It'll help."

"That's not good enough, Dad!"

"Good is no guarantee for your body. It's mainly for peace of mind—"

"But sometimes, Dad, aren't you so scared that even—"

"—the mind isn't peaceful?" His father nodded, his face uneasy.

"Dad," said Will, his voice very faint. "Are *you* a good person?"

"To you and your mother, yes, I try. But no man's a hero to himself. I've lived with me a lifetime, Will. I know everything worth knowing about myself—"

"And, adding it all up . . . ?"

"The sum? As they come and go, and I mostly sit very still and tight, yes, I'm all right."

"Then, Dad," asked Will, "why aren't you happy?"

"The front lawn at . . . let's see . . . one-thirty in the morning . . . is no place to start a philosophical . . ."

"I just wanted to know is all."

There was a long moment of silence. Dad sighed.

Dad took his arm, walked him over and sat him down on the porch steps, relit his pipe. Puffing, he said, "All right. Your mother's asleep. She doesn't know we're out here with our tomcat talk. We can go on. Now, look, since when did you think being good meant being happy?"

"Since always."

"Since now learn otherwise. Sometimes the man who looks happiest in town, with the biggest smile, is the one carrying the biggest load of sin. There are smiles and smiles; learn to tell the dark variety from the light. The seal-barker, the laugh-shouter, half the time he's covering up. He's had his fun and he's guilty. And men *do* love sin, Will, oh how they love it, never doubt, in all shapes, sizes, colors, and smells. Times come when troughs, not tables, suit our appetites. Hear a man too loudly praising others, and look to wonder if he didn't just get up from the sty. On the other hand, that unhappy, pale, put-upon man walking by, who looks all guilt and sin, why, often that's your good man with a capital G, Will. For being good *is* a fearful occupation; men strain at it and sometimes break in two. I've known a few. You work twice as hard to be a farmer as to be his hog. I suppose it's thinking about trying to be good makes the crack run up the wall one night. A man with high standards, too, the least hair falls on him sometimes wilts his spine. He can't let himself alone, won't lift himself off the hook if he falls just a breath from grace.

"Oh, it would be lovely if you could just *be* fine, *act* fine, not think of it all the time. But it's hard, right? with the last piece of lemon cake waiting in the icebox, middle of the night, not yours, but you lie awake in a hot sweat for it, eh? do I need tell you? Or, a hot spring day, noon, and there you are chained to your school desk and away off there goes the river, cool and fresh over the rock-fall. Boys can hear clear water like that miles away. So, minute by minute, hour by hour, a lifetime, it never ends, never stops, you got the choice this second, now this next, and the next after that, be good, be bad, that's what the clock ticks, that's what it says in the ticks. Run swim, or stay hot, run eat or lie hungry. So you stay, but once stayed, Will, you know the secret, don't you? don't think of the river again. Or the cake. Because if you do, you'll go crazy. Add up all the rivers never swum in, cakes never eaten, and by the time you get my age, Will, it's a lot missed out on. But then you console yourself, thinking, the more times in, the more times possibly drowned, or choked on lemon frosting. But then, through plain dumb cowardice, I guess, maybe you hold off from too much, wait, play it safe.

"Look at me: married at thirty-nine, Will, thirty-nine! But I was so busy wrestling myself two falls out of three, I figured I couldn't marry until I had licked myself good and forever. Too late, I found you can't wait to become perfect, you got to go out and fall down and get up with everybody else. So at last I looked up from my great self-wrestling match one night when your mother came to the library for a book, and got me, instead. And I saw then and there you take a man half-bad and a woman half-bad and put their two good halves together and you got one human all good to share between. That's you, Will, for my money. And the strange thing is, son, and sad, too, though you're always racing out there on the rim of the lawn, and me on the roof using books for shingles, comparing life to libraries, I soon saw you were wiser, sooner and better, than I will ever be. . . ."

Dad's pipe was dead. He paused to tap it out and reload it.

"No, sir," Will said.

"Yes," said his father, "I'd be a fool not to know I'm a fool. My one wisdom is: you're wise."

"Funny," Will said, after a long pause. "You've told me more, tonight, than I've told you. I'll think some more. Maybe I'll tell you everything, at breakfast. Okay?"

"I'll be ready, if you are."

"Because . . . I want you to be happy, Dad."

He hated the tears that sprang to his eyes.

"I'll be all right, Will."

"Anything I could say or do to make you happy, I would."

"Willy, William." Dad lit his pipe again and watched the smoke blow away in sweet dissolvings. "Just tell me I'll live forever. That would do nicely."

His voice, Will thought, I never noticed. It's the same color as his hair.

"Pa," he said, "don't sound so sad."

"Me? I'm the original sad man. I read a book and it makes me sad. See a film: sad. Plays? they really work me over."

"Is there anything," said Will, *"doesn't* make you sad?"

"One thing. Death."

"Boy!" Will started. "I should think *that* would!"

"No," said the man with the voice to match his hair. "Death makes everything else sad. But death itself only scares. If there wasn't death, all the other things wouldn't get tainted."

And, Will thought, here comes the carnival, Death like a rattle in one hand, Life like candy in the other; shake one to scare you, offer one to make your mouth water. Here comes the side show, both hands *full!*

He jumped to his feet.

"Dad, oh, listen! You'll live forever! Believe me, or you're sunk! Sure, you were sick a few years ago—but that's over. Sure, you're fifty-four, but that's young! And another thing—"

"Yes, Willy?"

His father waited for him. He swayed. He bit his lips, then blurted out:

"Don't go near the carnival."

"Strange," his father said, "that's what I was going to tell you."

"I wouldn't go back to that place for a billion dollars!"

But, Will thought, that won't stop the carnival searching through town to visit *me*.

"Promise, Dad?"

"Why don't you want me to go there, Will?"

"That's one of the things I'll tell tomorrow or next week or next year. You just got to trust me, Dad."

"I do, son." Dad took his hand. "It's a promise."

As if at a signal, both turned to the house. The time was up, the hour was late, enough had been said, they properly sensed they must go.

"The way you came out," said Dad, "is the way you go in."

Will walked silently to touch the iron rungs hidden under the rustling ivy.

"Dad. You won't pull these *off* . . . ?"

Dad probed one with his fingers.

"Some day, when you're tired of them, you'll take them off yourself."

"I'll never be tired of them."

"Is that how it seems? Yes, to someone your age, you figure you'll never get tired of anything. All right, son, up you go."

He saw how his father looked up along the ivy and the hidden path.

"You want to come up this way, too?"

"No, no," his father said, quickly.

"Because," said Will, "you're welcome."

"That's all right. Go on."

But still he looked at the ivy stirring in the dark morning light.

Will sprang up, grabbed the first, the second, the third rungs and looked down.

From just this distance, Dad looked as if he were shrinking, there on the ground. Somehow he didn't want to leave him behind, there in the night, like someone ditched by someone else, one hand up to move, but not moving.

"Dad!" he whispered. "You ain't got the *stuff!*"

Who says!? cried Dad's mouth, silently.

And he jumped.

And laughing without sound, the boy, the man swung up the side of the house, unceasingly, hand over hand, foot after foot.

He heard Dad slip, scrabble, grab.

Hold tight! he thought.

"Ah . . . !"

The man breathed hard.

Eyes tight, Will prayed: hold . . . *there* . . . now . . . !!

The old man gusted out, sucked in, swore in a fierce whisper, then climbed again.

Will opened his eyes and climbed and the rest was smooth, high, higher, fine, sweet, wondrous, done! They swung in and sat upon the sill, same size, same weight, colored same by the stars, and sat embraced once more with grand fine exhaustion, gasping on huge ingulped laughs which swept their bones together, and for fear of waking God, country, wife, Mom, and hell, they snug-clapped hands to each other's mouths, felt the vibrant warm hilarity fountained there, and sat one instant longer, eyes bright with each other and wet with love.

Then, with a last strong clasp, Dad was gone, the bedroom door shut.

Drunk on the long night's doings, lolled away from fear toward better, grander things found in Dad, Will slung off limp-falling clothes with tipsy arms and delightfully aching legs, and like a fall of timber chopped himself to bed. . . .

CHAPTER TWENTY-NINE

He slept for exactly one hour.

And then, as if remembering something he had only half seen, he woke, sat up, and peered out at Jim's rooftop.

"The lightning rod!" he yelped. "It's *gone!*"

Which indeed it was.

Stolen? No. Jim take it down? Yes! Why? For the shucks of it. Smiling, he had climbed to scuttle the iron, dare any storm to strike *his* house! Afraid? No. Fear was a new electric-power suit Jim must try for size.

Jim! Will wanted to smash his confounded window. Go nail the rod back! Before morn, Jim, the blasted carnival'll send someone to find where we live, don't know how they'll come or what they'll look like, but, Lord, your roof's so *empty!* the clouds are moving fast, that storm's rushing at us and . . .

Will stopped.

What sort of noise does a balloon make, adrift?

None.

No, not quite. It noises itself, it soughs, like the wind billowing your curtains all white as breaths of foam. Or it makes a sound like the stars turning over in your sleep. Or it announces itself like moonrise and moonset. That last is best: like the moon sailing the universal deeps, so rides a balloon.

How do you hear it, how are you warned? The ear, does it hear? No. But the hairs on the back of your neck, and the peach-fuzz in your ears, *they* do, and the hair along your arms sings like grasshopper legs frictioned and trembling with strange music. So you know, you feel, you are sure, lying abed, that a balloon is submerging the ocean sky.

Will sensed a stir in Jim's house; Jim, too, with his

fine dark antennae, must have felt the waters part high over town to let a Leviathan pass.

Both boys felt a shadow bulk the drive between houses, both flung up their windows, both poked their heads out, both dropped their jaws in surprise at this friendly, this always exquisite timing, this delightful pantomime of intuition, of apprehension, their tandem teamwork over the years. Then, silver-faced, for the moon was rising, both glanced up.

As a balloon wafted over and vanished.

"Holy cow, what's a balloon doing *here!?*" Jim asked, but wished no answer.

For, peering, they both knew the balloon was searching the best search ever; no car-motor racket, no tires whining asphalt, no footstepped street, just the wind clearing a great amazon through the clouds for a solemn voyage of wicker basket and storm sail riding over.

Neither Jim nor Will crashed his window or pulled his shade, they simply *had* to stay motionless waiting, for they *heard* the noise again like a murmur in someone else's dream. . . .

The temperature dropped forty degrees.

Because now the storm-bleached balloon whisper-purled, plummet-sank softly down, its elephant shadow cooling gemmed lawns and sundials as they flaunted their swift gaze high through that shadow.

And what they saw was something akimbo and arustle in the down-hung wicker carriage. Was that head and shoulders? Yes, with the moon like a silver cloak thrown up behind. Mr. Dark! thought Will. The Crusher! thought Jim. The Wart! thought Will. The Skeleton! The Lava Sipper! The Hanging Man! Monsieur Guillotine!

No.

The Dust Witch.

The Witch who might draw skulls and bones in the dust, then sneeze it away.

Jim looked to Will and Will to Jim; both read their lips: *the Witch!*

But why a wax crone flung out in a night balloon to search? thought Will, why none of the others, with their lizard-venom, wolf-fire, snake-spit eyes? Why send a crumbled statue with blind-newt lashes sewn tight with black-widow thread?

And then, looking up, they knew.

For the Witch, though peculiar wax, was peculiarly alive. Blind, yes, but she thrust down rust-splotched fingers which petted, stroked the sluices of air, which cut and splayed the wind, peeled layers of space, blinded stars, which hovered and danced, then fixed and pointed as did her nose.

And the boys knew even more.

They knew that she was blind, but special blind. She could dip down her hands to feel the bumps of the world, touch house roofs, probe attic bins, reap dust, examine draughts that blew through halls and souls that blew through people, draughts vented from bellows to thump-wrist, to pound-temples, to pulse-throat, and back to bellows again. Just as they felt that balloon sift down like an autumn rain, so she could feel their souls disinhabit, reinhabit their tremulous nostrils. Each soul, a vast warm fingerprint, *felt* different, she could roil it in her hand like clay; smelled different, Will could hear her snuffing his life away; *tasted* different, she savored them with her raw-gummed mouth, her puff-adder tongue; *sounded* different, she stuffed their souls in one ear, tissued them out the other!

Her hands played down the air, one for Will, one for Jim.

The balloon shadow washed them with panic, rinsed them with terror.

The Witch exhaled.

The balloon, freed of this small sour ballast, uprose. The shadow passed.

"Oh God!" said Jim. "Now they know where we live!"

Both gasped. Some monstrous baggage brushed and dragged across the shingles of Jim's house.

"Will! She's *got* me!"

"No! I think—"

The drag, brush, rustle scurried from bottom to top of Jim's roof. Then Will saw the balloon whirl up, fly off toward the hills.

"She's gone, there she goes! Jim, she *did* something to your roof. Shove the monkey pole over!"

Jim slid the long slender clothesline pole over, Will fixed it on his sill, then swung out, hand over hand, swung until Jim pulled him through his window and they barefooted it into Jim's clothes closet and boosted and hoisted each other up inside the attic that smelled like lumber mills, old, dark, and too silent. Perched out on the high roof, shivering, Will cried: "Jim, there it *is.*"

And there it was, in the moonlight.

It was a track like a snail paints on a sidewalk. It glistered. It was silver-slick. But this was a path left by a *gigantic* snail that, if it existed at all, weighed a hundred pounds. The silver ribbon was a yard across. Starting down at the leaf-filled rain trough, the silver track shimmered to the rooftop, then tremored down the other side.

"Why?" gasped Jim. "Why?"

"Easier than looking for house numbers or street names. She marked your roof so you can see it for miles around, night *or* day!"

"Ohmigosh." Jim bent to touch the track. A faint evil-smelling glue covered his finger. "Will, what'll we do?"

"I got a hunch," the other whispered, "they won't be back till morning. They can't just start a rumpus. They got some plan. Right now—*there's* what we do!"

Coiled across the lawn below like a vast boa constrictor, waiting for them, was the garden hose.

Will was gone, down, fast, and didn't knock anything over or wake anyone up. Jim, on the roof, was surprised, in no time at all, when Will came scuttling up all panting teeth, the water-fizzing hose in his fist.

"Will, you're a genius!"

"Sure! Quick!"

They dragged the hose to drench the shingles, to wash the silver, flood the evil mercury paint away.

Working, Will glanced off at the pure color of night turning toward morn and saw the balloon trying to make decisions on the wind. Did it sense, would it come back? Would she mark the roof again, and they have to wash it off, and she mark it, and they wash it, until dawn? Yes, if need be.

If only, thought Will, I could stop the Witch for good. They don't know our names or where we live, Mr. Cooger's too near dead to remember or tell. The Dwarf—if he *is* the lightning-rod man—is mad—and, God willing, won't recollect! And they won't dare bother Miss Foley until morning. So, grinding their teeth way out in the meadows, they've sent the Dust Witch to search. . . .

"I'm a fool," grieved Jim, quietly, rinsing the roof where the lightning rod had been. "Why didn't I leave it *up?*"

"Lightning hasn't struck yet," Will said. "And if we jump lively, it won't. Now—over here!"

They showered the roof.

Below, someone put down a window.

"Mom." Jim laughed, bleakly. "She thinks it's raining."

CHAPTER THIRTY

The rain ceased.

The roof was clean.

They let the hose snake away to thump on the night grass a thousand miles below.

Beyond town, the balloon still paused between unpromising midnight and promised and hoped-for sun.

"Why's she waiting?"

"Maybe she *smells* what we're up to."

They went back down through the attic and soon were in separate rooms and beds after many fevers and chills of talk and now lay quietly separate listening to hearts and clocks beat too quickly toward dawn.

Whatever they do, thought Will, we *must* do it first. He wished the balloon might fly back, the Witch might guess they had washed her mark off and soar down to trace the roof again. Why?

Because.

He found himself staring at his Boy Scout archery set, the big beautiful bow and quiver of arrows arranged on the east wall of his room.

Sorry, Dad, he thought, and sat up, smiling. This time it's me out, alone. I don't want *her* going back to report on us for hours, maybe days.

He grabbed the bow and quiver from the wall, hesitated, thinking, then stealthily ran the window up and leaned out. No need to holler loud and long, no. But just think real hard. *They* can't read thoughts, I know, that's sure, or they wouldn't send her, and *she* can't read thoughts, but she *can* feel body heat and special temperatures and special smells and excitements, and if I jump up and down and let her know just by my feeling good about having tricked her, maybe, maybe . . .

Four o'clock in the morning, said a drowsy clock chime, off in another land.

Witch, he thought, *come back.*

Witch, he thought louder and let his blood pound, the roof's clean, hear!? We made our own rain! You got to come back and re-mark it! Witch . . . ?

And the Witch moved.

He felt the earth turn under the balloon.

Okay, Witch, come on, there's just me, the no-name boy, you can't read my mind, but here's me spitting on you! and here's me yelling we tricked you, and the general idea gets through, so come on, come on! dare! double-dare you!

Miles away, there was a gasp of assent rising, coming near.

Holy cow, he thought suddenly, I don't want her back to *this* house! Come on! He thrashed into his clothes.

Clutching his weapons, he aped down the hidden ivy rungs and dogged the wet grass.

Witch! Here! He ran leaving patterns, ran feeling crazy fine, wild as a hare who has chewed some secret, delicious, sweetly poisonous root that now gallops him berserk. Knees striking his chin, shoes crushing wet leaves, he soared over a hedge, his hands full of bristly porcupine weapons, fear and joy a tumble of mixed marbles in his mouth.

He looked back. The balloon swung near! It inhaled, exhaled itself along from tree to tree, from cloud to cloud.

Where am I *going?* he thought. Wait! The Redman house! Not lived in in years! Two blocks more!

There was the swift shush of his feet in the leaves and the big shush of the creature in the sky, while moonlight snowed everything and stars glittered.

He pulled up in front of the Redman house, a torch in each lung, tasting blood, crying out silently: here! this is *my* house!

He felt a great river change its bed in the sky.

Good! he thought.

His hand turned the doorknob of the old house. Oh God, he thought, what if *they* are inside, waiting for me?

He opened a door on darkness.

Dust came and went in that dark, and a harpstring gesticulation of spiders. Nothing else.

Will jumped two at a time up the crumbling stairs, around and out on the roof where he stashed his weapons behind the chimney and stood tall.

The balloon, green as slime, printed with titan pictures of winged scorpions, ancient phoenixes, smokes, fires, clouded weathers, swung its wicker basket wheezing, down.

Witch, he thought, *here!*

The dank shadow struck him like a batwing.

Will toppled. He flung up his hands. The shadow was almost black flesh, striking.

He fell. He clutched the chimney.

The shadow draped him, hushing down.

It was cold as a sea cave in that cloud-dark.

But suddenly the wind, of itself, veered.

The Witch hissed in frustration. The balloon swam a washing circle up around.

The wind! thought the boy wildly, it's on *my* side!

No, don't go! he thought. Come back.

For he feared she had smelled his plan.

She had. She itched for his scheme. She snuffed, she gasped at it. He saw the way her nails filed and scraped the air as if running over grooved wax to seek patterns. She turned her palms out and down as if he were a small stove burning softly somewhere in a nether world and she came to warm her hands at him. As the basket swung

in an upglided pendulum he saw her squinched blind-
sewn eyes, the ears with moss in them, the pale
wrinkled apricot mouth mummifying the air it drew in,
trying to taste what was wrong with his act, his thought.
He was too good, too rare, too fine, too available to be
true! surely she knew that!

And knowing it, she held her breath.

Which made the balloon suspend itself, half between
inhale and exhale.

Now, tremulously, experimentally, daring to test, the
Witch inhaled. The balloon, so weighted, sank. Exhaled
—so freed of vapor—the craft ascended!

Now, now, the waiting, the holding of dank sour breath
in the wry tissues of her childlike body.

Will waggled his fingers, thumb to nose.

She sucked air. The weight of this one breath skimmed
the balloon down.

Closer! he thought.

But, careful, she circled her craft, scenting the sharp
adrenalin wafted from his pores. He wheeled, following
as the balloon spun, and him reeling. You! he thought,
you want me sick! Spin me, will you? Make me dizzy?

There was one last thing to try.

He stood very still with his back to the balloon.

Witch, he thought, you can't resist.

He felt the sound of the green slime cloud, the kept
bag of sour air, the squeal and stir of mouse-wicker on
wicker as the shadow cooled his legs, his spine, his neck.

Close!

The Witch took air, weight, night burden, star-and-
cold-wind ballast.

Closer!

Elephant shadow stroked his ears.

He nudged his weapons.

The shadow engulfed him.

A spider flicked his hair—her *hand?*

Choking a scream, he spun.

The Witch, leaned out, was a mere foot away.

He bent. He snatched.

The Witch tried to scream out breath when she
smelled, felt, knew what he held tight.

But, in reaction, horrified, she seized a breath, sucked weight, burdened the balloon. It dragged the roof.

Will pulled the bowstring back, freighted with single destruction.

The bow broke in two pieces. He stared at the unshot arrow in his hands.

The Witch let out her breath in one great sigh of relief and triumph.

The balloon swung up. It struck him with its dry rattle-chuckling heavy-laden basket.

The Witch shouted again with insane happiness.

Clutched to the basket rim, Will with one free hand drew back and with all his strength threw the arrowhead flint up at the balloon flesh.

The Witch gagged. She tore at his face.

Then the arrow, a long hour it seemed in flight, razored a small vent in the balloon. Rapidly the shaft sank as if cutting a vast green cheese. The surface slit itself further in a wide ripping smile across the entire surface of the gigantic pear, as the blind Witch gabbled, moaned, blistered her lips, shrieked in protest, and Will hung fast, hands gripped to wicker, kicking legs, as the balloon wailed, whiffled, guzzled, mourned its own swift gaseous death, as dungeon air raved out, as dragon breath gushed forth and the bag, thus driven, retreated up.

Will let go. Space whistled about him. He turned, hit shingles, fell skidding down the inclined ancient roof, over down to rim, to rainspout where, feet first, he spilled into further emptiness, yelling, clawed at the rain gutter, held, felt it groan, give way, as he swept the sky to see the balloon whistling, wrinkling, flying up like a wounded beast to evacuate its terrified exhalations in the clouds; a gunshot mammoth, not wanting to expire, yet in terrible flux coughing out its stinking winds.

All this in a flash. Then Will flailed into space, with no time to be glad for a tree beneath when it netted him, cut him, but broke his fall with mattress twig, branch and limb. Like a kite he was held face up to the moon where, at his exhausted leisure, he might hear the last Witch lamentations for a wake in progress as the balloon

spiraled her away from house, street, town with in-
human mourns.

The balloon smile, the balloon rip was all-encom-
passing now as it wandered in deliriums to die in the
meadows from which it had come, sinking down now beyond all the sleeping, ignorant and unknowing houses.

For a long while Will could not move. Buoyed in the
tree branches, afraid he might slip through and kill himself on the black earth below, he waited for the sledge
hammer to subside in his head.

The blows of his heart might jar him loose, crash him
down, but he was glad to hear them, know himself alive.

But then at last, gone calm, he gathered his limbs,
most carefully searched for a prayer, and climbed himself down through the tree.

CHAPTER THIRTY-ONE

Nothing much else happened, all the rest of that night.

CHAPTER THIRTY-TWO

At dawn, a juggernaut of thunder wheeled over the stony
heavens in a spark-throwing tumult. Rain fell softly on
town cupolas, chuckled from rainspouts, and spoke in
strange subterranean tongues beneath the windows
where Jim and Will knew fitful dreams, slipping out of
one, trying another for size, but finding all cut from the
same dark, mouldered cloth.

In the rustling drumbeat, a second thing occurred:

From the sodden carnival grounds, the carousel suddenly spasmed to life. Its calliope fluted up malodorous
steams of music.

Perhaps only one person in town heard and guessed that the carousel was working again.

The door to Miss Foley's house opened and shut; her footsteps hurried away along the street.

Then the rain fell hard as lightning did a crippled dance down the now-totally-revealed, now-vanishing-forever land.

In Jim's house, in Will's house, as the rain nuzzled the breakfast windows, there was a lot of quiet talk, some shouting, and more quiet talk again.

At nine-fifteen, Jim shuffled out into the Sunday weather, wearing his raincoat, cap, and rubbers.

He stood gazing at his roof where the giant snail track was washed away. Then he stared at Will's door to make it open. It did. Will emerged. His father's voice followed: "Want me to come along?" Will shook his head, firmly.

The boys walked solemnly, the sky washing them, toward the police station where they would talk, to Miss Foley's where they would apologize again, but right now they only walked, hands in pockets, thinking of yesterday's fearful puzzles. At last, Jim broke the silence:

"Last night, after we washed off the roof, and I finally got to sleep, I dreamed a funeral. It came right down Main Street, like a visit."

"Or . . . a parade?"

"That's it! A thousand people, all dressed in black coats, black hats, black shoes, and a coffin *forty feet long!*"

"Criminently!"

"Right! What's forty feet long needs to be buried?! I thought. And in the dream I ran up and looked in. Don't laugh."

"I don't feel funny, Jim."

"In the long coffin was a big long wrinkled thing like a prune or a big grape lying in the sun. Like a big skin or a giant's head, drying."

"The *balloon!*"

"Hey." Jim stopped. "You must've had the same dream! But . . . balloons can't die, can they?"

Will was silent.

"And you don't have funerals for them, *do* you?"

"Jim, I . . ."

"Darn balloon laid out like a hippo someone leaked the wind out of—"

"Jim, last night . . ."

"Black plumes waving, band banging on black velvet-muffled drums with black ivory bones, boy, boy! Then on top of it, have to get up this morning and tell Mom, not everything, but enough so she cried and yelled and cried some more, women sure like to cry, don't they? and called me her criminal son but—we *didn't* do anything bad, did we, Will?"

"Someone *almost* took a ride on a merry-go-round."

Jim walked along in the rain. "I don't think I want any more of that."

"You don't *think!?* After all *this!?* Good grief, let me *tell* you! The Witch, Jim, the balloon! Last night, all alone, I—"

But there was no time to tell it.

No time to tell his stabbing the balloon so it gusted away to die in the lonely country sinking the blind woman with it.

No time because walking in the cold rain now, they heard a sad sound.

They were passing an empty lot, deep within which stood a vast oak tree. Under it were rainy shadows, and the sound.

"Jim," said Will, "someone's—*crying.*"

"No." Jim moved on.

"There's a little girl in there."

"No." Jim would not look. "What would a girl be doing out under a tree in the rain? Come on."

"Jim! You *hear* her!"

"No! I don't, I don't!"

But then the crying came stronger across the dead grass, flew like a sad bird through the rain, and Jim had to turn, for there was Will marching across the rubble.

"Jim—that voice—I know it!"

"Will, don't go there!"

And Jim did not move, but Will stumbled and walked until he entered the shade of the raining tree where the sky fell and was lost in autumn leaves and crept down at last in shining rivers along the branches and trunk and there was the little girl, crouched, face buried in her hands, weeping as if the town were gone and the people in it and herself lost in terrible woods.

And at last Jim came edging up and stood at the edge of the shadow and said, "Who is it?"

"I don't know." But Will felt tears start to his eyes, as if some part of him guessed.

"It's not Jenny Holdridge, is it . . . ?"

"No."

"Jane Franklin?"

"No." His mouth felt full of novocaine, his tongue merely stirred in his numb lips. ". . . no . . ."

The little girl wept, feeling them near, but not looking up yet.

". . . me . . . me . . . help me . . . nobody'll help me . . . me . . . me . . . I don't *like* this . . ."

Then when she had strength enough and was quieter she turned her face, her eyes almost swollen shut with weeping. She was shocked to see anyone near, then surprised.

"Jim! Will! Oh God, it's you!"

She seized Jim's hand. He writhed back, yelling. "No! I don't know you, let go!"

"Will, help me, Jim, oh don't go, don't leave!" she gasped, brokenly, new tears bursting from her eyes.

"No, no, don't!" screamed Jim, he thrashed, he broke free, fell, leaped to his feet, one fist raised to strike. He stopped, trembling, held it to his side. "Oh, Will, Will, let's get out of here, I'm sorry, oh God, God."

The little girl in the shadow of the tree, flung back, widened her eyes to fix the two in wetness, moaned, clutched herself and rocked back and forth, her own child-baby, comforting her elbows . . . soon she might sing to herself and sing that way, alone beneath the dark tree, forever, no one able to join or stop the song.

". . . someone must help me . . . someone must help *her* . . ." she mourned as for one dead, "someone must help her . . . nobody will . . . nobody has . . . help her if not me . . . terrible . . . terrible . . ."

"She knows us!" said Will, hopelessly, half bent down to her, half turned to Jim. "I can't leave her!"

"Lies!" said Jim, wildly. "Lies! She don't know us! Never saw her before!"

"She's gone, bring her back, she's gone, bring her back," mourned the girl, eyes shut.

"Find who?" Will got down on one knee, dared to touch her hand. She grabbed him. Almost immediately she knew this was wrong for he tried to tear free, so she let him go, and wept, while he waited near and Jim, far out in the dead grass, called in for them to go, he didn't like it, they must, they must go.

"Oh, she's lost," sobbed the little girl. "She ran off in that place and never came back. Will you find her, please, please . . . ?"

Shivering, Will touched her cheek. "Hey now," he whispered. "You'll be okay. I'll find help," he said, gently. She opened her eyes. "This is Will Halloway, okay? Cross my heart, we'll be back. Ten minutes. But you mustn't go away." She shook her head. "You'll wait here under the tree for us?" She nodded, mutely. He stood up. This simple motion frightened her and she flinched. So he waited and looked at her and said, "I know who you are." He saw the great familiar eyes open gray in the small wounded face. He saw the long rain-washed black hair and the pale cheeks. "I know who you are. But I got to check."

"Who'll believe?" she wailed.

"*I* believe," Will said.

And she lay back against the tree, her hands in her lap, trembling, very thin, very white, very lost, very small.

"Can I go now?" he said.

She nodded.

And he walked away.

At the edge of the lot, Jim stomped his feet in disbelief, almost hysterical with outrage and declamation.

"It can't be!"

"It *is*," said Will. "The eyes. That's how you tell. Like it was with Mr. Cooger and the evil boy— There's one way to be sure. Come on!"

And he took Jim through the town and they stopped at last in front of Miss Foley's house and looked at the unlit windows in the morning gloom and walked up the steps and rang the bell, once, twice, three times.

Silence.

Very slowly, the front door moved whining back on its hinges.

"Miss Foley?" Jim called, softly.

Somewhere off in the house, shadows of rain moved on far windowpanes.

"Miss Foley . . . ?"

They stood in the hall by the bead-rain in the entry door, listening to the great attic beams ashift and astir in the downpour.

"Miss Foley!" Louder.

But only the mice in the walls, warmly nested, made sgraffito sounds in answer.

"She's gone out to shop," said Jim.

"No," said Will. "We know where she is."

"Miss Foley, I know you're here!" shouted Jim suddenly, savagely, dashing upstairs. "Come on out, you!"

Will waited for him to search and drag slowly back down. As Jim reached the bottom of the steps, they both heard the music blowing through the front door with the smell of fresh rain and ancient grass.

The carousel calliope, among the hills, piping the "Funeral March" backwards.

Jim opened the door wider and stood in the music, as one stands in the rain.

"The merry-go-round. They fixed it!"

Will nodded. "She must've heard the music, gone out at sunrise. Something went wrong. Maybe the carousel wasn't fixed right. Maybe accidents happen all the time. Like to the lightning-rod man, him inside-out and crazy. Maybe the carnival *likes* accidents, gets a kick out of them. Or maybe they did something to her on purpose. Maybe they wanted to know more about us, our names, where we live, or wanted her to help them hurt us. Who knows *what?* Maybe she got suspicious or scared. Then they just gave her *more* than she ever wanted or asked for."

"I don't understand—"

But now, in the doorway, in the cold rain, there was

time to think of Miss Foley afraid of mirror mazes, Miss
Foley alone not so long ago at the carnival, and maybe
screaming when they did what they finally did to her,
around and around, around and around, too many years,
more years than she had ever dreamed of shucked away,
rubbing her raw, leaving her naked small, alone, and be-
wildered because unknown-even-to-herself, around and
around, until all the years were gone and the carousel
rocked to a halt like a roulette wheel, and nothing
gained and all lost and nowhere for her to go, no way to
tell the strangeness, and nothing to do but . . . weep
under a tree, alone, in the autumn rain. . . .

Will thought this. Jim thought it, and said:

"Oh, the poor . . . the poor . . ."

"We got to help her, Jim. Who else would believe? If
she tells anyone, 'I'm Miss Foley!' 'Get away!' they'd
say, 'Miss Foley's left town, disappeared!' Go on, little
girl!' Oh, Jim, I bet she's pounded a dozen doors this
morning, wanting help, scared people with her screaming
and yelling, then run off, gave up, and hid under that
tree. Police are probably looking for her now, but so
what? it's just a wild girl crying and they'll lock her away
and she'll go crazy. That carnival, boy, do they know how
to punish so you can't hit back. They just shake you up
and change you so no one ever knows you again and
let you run free, it's okay, go ahead, talk, 'cause folks
are too scared of you to listen. Only *we* hear, Jim, only
you and me, and right now I feel like I just ate a cold
snail raw."

They looked back a last time at the shadows of rain
crying on the windows inside the parlor where a teacher
had often served them cookies and hot chocolate and
waved to them from the window and moved tall through
the town. Then they stepped out and shut the door and
ran back toward the empty lot.

"We got to hide her, until we can help—"

"Help?" panted Jim. "We can't help *ourselves!*"

"There's got to be weapons, right in front of us, we're
just too blind—"

They stopped.

Beyond the thump of their own hearts, a greater heart

thumped. Brass trumpets wailed. Trombones blared. A herd of tubas made an elephant charge, alarmed for unknown reasons.

"The carnival!" gasped Jim. "We never thought! It can come *right into town*. A parade! Or that funeral I dreamt about, for the balloon?"

"Not a funeral and only what *looks* like a parade but's a search for us, Jim, for us, or Miss Foley, if they want her back! They can march down any old street, fine and dandy, and spy as they go, drum and bugle! Jim, we got to get her before they—"

And breaking off, they flung themselves down an alley, but stopped suddenly, and leaped to hide in some bushes.

At the far end of the alley, the carnival band, animal wagons, clowns, freaks and all, banged and crashed between them and the empty lot and the great oak tree.

It must have taken five minutes for the parade to pass. The rain seemed to move on away, the clouds moving with them. The rain ceased. The strut of drums faded. The boys loped down the alley, across the street, and stopped by the empty lot.

There was no little girl under the tree.

They circled it, looked up in it, not daring to call a name.

Then, very much afraid, they ran to hide themselves somewhere in the town.

CHAPTER THIRTY-THREE

The phone rang.

Mr. Halloway picked it up.

"Dad, this is Willy, we can't go to the police station, we may not be home today, tell Mom, tell Jim's mom."

"Willy, where are you?"

"We got to hide. *They're* looking for us."

"*Who*, for God's sake?"

"I don't want you in it, Dad. You got to believe, we'll just hide one day, two, until they go away. If we came home they'd follow and hurt you or Ma or Jim's mom. I got to go."

"Willy, don't!"

"Oh, Dad," said Will. "Wish me luck."

Click.

Mr. Halloway looked out at the trees, the houses, the streets, hearing a faraway music.

"Willy," he said to the dead phone. "Luck."

And he put on his coat and hat and went out into the strange bright rainy sunshine that filled the cold air.

CHAPTER THIRTY-FOUR

In front of the United Cigar Store on this before-noon Sunday with the bells of all churches ringing across here, colliding with each other there, showering sound from the sky now that the rain was spent, in front of the cigar store the Cherokee wooden Indian stood, his carved plumes pearled with water, oblivious to Catholic or Baptist bells, oblivious to the steadily approaching sun-bright cymbals, the thumping pagan heart of the carnival band. The flourished drums, the old-womanish shriek of calliope, the shadow drift of creatures far stranger than he, did not witch the Indian's yellow hawk-fierce gaze. Still, the drums did tilt churches and plummet forth mobs of boys curious and eager for any change mild or wild, so, as the church bells stopped up their silver and iron rain, pew-stiffened crowds became relaxed parade crowds as the carnival, a promotion of brass, a flush of velvet, all lion-pacing, mammoth-shuffling, flag-fluttered by.

The shadow of the Indian's wooden tomahawk lay on an iron grille imbedded in the sidewalk in front of the cigar store. Over this grille, with faint metallic reverberations, year after year, people passed, dropping tonnages of mint-gum wrapper, gold cigar band, matchstub, cigarette butt or copper penny which vanished below forever.

Now, with the parade, hundreds of feet rang and, clustered on the grille as the carnival strode by on stilts, roared by in tiger and volcano sounds and colors.

Under the grille, two shapes trembled.

Above, like a great baroque peacock striding the bricks and asphalt, the freaks' eyes opened out, to stare, to search office roofs, church spires, read dentists' and opticians' signs, check dime and dry goods stores as drums shocked plate glass windows and wax dummies quaked in facsimiles of fear. A multitude of hot and incredibly bright fierce eyes, the parade moved, desiring, but not quenching its desire.

For the things it most wanted were hidden in dark.

Jim and Will, under the cigar store sidewalk grille.

Crouch-pressed knee to knee, heads up, eyes alert, they sucked their breaths like iron Popsicles. Above, women's dresses flowered in a cold breeze. Above, men tilted on the sky. The band, in a collision of cymbals, knocked children against their mothers' knees with concussion.

"There!" exclaimed Jim. "The parade! It's right out front the cigar store! What're we *doing* here, Will? Let's go!"

"No!" cried Will, hoarsely, clenching Jim's knee. "It's the most *obvious* place, in front of everybody! They'll never think to check here! Shut up!"

Thrrrummmmm . . .

The grille, above, rang with the touch of a man's shoe, and the worn nails in that shoe.

Dad! Will almost cried.

He rose, sank back, biting his lips.

Jim saw the man above wheel this way, wheel that, searching, so near, yet so far, three feet away.

I could just reach up . . . thought Will.

But Dad, pale, nervous, hurried on.

And Will felt his soul fall over cold and white-jelly quivering inside.

Bang!

The boys jerked.

A chewed lump of pink bubble gum, falling, had hit a pile of old paper near Jim's foot.

A five-year-old boy, above, crouched on the grille, peered down with dismay after his vanished sweet.

Get! thought Will.

The boy knelt, hands to the grille.

Go on! thought Will.

He had a crazy wish to grab the gum and stuff it back up into the little boy's mouth.

A parade-drum thumped one huge time, then—silence.

Jim and Will glanced at each other.

The parade, both thought, it's *halted!*

The small boy stuck one hand half through the grille.

Above, in the street, Mr. Dark, the Illustrated Man, glanced back over his river of freaks, cages, at the sunburst tubas and python brass horns. He nodded.

The parade fell apart.

The freaks hurried half to one sidewalk, half to the other, mingling with the crowd, passing out handbills, eyes fire-crystal, quick, striking like snakes.

The small boy's shadow cooled Will's cheek.

The parade's over, he thought, now the search begins.

"Look, Ma!" The small boy pointed down through the grille. *"There!"*

CHAPTER THIRTY-FIVE

In Ned's Night Spot, half a block from the cigar store, Charles Halloway, exhausted from no sleep, too much thinking, far too much walking, finished his second coffee and was about to pay when the sharp silence from the street outside made him uneasy. He sensed rather than saw the mild intermingled disturbance as the parade melted among the sidewalk crowds. Not knowing why, Charles Halloway put his money away.

"Warm it up again, Ned?"

Ned was pouring coffee when the door swung wide,

someone entered, and splayed his right hand lightly on the counter.

Charles Halloway stared.

The hand stared back at him.

There was a single eye tattooed on the back of each finger.

"Mom! Down there! Look!"

The boy cried, pointing through the grille.

More shadows passed and lingered.

Including—the Skeleton.

Tall as a dead tree in winter, all skull, all scarecrow-stilted bones, the thin man, the Skeleton, Mr. Skull played his xylophone shadow upon hidden things, cold paper rubbish, warm flinching boys, below.

Go! thought Will. Go!

The plump fingers of the child gesticulated through the grille.

Go.

Mr. Skull walked away.

Thank God, thought Will, then gasped, "Oh, *no!*"

For the Dwarf as suddenly appeared, waddling along, a fringe of bells on his dirty shirt jingling softly, his toad-shadow tucked under him, his eyes like broken splinters of brown marble now bright-on-the-surface mad, now deeply mournfully forever-lost-and-gone-buried-away mad, looking for something could not be found, a lost self somewhere, lost boys for an instant, then the lost self again, two parts of the little squashed man fought to jerk his flashing eyes here, there, around, up, down, one seeking the past, one the immediate present.

"Mama!" said the child.

The Dwarf stopped and looked at the boy no bigger than himself. Their eyes met.

Will flung himself back, tried to gum his body into the concrete. He felt Jim do the same, not moving but moving his mind, his soul, thrusting it into darkness to hide from the little drama above.

"Come on, Junior!" A woman's voice.

The boy was pulled up and away.

Too late.

For the Dwarf was looking down.

And in his eyes were the lost bits and fitful pieces of a man named Fury who had sold lightning rods how many days how many years ago in the long, the easy, the safe and wondrous time before this fright was born.

Oh, Mr. Fury, thought Will, what they've done to you. Threw you under a pile driver, squashed you in a steel press, squeezed the tears and screams out of you, trapped you in a jack-in-a-box all pressed down until there's nothing left of you, Mr. Fury . . . nothing left but this . . .

Dwarf. And the Dwarf's face was less human, more machine now; in fact, a camera.

The shuttering eyes flexed, sightless, opening upon darkness. Tick. Two lenses expanded—contracted with liquid swiftness: a picture-snap of the grille.

A snap, also, of what lay beneath?

Is he staring at the metal, thought Will, or the spaces between the metal?

For a long moment, the ruined-squashed clay doll Dwarf squatted while standing tall. His flash-camera eyes were bulbed wide, perhaps still taking pictures?

Will, Jim, were not seen really at all, only their shape, their color and size were borrowed by these dwarf camera eyes. They were clapped away in the box-Brownie skull. Later—how much later?—the picture would be developed by the wild, the tiny, the forgetful, the wandering and lost lightning-rod mind. What lay under the grille would then be really seen. And after that? Revelation! Revenge! Destruction!

Click-snap-tick.

Children ran laughing by.

The Dwarf-child, drawn by their running joy, was swept along with them. Madly, he skipped off, remembered himself, and went looking for something, he knew not what.

The cloudy sun poured light through all the sky.

The two boys, boxed in light-slotted pit, hisstled their breath softly out through gritted teeth.

Jim squeezed Will's hand, tight, tight.

Both waited for more eyes to stride along and rake the steel grille.

The blue-red-green tattooed eyes, all five of them, fell away from the counter top.

Charles Halloway, sipping his third coffee, turned slightly on the revolving stool.

The Illustrated Man was watching him.

Charles Halloway nodded.

The Illustrated Man did not nod or blink, but stared until the janitor wanted to turn away, but did not, and simply *gazed* as calmly as possible at the impertinent intruder.

"What'll it be?" asked the cafe proprietor.

"Nothing." Mr. Dark watched Will's father. "I'm looking for two boys."

Who *isn't?* Charles Halloway rose, paid, walked off. "Thanks, Ned." In passing, he saw the man with the tattoos hold his hands out, palms up toward Ned.

"Boys?" said Ned. "How old?"

The door slammed.

Mr. Dark watched Charles Halloway walk off outside the window.

Ned talked.

But the Illustrated Man did not hear.

Outside, Will's father moved toward the library, stopped, moved toward the courthouse, stopped, waited for some better sense to direct him, felt his pocket, missed his smokes, and turned toward the United Cigar Store.

Jim looked up, saw familiar feet, pale face, salt and pepper hair. "Will! Your dad! Call to him. He'll help us!"

Will could not speak.

"I'll call to him!"

Will hit Jim's arm, shook his head, violently, No!

Why not? mouthed Jim.

Because, said Will's lips.

Because . . . he gazed up . . . Dad looked even smaller up there than he had last night, seen from the side of the house. It would be like calling to one more boy passing. They didn't need one more boy, they needed a general, no, a major general! He tried to see Dad's face at the cigar counter window, and discover whether it looked really older, firmer, stronger, than it did last night washed with all the milk colors of the moon. But all he saw was Dad's fingers twitching nervously, his mouth working, as if he didn't dare ask his needs from Mr. Tetley. . . .

"One . . . that is . . . one twenty-five cent cigar."

"My God," said Mr. Tetley, above. "The man's rich!"

Charles Halloway took his time removing the cellophane, waiting for some hint, some move on the part of the universe to show him where he was going, why he had come back this way for a cigar he did not really want. He thought he heard himself called, twice, glanced swiftly at the crowds, saw clowns passing with handbills, then lit the cigar he did not want from the eternal blue-gas flame that burned in a small silver jet pipe on the counter, and, puffing smoke, dropped the cigar band with his free hand, saw the band bounce on the metal grille, and vanish, his eyes following it farther down to where . . .

It lit at the feet of Will Halloway, his son.

Charles Halloway choked on cigar smoke.

Two shadows there, yes! And the eyes, terror gazing up out of the dark well under the street. He almost bent to seize the grate, yelling.

Instead, incredulous, he only blurted softly, with the crowd around, and the weather clearing:

"Jim? Will! What the hell's going on?"

At which moment, one hundred feet away, the Illustrated Man came out of Ned's Night Spot.

"Mr. Halloway—" said Jim.

"Come up out of there," said Charles Halloway.

The Illustrated Man, a crowd among crowds, pivoted slowly, then walked toward the cigar store.

"Dad, we can't! Don't look at us down here!"

The Illustrated Man was some eighty feet away.

"Boys," said Charles Halloway. "The police—"

"Mr. Halloway," said Jim, hoarsely, "we're dead if you don't look up! The Illustrated Man, if he—"

"The *what?*" asked Mr. Halloway.

"The man with the tattoos!"

From the café counter, five electric blue-inked eyes fixed Mr. Halloway's memory.

"Dad, look over at the courthouse clock, while we tell you what happened—"

Mr. Halloway straightened up.

And the Illustrated Man arrived.

He stood studying Charles Halloway.

"Sir," said the Illustrated Man.

"Eleven-fifteen." Charles Halloway judged the court-house clock, adjusted his wrist watch, cigar in mouth. "One minute slow."

"Sir," said the Illustrated Man.

Will held Jim, Jim held Will fast in the gum-wrapper, tobacco-littered pit, as the four shoes rocked, shuffled, tilted above.

"Sir," said the man named Dark, probing Charles Halloway's face for the bones there to compare to other bones in other half-similar people, "the Cooger-Dark Combined Shows have picked two local boys, two! to be our special guests during our celebratory visit!"

"Well, I—" Will's father tried not to glance at the sidewalk.

"These two boys—"

Will watched the tooth-sharp shoe nails of the Illustrated Man flash, sparking the grille.

"—these boys will ride all rides, see each show, shake hands with every performer, go home with magic kits, baseball bats—"

"Who," interrupted Mr. Halloway, "are these lucky boys?"

"Two selected from photos snapped on our midway yesterday. Identify them, sir, and you will share their fortune. *There* are the boys!"

He *sees* us down here! thought Will. Oh, God!

The Illustrated Man thrust out his hands.

Will's father lurched.

Tattooed in bright blue ink, Will's face gazed up at him from the palm of the right hand.

Ink-sewn to the left palm, Jim's face was indelible and natural as life.

"You know them?" The Illustrated Man saw Mr. Halloway's throat clench, his eyelids squinch, his bones struck vibrant as from a sledge-hammer blow. "Their names?"

Dad, careful! Will thought.

"I don't—" said Will's father.

"You know them."

The Illustrated Man's hands shook, held out to view, asking for the gift of names, making Jim's face on the flesh, Will's face on the flesh, Jim's face hidden beneath the street, Will's face hidden beneath the street, tremble, writhe, pinch.

"Sir, you wouldn't want them to lose out . . . ?"

"No, but—"

"But, but, but?" Mr. Dark loomed closer, magnificent in his picture-gallery flesh, his eyes, the eyes of all his beasts and hapless creatures cutting through his shirt, coat, trousers, fastening the old man tight, biting him with fire, fixing him with thousandfold attentions. Mr. Dark shoved his two palms near. *"But?"*

Mr. Halloway needing something to excruciate, bit his cigar. "I thought for a moment—"

"Thought what?" Grand delight from Mr. Dark.

"One of them looked like—"

"Like *who?*"

Too eager, thought Will. You see that, Dad, don't you?

"Mister," said Will's father. "Why are you so jumpy about two boys?"

"Jumpy . . . ?"

Mr. Dark's smile melted like cotton candy.

Jim scootched himself down into a dwarf, Will crammed himself down into a midget, both looking up, waiting.

"Sir," said Mr. Dark, "is my enthusiasm *that* to you? *Jumpy?*"

Will's father noted the muscles cord along the arms, roping and unroping themselves with a writhe like the puff adders and sidewinders doubtless inked and venomous there.

"One of those pictures," drawled Mr. Halloway, "looks like Milton Blumquist."

Mr. Dark clenched a fist.

A blinding ache struck Jim's head.

"The other," Will's father was almost bland, "looks like Avery Johnson."

Oh, Dad, thought Will, you're great!

The Illustrated Man clenched his other fist.

Will, his head in a vise, almost screamed.

"Both boys," finished Mr. Halloway, "moved to Milwaukee some weeks ago."

"You," said Mr. Dark, coldly, "lie."

Will's father was truly shocked.

"Me? And spoil the prizewinners' fun?"

"Fact is," said Mr. Dark, "we found the names of the boys ten minutes ago. Just want to double-check."

"So?" said Will's father, disbelieving.

"Jim," said Mr. Dark. "Will."

Jim writhed in the dark. Will sank his head deep in his shoulder blades, eyes tight.

Will's father's face was a pond into which the two dark stone names sank without a ripple.

"First names? Jim? Will? Lots of Jims and Wills, couple hundred, town like this."

Will, crouched and squirming, thought, who told? Miss Foley? But she was gone, her house empty and full of rain shadows. Only one other person . . .

The little girl who looked like Miss Foley weeping under the tree? The little girl who frightened us so bad? he wondered. In the last half hour the parade, going by, found her, and her crying for hours, afraid, and ready to do anything, say anything, if only with music, horses plunging, world racing, they would grow her old again, grow her around again, lift her, shut up her crying, stop up the awful thing and make her as she was. Did the carnival promise, lie to her, when they found her under the tree and ran her off? The little girl crying, but not telling all, because—

"Jim. Will," said Will's father. "First names. What about the last?"

Mr. Dark did not know the last names.

His universe of monsters sweated phosphorus on his hide, soured his armpits, reeked, slammed between his iron-sinewed legs.

"Now," said Will's father, with a strange, and to him almost-delightful-because-new, calm, "I think you're lying. You don't know the last names. Now, why should you, a carnival stranger, lie to me here on a street in some town on the backside of nowhere?"

The Illustrated Man clenched his two calligraphic fists very hard.

Will's father, his face pale, considered these mean, constricted fingers, knuckles, digging nails, inside which two boys' faces, crushed hard in dark vise, tight, very tight in prison flesh, were kept in fury.

Two shadows, below, thrashed in agony.

The Illustrated Man erased his face to serenity.

But a bright drop fell from his right fist.

A bright drop fell from his left fist.

The drops vanished through the steel sidewalk grille.

Will gasped. Wetness had struck his face. He clapped his hand to it, then looked at his palm.

The wetness that had hit his cheek was bright red.

He glanced from it to Jim, who lay still now also, for the scarification, real or imagined, seemed over and both flicked their eyes up to where the Illustrated Man's shoes flint-sparked the grille, grinding steel on steel.

Will's father saw the blood ooze from the clenched fists, but forced himself to look only at the Illustrated Man's face, as he said:

"Sorry I can't be more help."

Beyond the Illustrated Man, rounding the corner, hands weaving the air, dressed in harlequin Gypsy colors, face waxen, eyes hid behind plum-dark glasses, the Fortune Teller, the Dust Witch came mumbling.

A moment later, looking up, Will saw her. Not dead! he thought. Carried off, bruised, fallen, yes, but now back, and mad! Lord, yes, mad, looking *especially* for *me!*

Will's father saw her. His blood slowed, by instinct alone, to a pudding in his chest.

The crowd opened happily, laughing and commenting on her bright if tattered costume, trying to remember what she rhymed, so as to tell it later. She moved, fingers feeling the town as if it were an immensely complicated and lush tapestry. And she sang:

"Tell you your husbands. Tell you your wives. Tell you your fortunes. Tell you your lives. See me, I know. See me at the show. Tell you the color of his eyes. Tell you the color of her lies. Tell you the color of his goal. Tell you the color of her soul. Come now, don't go. See me, see me at the show."

Children appalled, children impressed, parents delighted, parents in high good humor, and still the Gypsy from the dusts of living sang. Time walked in her murmuring. She made and broke microscopic webs between her fingers wherewith to feel soot fly up, breath fly out. She touched the wings of flies, the souls of invisible bacteria, all specks, mites, and mica-snowings of sunlight filtrated with motion and much more hidden emotion.

Will and Jim cracked their bones, cowered down, hearing:

"Blind, yes, blind. But I see what I see, I see where I be," said the Witch, softly. "There's a man with a straw hat in autumn. Hello. And—why there's Mr. Dark, and . . . an old man . . . an *old* man."

He's not that old! cried Will to himself, blinking up at the three, as the Witch stopped, her shadow falling moist-frog cool on the hidden boys.

". . . old man . . ."

Mr. Halloway was jolted as by a series of cold knives thrust in his stomach.

". . . old man . . . old man . . ." said the Witch.

She stopped this. "Ah . . ." The hairs in her nostrils bristled. She gaped her mouth to savor air. "Ah . . ."

The Illustrated Man quickened.

"Wait . . . !" sighed the Gypsy.

Her fingernails scraped down an unseen blackboard of air.

Will felt himself yip, bark, whimper like an aggravated hound.

Slowly her fingers climbed down, feeling the spectrums, weighing the light. In another moment, a forefinger might thrust to the sidewalk grille, implying: there! there!

Dad! thought Will. *Do* something!

The Illustrated Man, gone sweetly patient now that his

blind but immensely aware dust lady was here, watched her with love.

"Now . . ." The Witch's fingers itched.

"Now!" said Will's father, loud.

The Witch flinched.

"Now, *this* is a fine cigar!" yelled Will's father, turning with great pomp back to the counter.

"Quiet . . ." said the Illustrated Man.

The boys looked up.

"Now—" The Witch sniffed the wind.

"Got to light it again!" Mr. Halloway stuck the cigar in the eternal blue flame.

"Silence . . ." suggested Mr. Dark.

"Ever smoke, yourself?" asked Dad.

The Witch, from the concussion of his fiercely erupted and overly jovial words, dropped one wounded hand to her side, wiped sweat from it, as one wipes an antenna for better reception, and drifted it up again, her nostrils flared with wind.

"Ah!" Will's father blew a dense cloud of cigar smoke. It made a fine thick cumulus surrounding the woman.

"Gah!" she choked.

"Fool!" The Illustrated Man barked, but whether at man or woman, the boys below could not tell.

"Here, let's buy you one!" Mr. Halloway blew more smoke, handing Mr. Dark a cigar.

The Witch exploded a sneeze, recoiled, staggered away. The Illustrated Man snatched Dad's arm, saw that he had gone too far, let go, and could only follow his Gypsy woman off, in some clumsy and totally unexpected defeat. But then, in going, he heard Will's father say, "A *fine* day to you, sir!"

No, Dad! thought Will.

The Illustrated Man came back.

"Your name, sir?" he asked, directly.

Don't tell him! thought Will.

Will's father debated a moment, took the cigar from his mouth, tapped ash and said, quietly:

"Halloway. Work in the library. Drop by some time."

"You can be sure, Mr. Halloway. I will."

The Witch was waiting near the corner.

Mr. Halloway whetted his forefinger, tested the wind, and sent a cumulus her way.

She flailed back, gone.

The Illustrated Man went rigid, spun about, and strode off, the ink portraits of Jim and Will crushed hard iron tight in his fists.

Silence.

It was so quiet under the grille, Mr. Halloway thought the two boys had died of fright.

And Will, below, gazing up, eyes wet, mouth wide, thought, Oh my gosh, why didn't I see it before?

Dad's tall. Dad's very tall indeed.

Still Charles Halloway did not look down at the grille but only at the small comets of splashed red color left on the sidewalk, trailed around the corner, dropped from the clenched hands of the vanished Mr. Dark. He was also gazing with surprise at himself, accepting the surprise, the new purpose, which was half despair, half serenity, now that the incredible deed was done. Let no one ask why he had given his true name; even he could not assay and give its real weight. Now he could only read the numerals on the courthouse clock and speak to it, while the boys below, listened.

"Oh, Jim, Will, something *is* going on. Can you hide, keep out from under, the rest of the day? We got to have time. With things like this, where do you begin? No law's been broken, none on the books, anyway. But I feel dead and buried a month. My flesh ripples. Hide, Jim, Will, hide. I'll tell your mothers you've got jobs at the carnival, good excuse for you not coming home. Stay hid until dark, then come to the library at seven. Meantime, I'll check police records on carnivals, newspaper files at the library, books, old folios, everything that might fit. God willing, by the time you show up, after dark, I'll have a plan. Walk easy until then. Bless you, Jim. Bless you, Will."

The small father who was very tall now walked slowly away.

His cigar, unnoticed, fell from his hand, dropped in a spark shower through the grate.

It lay in the square pit glowing its single fiery pink eye at Jim and Will, who looked back and at last snatched to blind and put it out.

CHAPTER THIRTY-SIX

The Dwarf, bearing his demented and wildly lighted eyes, made his way south on Main Street.

Stopping suddenly, he developed a film strip in his head, scanned it, bleated, and blundered back through the forest of legs to reach for and pull the Illustrated Man down where a whisper was as good as a shout. Mr. Dark listened, then fled, leaving the Dwarf far behind.

Reaching the cigar store Indian, the Illustrated Man sank to his knees. Clutching the steel lattice-grille, he peered down in the pit.

Below lay yellow newspapers, wilted candy wrappers, burnt cigars, and gum.

Mr. Dark's cry was muffled fury.

"*Lose* something?"

Mr. Tetley blinked over his counter.

The Illustrated Man clenched the grate, nodding once.

"I clean under the grate once a month for the money," said Mr. Tetley. "How much you lose? Dime? Quarter? Half dollar?"

Bing!

The Illustrated Man glared up.

In the cash-register window a small fire-red sign jumped high:

NO SALE.

CHAPTER THIRTY-SEVEN

The town clock struck seven.

The echoes of the great chime wandered in the unlit halls of the library.

An autumn leaf, very crisp, fell somewhere in the dark.

But it was only the page of a book, turning.

Off in one of the catacombs, bent to a table under a grass-green-shaded lamp, lips pursed, eyes narrowed, sat Charles Halloway, his hands trembling the pages, lifting, rearranging the books. Now and then he hurried off to peer into the autumn night, watchful of the streets. Then again he came back to paper-clip pages, to insert papers, to scribble out quotations, whispering to himself. His voice brought forth quick echoes from the library vaults:

"Look here!"

". . . here . . . !" said the night passages.

"This picture . . . !"

". . . picture . . . !" said the halls.

"And *this!*"

". . . this . . ." The dust settled.

It had been the longest day of all the days he could remember in his life. He had mingled with strange and not-so-strange crowds, he had searched after the searchers, in the wake of the wide-scattering parade. He had resisted telling Jim's mother, Will's mother, more than they needed to know for a happy Sunday, and meantime crossed shadows with Dwarf, traded nods with Pinhead and Fire-eater, kept free of shadowed alleys, and controlled his panic when, doubling back, he saw the basement pit empty under the cigar store grille and knew that the boys were at hide-and-seek somewhere nearby or somewhere, praise God, very far away.

Then, in the crowds, he moved to the carnival ground, stayed out of tents, stayed free of rides, observed,

135

watched the sun go down, and just at twilight, surveyed the cold glass waters of the Mirror Maze and saw just enough on the shore to pull him back before he drowned. Wet all over, cold to the bone, before night caught him he let the crowd protect, warm, and bear him away up into town, to the library, and to most important books . . . which he arranged in a great literary clock on a table, like someone learning to tell a new time. So he paced round and round the huge clock squinting at the yellowed pages as if they were mothwings pinned dead to the wood.

Here lay a portrait of the Prince of Darkness. Next a series of fantastic sketches of the Temptations of St. Anthony. Next some etchings from the *Bizarie* by Giovanbatista Bracelli, depicting a set of curious toys, humanlike robots engaged in various alchemical rites. At five minutes to twelve stood a copy of *Dr. Faustus,* at two lay an *Occult Iconography;* at six, under Mr. Halloway's trailed fingers now, a history of circuses, carnivals, shadow shows, puppet menageries inhabited by mountebanks, minstrels, stilt-walking sorcerers and their fantoccini. More: *A Manual of the Air Kingdoms* (Things That Fly Down History). At nine sharp: *By Demons Possessed,* lying atop *Egyptian Philtres,* lying atop the *Torments of the Damned,* which in turn crushed flat *The Spell of Mirrors.* Very late up the literary clock one named *Locomotives and Trains, The Mystery of Sleep, Between Midnight and Dawn, The Witches' Sabbath,* and *Pacts With Demons.* It was all laid out. He could see the face.

But there were no hands on this clock.

He could not tell what hour of the night of life it was for himself, the boys, or the unknowing town.

For, in sum, what had he to go by?

A three-o'clock-in-the-morning arrival, a grotesque looking-glass maze, a Sunday parade, a tall man with a swarm of electric-blue pictures itching on his sweaty hide, a few drops of blood falling down through a pavement grille, two frightened boys staring up out of the earth, and himself, alone in mausoleum quiet, nudging the puzzle together.

What was there about the boys that made him believe

the simplest word they whispered up through the grille? Fear itself was proof here, and he had seen enough fear in his life to know it, like the smell from a butcher's shop in summer twilight.

What was there about the illustrated carnival owner's silences that spoke thousands of violent, corrupt, and crippling words?

What was there in that old man he had seen through a tent flap late this afternoon, seated in a chair with the words MR. ELECTRICO bannered over him, power webbing and crawling on his flesh like green lizards?

All, all, all of it. And now, these books. This. He touched *Physiognomonie. The secrets of the individual's character as found in his face.*

Were Jim and Will, then, featured all angelic, pure, half-innocent, peering up through the sidewalk at marching terror? Did the boys represent the ideal for your Woman, Man, or Child of Excellent Bearing, Color, Balance, and Summer Disposition?

Conversely . . . Charles Halloway turned a page . . . did the scurrying freaks, the Illustrated Marvel, bear the foreheads of the Irascible, the Cruel, the Covetous, the mouths of the Lewd and Untruthful? the teeth of the Crafty, the Unstable, the Audacious, the Vainglorious, and your Murderous Beast?

No. The book slipped shut. If faces were judged, the freaks were no worse than many he'd seen slipping from the library late nights in his long career.

There was only one thing sure.

Two lines of Shakespeare said it. He should write them in the middle of the clock of books, to fix the heart of his apprehension:

> *By the pricking of my thumbs,*
> *Something wicked this way comes.*

So vague, yet so immense.

He did not want to live with it.

Yet he knew that, during this night, unless he lived with it very well, he might have to live with it all the rest of his life.

At the window he looked out and thought, Jim, Will, are you coming? will you *get* here?

Waiting, his flesh took paleness from his bones.

CHAPTER THIRTY-EIGHT

The library, then, at seven-fifteen, seven-thirty, seven-forty-five of a Sunday night, cloistered with great drifts of silence and transfixed avalanche of books poised like the cuneiform stones of eternity on shelves, so high the unseen snows of time fell all year there.

Outside, the town breathed back and forth to the carnival, hundreds of people passing near where Jim and Will lay strewn in bushes to one side of the library, now ducking up, now ducking down to nose raw earth.

"Cheezit!"

Both smothered in grass. Across the street there passed what could have been a boy, could have been a dwarf, could have been a boy-with-dwarf-mind, could have been anything blown along like the scuttle-crab leaves on the frost-mica sidewalks. But then whatever it was went away; Jim sat up, Will still lay face buried in good safe dirt.

"Come on, what's wrong?"

"The library," said Will. "I'm even afraid of *it*, now." All the books, he thought, perched there, hundreds of years old, peeling skin, leaning on each other like ten million vultures. Walk along the dark stacks and all the gold titles shine their eyes at you. Between old carnival, old library and his own father, everything old . . . well . . .

"I know Dad's in there, but *is* it Dad? I mean, what if *they* came, changed him, made him bad, promised him something they can't give but he thinks they can, and we go in there and some day fifty years from now someone opens a book in there and you and me drop out, like two dry moth wings on the floor, Jim, someone pressed and hid us between pages, and no one ever guessed where we went—"

This was too much for Jim, who had to do something to flog his spirits. Next thing Will knew, Jim was hammering on the library door. Both hammered, frantic to jump from this night to that warmer book-breathing night inside. Given a choice of darknesses, this one was the better: the oven smell of books, as the door opened and Dad stood with his ghost-colored hair. They tiptoed back through the deserted corridors, Will feeling a crazy urge to whistle as he often did past the graveyard at sundown, Dad asking what made them late, and they trying to remember all the places they hid in one day.

They had hid in old garages, they had hid in old barns, they had hid in the highest trees they could climb and got bored and boredom was worse than fear so they came down and reported in to the Police Chief and had a fine chat which gave them twenty safe minutes right in the station and Will got the idea of touring churches and they climbed all the steeples in town and scared pigeons off the belfries and whether or not it was safer in churches and especially up with the bells or not, no one could claim, but it *felt* safe. But there again they began to get starchy with boredom and fatigued with sameness, and were almost on the point of giving themselves up to the carnival in order to have something to do, when quite fortunately the sun went down. From sundown to now it had taken a wonderful time, creeping upon the library, as if it were a once friendly fort that might now be manned by Arabs.

"So here we are," whispered Jim, and stopped.

"Why am I whispering? It's after hours. Heck!"

He laughed, then stopped.

For he thought he heard a soft tread off in the subterranean vaults.

But it was only his laughter walking back through the deep stacks on panther feet.

So when they talked again, it was still in whispers. Deep forests, dark caves, dim churches, half-lit libraries were all the same, they tuned you down, they dampened your ardor, they brought you to murmurs and soft cries for fear of raising up phantom twins of your voice which might haunt corridors long after your passage.

They reached the small room and circled the table on

which Charles Halloway had laid out the books, where he
had read many hours, and for the first time looked in each
other's faces and saw a dreadful paleness, so did not
comment.

"From the beginning." Will's father pulled out chairs.
"Please."

So, each taking his part, in their own good time, the
boys told of the wandering-by lightning-rod salesman,
the predictions of storms to come, the long-after-midnight
train, the suddenly inhabited meadow, the moonblown
tents, the untouched but full-wept calliope, then the
light of noon showering over an ordinary midway with
hundreds of Christians wandering through but no lions
for them to be tossed to, only the maze where time lost
itself backward and forward in waterfall mirrors, only the
OUT OF ORDER carousel, the dead supper hour, Mr. Cooger,
and the boy with the eyes that had seen all the glistery
tripes of the world shaped like hung-and-dripping sins
and all the sins tenterhooked and running red and ver-
minous, this boy with the eyes of a man who has lived
forever, seen too much, might like to die but doesn't
know how. . . .

The boys stopped for breath.

Miss Foley, the carnival again, the carousel run wild,
the ancient Cooger mummy gasping moonlight, exhaling
silver dust, dead, then resurrected in a chair where green
lightning struck his skeleton alight, all of it a storm minus
rain, minus thunder, the parade, the cigar store basement,
the hiding, and at last them here, finished, done with the
telling.

For a long moment, Will's father sat staring blindly
into the center of the table. Then, his lips moved.

"Jim. Will," he said. "I believe."

The boys sank in their chairs.

"All of it?"

"All."

Will wiped his eyes. "Boy," he said gruffly. "I'm going
to start bawling."

"We got no time for that!" said Jim.

"No time." And Will's father stood up, stuffed his pipe
with tobacco, rummaged his pockets for matches, brought

out a battered harmonica, a penknife, a cigarette lighter that wouldn't work, and a memo pad he had always meant to write great thoughts down on but never got around to, and lined up these weapons for a pygmy war that could be lost before it even started. Probing this idle refuse, shaking his head, he finally found a tattered matchbox, lit his pipe and began to muse, pacing the room.

"Looks like we're going to do a lot of talking about one particular carnival. Where's it come from, where's it going, what's it up to? We thought it never hit town before. Yet, by God, look here."

He tapped a yellowed newspaper ad dated October 12, 1888, and ran his fingernail along under this:

J. C. COOGER AND G. M. DARK PRESENT THE PANDE-MONIUM THEATER CO. COMBINED SIDE SHOWS AND UN-NATURAL MUSEUMS, INTERNATIONAL!

"J.C. G.M." said Jim. "Those are the same initials as on the throwaways around town this week. But—it couldn't be the *same* men. . . ."

"No?" Will's father rubbed his elbows. "My goose pimples run counter to that."

He laid forth other old newspapers.

"1860. 1846. Same ad. Same names. Same initials. Dark and Cooger, Cooger and Dark, they came and went, but only once every twenty, thirty, forty years, so people forgot. Where were they all the other years? Traveling. And *more* than traveling. Always in October: October 1846, October 1860, October 1888, October 1910, and October now, tonight." His voice trailed off. ". . . Beware the autumn people. . . ."

"What?"

"An old religious tract. Pastor Newgate Phillips, I think. Read it as a boy. How does it go again?"

He tried to remember. He licked his lips. He did remember.

" 'For some, autumn comes early, stays late through life where October follows September and November touches October and then instead of December and Christ's birth, there is no Bethlehem Star, no rejoicing, but September comes again and old October and so on down the years, with no winter, spring, or revivifying summer.

For these beings, fall is the ever normal season, the only weather, there be no choice beyond. Where do they come from? The dust. Where do they go? The grave. Does blood stir their veins? No: the night wind. What ticks in their head? The worm. What speaks from their mouth? The toad. What sees from their eye? The snake. What hears with their ear? The abyss between the stars. They sift the human storm for souls, eat flesh of reason, fill tombs with sinners. They frenzy forth. In gusts they beetle-scurry, creep, thread, filter, motion, make all moons sullen, and surely cloud all clear-run waters. The spider-web hears them, trembles—breaks. Such are the autumn people. Beware of them.' "

After a pause, both boys exhaled at once.

"The autumn people," said Jim. "That's them. *Sure!*"

"Then—" Will swallowed—"does that makes us . . . *summer* people?"

"Not quite." Charles Halloway shook his head. "Oh, you're nearer summer than me. If I was ever a rare fine summer person, that's long ago. Most of us are half-and-half. The August noon in us works to stave off the November chills. We survive by what little Fourth of July wits we've stashed away. But there are times when we're all autumn people."

"Not you, Dad!"

"Not *you,* Mr. Halloway!"

He turned quickly to see both appraising him, paleness next to paleness, hands on knees as if to bolt.

"It's a way of speaking. Easy, boys. I'm after the facts. Will, do you really *know* your Dad? Shouldn't you know me, and me you, if it's going to be us'ns against them'ns?"

"Hey, yeah," breathed Jim. "Who *are* you?"

"We *know* who he is, darn it!" Will protested.

"Do we?" said Will's father. "Let's see. Charles William Halloway. Nothing extraordinary about me except I'm fifty-four, which is always extraordinary to the man inside it. Born in Sweet Water, lived in Chicago, survived in New York, brooded in Detroit, floundered in lots of places, arrived here late, after living in libraries around the country all those years because I liked being alone, liked matching up in books what I'd seen on the roads.

Then in the middle of all the running-away, which I called travel, in my thirty-ninth year, your mother fixed me with one glance, been here ever since. Still most comfortable in the library nights, in out of the rain of people. Is this my last stop? Chances are. Why am I here at all? Right now, it seems, to help you."

He paused and looked at the two boys and their fine young faces.

"Yes," he said. "Very late in the game. To help you."

CHAPTER THIRTY-NINE

Every night-blind library window chattered with cold.

The man, the two boys, waited for the wind to pass away.

Then Will said: "Dad. You've always helped."

"Thanks, but it's not true." Charles Halloway examined one very empty hand. "I'm a fool. Always looking over your shoulder to see what's coming instead of right at you to see what's *here*. But then, for what salve it gives me, every man's a fool. Which means you got to pitch in all your life, bail out, board over, tie rope, patch plaster, pat cheeks, kiss brows, laugh, cry, make do, against the day you're the worst fool of all and shout 'Help!' Then all you need is one person's answer. I see it so clear, across the country tonight lie cities, towns and mere jerkwater stops of fools. So the carnival steams by, shakes *any* tree: it rains jackasses. Separate jackasses, I should say, individuals with no one, they think, or no one actual, to answer their 'Help!' Unconnected fools, that's the harvest the carnival comes smiling after with its threshing machine."

"Oh gosh," said Will. "It's hopeless!"

"No. The very fact we're here worrying about the difference between summer and autumn, makes me sure there's a way out. You don't have to *stay* foolish and you don't *have* to be wrong, evil, sinful, whatever you want to

call it. There's more than three or four choices. *They*, that
Dark fellow and his friends don't hold all the cards, I
could tell that today, at the cigar store. I'm afraid of him
but, I could see, he was afraid of me. So there's fear on
both sides. Now *how* can we use it to advantage?"

"How?"

"First things first. Let's bone up on history. If men
had wanted to stay bad forever, they could have, agreed?
Agreed. *Did* we stay out in the fields with the beasts?
No. In the water with the barracuda? No. Somewhere
we let go of the hot gorilla's paw. Somewhere we turned
in our carnivore's teeth and started chewing blades of
grass. We been working mulch as much as blood, into
our philosophy, for quite a few lifetimes. Since then we
measure ourselves up the scale from apes, but not half
so high as angels. It was a nice new idea and we were
afraid we'd lose it, so we put it on paper and built buildings like this one around it. And we been going in and
out of these buildings chewing it over, that one new
sweet blade of grass, trying to figure how it all started,
when we made the move, when we decided to be different. I suppose one night hundreds of thousands of years
ago in a cave by a night fire when one of those shaggy
men wakened to gaze over the banked coals at his
woman, his children, and thought of their being cold,
dead, gone forever. Then he must have wept. And he
put out his hand in the night to the woman who must
die some day and to the children who must follow her.
And for a little bit next morning, he treated them somewhat better, for he saw that they, like himself, had the
seed of night in them. He felt that seed like slime in his
pulse, splitting, making more against the day they would
multiply his body into darkness. So that man, the first
one, knew what we know now: our hour is short, eternity is long. With this knowledge came pity and mercy,
so we spared others for the later, more intricate, more
mysterious benefits of love.

"So, in sum, what are we? We are the creatures that
know and know too much. That leaves us with such a
burden again we have a choice, to laugh or cry. No other
animal does either. We do both, depending on the season

and the need. Somehow, I feel the carnival watches, to see which we're doing and how and why, and moves in on us when it feels we're ripe."

Charles Halloway stopped, for the boys were watching him so intently he suddenly had to turn, flushing, away.

"Boy, Mr. Halloway," cried Jim, softly. "That's great. Go on!"

"Dad," said Will, amazed. "I never knew you could *talk.*"

"You should hear me here late nights, nothing *but* talk!" Charles Halloway shook his head. "Yes, you should've heard. I should've said more to you any day you name in the past. Hell. Where *was* I? Leading up to love, I think. Yes . . . love."

Will looked bored, Jim looked wary of the word.

And these looks gave Charles Halloway pause.

What could he say that might make sense to them? Could he say love was, above all, common cause, shared experience? That *was* the vital cement, wasn't it? Could he say how he felt about their all being here tonight on this wild world running around a big sun which fell through a bigger space falling through yet vaster immensities of space, maybe toward and maybe away from Something? Could he say: we share this billion-mile-an-hour ride. We have common cause against the night. You start with little common causes. Why love the boy in a March field with his kite braving the sky? Because our fingers burn with the hot string singeing our hands. Why love some girl viewed from a train, bent to a country well? The tongue remembers iron water cool on some long lost noon. Why weep at strangers dead by the road? They resemble friends unseen in forty years. Why laugh when clowns are hit by pies? We taste custard, we taste life. Why love the woman who is your wife? Her nose breathes in the air of a world that I know; therefore I love that nose. Her ears hear music I might sing half the night through; therefore I love her ears. Her eyes delight in seasons of the land; and so I love those eyes. Her tongue knows quince, peach, chokeberry, mint and lime; I love to hear it speaking. Because her flesh knows heat, cold, affliction, I know fire, snow, and pain. Shared and once again shared experience. Billions of prickling textures. Cut one sense away, cut part of life away. Cut two senses; life halves itself on the instant. We love what we know, we love what we are. Common cause, common cause, common cause of mouth, eye, ear, tongue, hand, nose, flesh, heart, and soul.

But . . . how to say it?

"Look," he tried, "put two men in a rail car, one a soldier, the other a farmer. One talks war, the other wheat; and bore each other to sleep. But let one spell long-distance running, and if the other once ran the mile, why, those men will run all night, like boys, sparking a friendship up from memory. So, all men have *one* business in common: women, and can talk that till sunrise and beyond. Hell."

Charles Halloway stopped, flushed, self-conscious again, knowing vaguely there was a target up ahead but not quite how to get there. He chewed his lips.

Dad, don't stop, thought Will. When you talk, it's swell in here. You'll save us. Go on.

The man read his son's eyes, saw the same look in Jim, and walked slowly around the table, touching a night beast here, a clutch of ragged crones there, a star, a crescent moon, an antique sun, an hourglass that told time with bone dust instead of sand.

"Have I said anything I started out to say about being good? God, I don't know. A stranger is shot in the street, you hardly move to help. But if, half an hour before, you spent just ten minutes with the fellow and knew a little about him and his family, you might just jump in front of his killer and try to stop it. Really knowing is good. Not knowing, or refusing to know, is bad, or amoral, at least. You can't act if you don't know. Acting without knowing takes you right off the cliff. God, God, you must think I'm crazy, this talk. Probably think we should be out duck-shooting, elephant-gunning balloons, like you did, Will, but we got to know all there is to know about those freaks and that man heading them up. We can't be good unless we know what bad is, and it's a shame we're working against time. Show'll close and the crowds go home early on a Sunday night. I feel we'll have a visit from the autumn people, then. That gives us maybe two hours."

Jim was at the window now, looking out across the town to the far black tents and the calliope that played by the turning of the world in the night.

"*Is* it bad?" he asked.

"Bad?" cried Will, angrily. "Bad! You ask that!?"

"Calmly," said Will's father. "A good question. Part of that show looks just great. But the old saying really applies: you can't get something for nothing. Fact is, from them, you get nothing for something. They make you empty promises, you stick out your neck and—wham!"

"Where'd they come from?" asked Jim. "Who are they?"

Will went to the window with his father and they both looked out and Charles Halloway said, to those far tents:

"Maybe once it was just one man walking across Europe, jingling his ankle bells, a lute on his shoulder making a hunchbacked shadow, before Columbus. Maybe a man walked around in a monkey skin a million years ago, stuffing himself with other people's unhappiness, chewed their pain all day like spearmint gum, for the sweet savor, and trotted faster, revivified by personal disaster. Maybe his son after him refined his father's deadfalls, mantraps, bone-crunchers, head-achers, flesh-twitchers, soul-skinners. These laid the scum on lonely ponds from which came vinegar gnats to snuff up noses, mosquitoes to ride summer-night flesh and sting forth those bumps that carnival phrenologists dearly love to fondle and prophesy upon. So from one man here, one man there, walking as swift as his oily glances, it became scuttles of dogmen begging gifts of trouble, pandering misery, seeking under carpets for centipede treads, watchful of night sweats, harkening by all bedroom doors to hear men twist basting themselves with remorse and warm-water dreams.

"The stuff of nightmare is their plain bread. They butter it with pain. They set their clocks by death-watch beetles, and thrive the centuries. They were the men with the leather-ribbon whips who sweated up the Pyramids seasoning it with other people's salt and other people's cracked hearts. They coursed Europe on the White Horses of the Plague. They whispered to Caesar that he

was mortal, then sold daggers at half-price in the grand
March sale. Some must have been lazing clowns, foot
props for emperors, princes, and epileptic popes. Then
out on the road, Gypsies in time, their populations grew
as the world grew, spread, and there was more delicious
variety of pain to thrive on. The train put wheels under
them and here they run down the long road out of the
Gothic and baroque; look at their wagons and coaches,
the carving like medieval shrines, all of it stuff once
drawn by horses, mules, or, maybe, men."

"All those years." Jim's voice swallowed itself. "The
same people? You think Mr. Cooger, Mr. Dark are both
a couple hundred years old?"

"Riding that merry-go-round they can shave off a year
or two, any time they want, right?"

"Why, then—" The abyss opened at Will's feet—"they
could live *forever!*"

"And *hurt* people." Jim turned it over, again and again.
"But why, why all the hurt?"

"Because," said Mr. Halloway. "You need fuel, gas,
something to run a carnival on, don't you? Women live
off gossip, and what's gossip but a swap of headaches,
sour spit, arthritic bones, ruptured and mended flesh, in-
discretions, storms of madness, calms after the storms?
If some people didn't have something juicy to chew on,
their choppers would prolapse, their souls with them.
Multiply *their* pleasure at funerals, their chuckling
through breakfast obituaries, add all the cat-fight marriages where folks spend careers ripping skin off each
other and patching it back upside around, add quack
doctors slicing persons to read their guts like tea leaves,
then sewing them tight with fingerprinted thread, square
the whole dynamite factory by ten quadrillion, and you
got the black candlepower of this one carnival.

"All the meannesses we harbor, they borrow in re-
doubled spades. They're a billion times itchier for pain,
sorrow, and sickness than the average man. We salt our
lives with other people's sins. Our flesh to us tastes sweet.
But the carnival doesn't care if it stinks by moonlight instead of sun, so long as it gorges on fear and pain. That's
the fuel, the vapor that spins the carousel, the raw stuffs

of terror, the excruciating agony of guilt, the scream from real or imagined wounds. The carnival sucks that gas, ignites it, and chugs along its way."

Charles Halloway took a breath, shut his eyes, and said:

"How do I know this? I don't! I *feel* it. I *taste* it. It was like old leaves burning on the wind two nights ago. It was a smell like mortuary flowers. I hear that music. I hear what you tell me, and half what you *don't* tell me. Maybe I've *always* dreamt about such carnivals, and was just waiting for it to come so's to see it once, and nod. Now, that tent show plays my bones like a marimba.

"My skeleton *knows*.

"*It* tells me.

"*I* tell you."

CHAPTER FORTY

"Can they . . ." said Jim. "I mean . . . do they . . . buy souls?"

"Buy, when they can get them free?" said Mr. Halloway. "Why, most men jump at the chance to give up everything for nothing. There's nothing we're so slapstick with as our own immortal souls. Besides, you're inferring that's the Devil out there. I only say it's a type of creature has learned to live off souls, not the souls themselves. That always worried me in the old myths. I asked myself, why would Mephistopheles want a soul? What does he *do* with it when he gets it, of what use is it? Stand back while I throw my own theory over the plate. Those creatures want the flaming gas off souls who can't sleep nights, that fever by day from old crimes. A dead soul is no kindling. But a live and raving soul, crisped with self-damnation, oh that's a pretty snoutful for such as them.

"How do I know this? I observe. The carnival is like people, only more so. A man, a woman, rather than walk away from, or kill, each other, ride each other a lifetime, pulling hair, extracting fingernails, the pain of each to the other like a narcotic that makes existence worth the day. So the carnival feels ulcerated egos miles off and lopes to toast its hands at that ache. It smells boys ulcerating to be men, paining like great unwise wisdom teeth, twenty thousand miles away, summer abed in winter's night. It feels the aggravation of middle-aged men like myself, who gibber after long-lost August afternoons to no avail. Need, want, desire, we burn those in our fluids, oxidize those in our souls, which jet streams out lips, nostrils, eyes, ears, broadcasts from antennae-fingers, long or short wave, God only knows, but the freakmasters perceive Itches and come crab-clustering to Scratch. It's traveled a long way on an easy map, with people handy by every crossroad to lend it lustful pints of agony to power it on. So maybe the carnival survives, living off the poison of the sins we do each other, and the ferment of our most terrible regrets."

Charles Halloway snorted.

"Good grief, how much have I said out loud, how much to myself, the last ten minutes?"

"You," said Jim, "talk a lot."

"In what language, dammit!?" cried Charles Halloway, for suddenly it seemed he had done no more than other nights walking exquisitely alone, deliciously propounding his ideas to halls which echoed them once, then made them vanish forever. He had written books a lifetime, on the airs of vast rooms in vast buildings, and had it all fly out the vents. Now it all seemed fireworks, done for color, sound, the high architecture of words, to dazzle the boys, powder his ego, but with no mark left on retina or mind after the color and sound faded; a mere exercise in self-declamation. Sheepishly he accosted himself.

"How much of all this got through? One sentence out of five, two out of eight?"

"Three in a thousand," said Will.

Charles Halloway could not but laugh and sigh in one. Then Jim cut across with:

"Is . . . is it . . . Death?"

"The carnival?" The old man lit his pipe, blew smoke, seriously studied the patterns. "No. But I think it uses Death as a threat. Death doesn't exist. It never did, it never will. But we've drawn so many pictures of it, so many years, trying to pin it down, comprehend it, we've got to thinking of it as an entity, strangely alive and greedy. All it is, however, is a stopped watch, a loss, an end, a darkness. Nothing. And the carnival wisely knows we're more afraid of Nothing than we are of Something. You can fight Something. But . . . Nothing? Where do you hit it? Has it a heart, soul, butt-behind, brain? No, no. So the carnival just shakes a great croupier's cupful of Nothing at us, and reaps us as we tumble back head-over-heels in fright. Oh, it shows us Something that might eventually lead to Nothing, all right. That flourish of mirrors out there in the meadow, that's a raw Something, for sure. Enough to knock your soul sidewise in the saddle. It's a hit below the belt to see yourself ninety years gone, the vapors of eternity rising from you like breath off dry ice. Then, when it's frozen you stiff, it plays that fine sweet soul-searching music that smells of fresh-washed frocks of women dancing on back-yard lines in May, that sounds like haystacks trampled into wine, all that blue sky and summer night-on-the-lake kind of tune until your head bangs with the drums that look like full moons beating around the calliope. Simplicity. Lord, I do admire their direct approach. Hit an old man with mirrors, watch his pieces fall in jigsaws of ice only the carnival can put together again. How? Waltz around back on the carousel to 'Beautiful Ohio' or 'Merry Widow.' But they're careful not to tell one thing to people who go riding to its music."

"What?" asked Jim.

"Why, that if you're a miserable sinner in one shape, you're a miserable sinner in another. Changing size doesn't change the brain. If I made you twenty-five tomorrow, Jim, your thoughts would still be boy thoughts, and it'd show! Or if they turned *me* into a boy of ten this instant, my brain would still be fifty and that boy would act funnier and older and weirder than any boy ever. Then, too, time's out of joint another way."

"Which way?" asked Will.

"If I became young again, all my friends would still be fifty, sixty, wouldn't they? I'd be cut off from them,

forever, for I couldn't tell them what I'd up and done,
could I? They'd resent it. They'd hate me. Their interests
would no longer be mine, would they? Especially their
worries. Sickness and death for them, new life for me.
So where's the place in this world for a man who looks
twenty but who is older than Methuselah, what man
could stand the shock of a change like that? Carnival
won't warn you it's equal to postoperative shock, but, by
God, I bet it is, and more!

"So, what happens? You get your reward: madness.
Change of body, change of personal environment, for one
thing. Guilt, for another, guilt at leaving your wife, husband, friends to die the way all men die—Lord, that
alone would give a man fits. So more fear, more agony
for the carnival to breakfast on. So with the green vapors
coming off your stricken conscience you say you want to
go back the way you were! The carnival nods and listens.
Yes, they promise, if you behave as they say, in a short
while they'll give you back your twoscore and ten or
whatever. On the promise alone of being returned to
normal old age, that train travels with the world, its side
show populated with madmen waiting to be released from
bondage, meantime servicing the carnival, giving it coke
for its ovens."

Will murmured something.

"What?"

"Miss Foley," mourned Will. "Oh, poor Miss Foley,
they got her now, just like you say. Once she got what
she wanted it scared her, she didn't like it, oh, she was
crying so hard, Dad, so hard; now I bet they promise her
someday she can be fifty again if she'll mind. I wonder
what they're doing with her, right now, oh, Dad, oh, Jim!"

"God help her." Will's father put a heavy hand out to
trace the old carnival portraits. "They've probably
thrown her in with the freaks. And what are they? Sinners who've traveled so long, hoping for deliverance,
they've taken on the shape of their original sins? The Fat
Man, what was he once? If I can guess the carnival's
sense of irony, the way they like to weight the scales, he
was once a ravener after all kinds and varieties of lust.
No matter, there he lives now, anyway, collected up in

his bursting skin. The Thin Man, Skeleton, or whatever, did he starve his wife's, children's spiritual as well as physical hungers? The Dwarf? Was he or was he not your friend, the lightning-rod salesman, always on the road, never settling, ever-moving, facing no encounters, running ahead of the lightning and selling rods, yes, but leaving others to face the storm, so maybe, through accident, or design, when he fell in with the free rides, he shrank not to a boy but a mean ball of grotesque tripes, all self-involved. The fortune-telling, Gypsy Dust Witch? Maybe someone who lived always tomorrow and let today slide, like myself, and so wound up penalized, having to guess other people's wild sunrises and sad sunsets. You tell me, you've seen her *near*. The Pinhead? The Sheep Boy? The Fire Eater? The Siamese Twins, good God, what were they? twins all bound up in tandem narcissism? We'll never know. They'll never tell. We've guessed, and probably guessed wrong, on ten dozen things the last half hour. Now—some plan. Where do we go from here?"

Charles Halloway placed forth a map of the town and drew in the location of the carnival with a blunt pencil.

"Do we keep hiding out? No. With Miss Foley, and so many others involved, we just can't. Well, then, how do we attack so we won't be picked off first thing? What kind of weapons—"

"Silver bullets!" cried Will, suddenly.

"Heck, no!" snorted Jim. "They're not vampires!"

"If we were Catholic, we could borrow church holy water and—"

"Nuts," said Jim. "Movie stuff. It don't happen that way in real life. Am I wrong, Mr. Halloway?"

"I wish you were, boy."

Will's eyes glowed fiercely. "Okay. Only one thing to do: trot down to the meadow with a couple gallons of kerosene and some matches—"

"That's against the law!" Jim exclaimed.

"Look who's *talking!*"

"Hold on!"

But everyone stopped right then.
Whisper.

A faint tide of wind flowed up along through the library corridors and into this room.

"The front door," Jim whispered. "Someone just opened it."

Far away, a gentle click. The draft that had for a moment stirred the boys' trouser cuffs and blown the man's hair, ceased.

"Someone just *closed* it."

Silence.

Just the great dark library with its labyrinths and hedgerow mazes of sleeping books.

"Someone's *inside*."

The boys half rose, bleating in the backs of their mouths.

Charles Halloway waited, then said one word, softly:

"Hide."

"We can't leave you—"

"Hide."

The boys ran and vanished in the dark maze.

Charles Halloway then rigidly, slowly, breathing in, breathing out, forced himself to sit back down, his eyes on the yellowed newspapers, to wait, to wait, then again . . . to wait some more.

CHAPTER FORTY-ONE

A shadow moved among shadows.

Charles Halloway felt his soul submerge.

It took a long time for the shadow and the man it escorted to come stand in the doorway of the room. The shadow seemed deliberate in its slowness so as to shingle his flesh and cheesegrate his steadily willed calm. And when at last the shadow reached the door it brought not one, not a hundred, but a thousand people with it to look in.

"My name is Dark," said the voice.

Charles Halloway let out two fistfuls of air.

"Better known as the Illustrated Man," said the voice. "Where are the boys?"

"Boys?" Will's father turned at last to appraise the tall man who stood in the door.

The Illustrated Man sniffed the yellow pollen that whiffed up from the ancient books as quite suddenly Will's father saw them laid out in full sight, leaped up, stopped, then began to close them, one by one, as casually as possible.

The Illustrated Man pretended not to notice.

"The boys are not home. The two houses are empty. What a shame, they'll miss those free rides."

"I wish I knew where they were." Charles Halloway started carrying the books to the shelves. "Hell, if they knew you were here with free tickets, they'd shout for joy."

"Would they?" Mr. Dark let his smile melt like a white and pink paraffin candy toy he no longer had appetite for. Softly, he said, "I could kill you."

Charles Halloway nodded, walking slowly.

"Did you hear what I said?" barked the Illustrated Man.

"Yes." Charles Halloway weighed the books, as if they were his judgment. "But you won't kill now. You're too smart. You've kept the show on the road a long time, being smart."

"So you've read a few papers and think you know all about us?"

"No, not all. Just enough to scare me."

"Be more scared, then," said the crowd of night-crawling illustrations locked under black suiting, speaking through the thin lips. "One of my friends, outside, can fix you so it seems you died of most natural heart failure."

The blood banged at Charles Halloway's heart, knocked at his temples, tapped twice at his wrists.

The Witch, he thought.

His lips must have formed the words.

"The Witch." Mr. Dark nodded.

The other shelved the books, withholding one.

"Well, what have you there?" Mr. Dark squinted. "A Bible? How very charming, how childish and refreshingly old-fashioned."

"Have you ever read it, Mr. Dark?"

"Read it! I've had every page, paragraph, and word read *at* me, sir!" Mr. Dark took time to light a cigarette and blow smoke toward the NO SMOKING sign, then at Will's father. "Do you really imagine that books can harm me? Is naiveté *really* your armor? Here!"

And before Charles Halloway could move, Mr. Dark ran lightly forward and took the Bible. He held it in his two hands.

"Aren't you surprised? See, I touch, hold, even *read* from it."

Mr. Dark blew smoke on the pages as he riffled them.

"Do you expect me to fall away into so many Dead Sea scrolls of flesh before you? Myths, unfortunately, are just that. Life, and by life I could mean so many fascinating things, goes on, makes shift for itself, survives wildly, and I not the least wild among many. Your King James and his literary version of some rather stuffy poetic materials is worth just about *this* much of my time and sweat."

Mr. Dark hurled the Bible into a wastepaper basket and did not look at it again.

"I hear your heart beating rapidly," said Mr. Dark. "My ears are not so finely tuned as the Gypsy's, but they hear. Your eyes jump beyond my shoulder. The boys hide out there in the warrens? Good. I would not wish for their escape. Not that anyone will believe their gibberings, in fact it's good advertisement for our shows, people titillate, night-sweat, then come prowling down to look us over, lick their lips, and wonder about investing in our special securities. You came, you prowled, and it wasn't just for curiosity. How old are you?"

Charles Halloway pressed his lips shut.

"Fifty?" purred Mr. Dark. "Fifty-one?" he murmured. "Fifty-two? Like to be younger?"

"No!"

"No need to yell. Politely, please." Mr. Dark hummed, strolling the room, running his hand over the books as if they were years to be counted. "Oh, it's nice to be young, really. Wouldn't forty be nice, again? Forty's ten years nicer than fifty, and thirty's twenty years nicer by an incredible long shot."

"I won't listen!" Charles Halloway shut his eyes.

Mr. Dark tilted his head, sucked on his cigarette, and observed. "Strange, you shut your eyes, not to listen. Clapping your hands over your ears would be better—"

Will's father clapped his hands to his ears, but the voice came through.

"Tell you what," said Mr. Dark, casually, waving his cigarette. "If you help me within fifteen seconds I'll give you your fortieth birthday. Ten seconds and you can celebrate thirty-five. A rare young age. A stripling, almost, by comparison. I'll start counting by my watch and by God, if you should jump to it, lend a hand, I might just cut thirty years off your life! Bargains galore, as the posters say. Think of it! Starting all over again, everything fine and new and glorious, all the things to be done and thought and savored again. Last chance! Here goes. One, Two. Three. Four—"

Charles Halloway hunched away, half crouched, propped hard against the shelves, grinding his teeth to drown the sound of counting.

"You're losing out, old man, my dear old fellow," said Mr. Dark. "Five. Losing. Six. Losing very much. Seven. Really losing. Eight. Frittering away. Nine. Ten. My God, you fool! Eleven. Halloway! Twelve. Almost gone. Thirteen! Gone! Fourteen! Lost! Fifteen! Lost forever!"

Mr. Dark put down his arm with the watch on it.

Charles Halloway, gasping, had turned away to bury his face in the smell of ancient books, the feel of old and comfortable leather, the taste of funeral dust and pressed flowers.

Mr. Dark stood in the door now, on his way out.

"Stay there," he directed. "Listen to your heart. I'll send someone to fix it. But, first, the boys . . ."

The crowd of unsleeping creatures, saddled upon tall flesh, strode quietly forth into darkness, borne with and all over upon Mr. Dark. Their cries and whines and utterances of vague but excruciating excitements sounded in his husky summoning:

"Boys? Are you there? Wherever you are . . . answer."

Charles Halloway sprang forward, then felt the room spin and whirl him, as that soft, that easy, that most pleasant voice of Mr. Dark went calling through the dark. Charles Halloway fell against a chair, thought: Listen, my heart! sank down to his knees, he said, Listen to my heart! it explodes! Oh God, it's tearing free!—and could not follow.

The Illustrated Man trod cat-soft in the labyrinths of shelved and darkly waiting books.

"Boys . . . ? Hear me . . . ?"

Silence.

"Boys . . . ?"

CHAPTER FORTY-TWO

Somewhere in the recumbent solitudes, the motionless but teeming millions of books, lost in two dozen turns right, three dozen turns left, down aisles, through corridors, toward dead ends, locked doors, half-empty shelves, somewhere in the literary soot of Dickens's London, or Dostoevsky's Moscow or the steppes beyond, somewhere in the vellumed dust of atlas or *Geographic,* sneezes pent but set like traps, the boys crouched, stood, lay sweating a cool and constant brine.

Somewhere hidden, Jim thought: *He's coming!*

Somewhere hidden, Will thought: *He's near!*

"Boys . . . ?"

Mr. Dark came carrying his panoply of friends, his jewel-case assortment of calligraphical reptiles which lay sunning themselves at midnight on his flesh. With him strode the stitch-inked *Tyrannosaurus rex,* which lent to his haunches a machined and ancient wellspring mineral-oil glide. As the thunder lizard strode, all glass-bead pomp, so strode Mr. Dark, armored with vile lightning scribbles of carnivores and sheep blasted by that thunder and arun before storms of juggernaut flesh. It was the pterodactyl kite and scythe which raised his arms almost to fly the marbled vaults. And with the inked and stencilled flashburnt shapes of pistoned or bladed doom came his usual crowd of hangers-on, spectators gripped to each limb, seated on shoulder blades, peering from his jungled chest, hung upside down in microscopic millions in his armpit vaults screaming bat-screams for encounters, ready for the hunt and if need be the kill. Like a black tidal wave upon a bleak shore, a dark tumult infilled with phosphorescent beauties and badly spoiled dreams, Mr. Dark sounded and hissed his feet, his legs, his body, his sharp face forward.

"Boys . . . ?"

Immensely patient, that soft voice, ever the warmest friend to chilly creatures burrowed away, nested amongst dry books; so he scuttered, crept, scurried, stalked, tiptoed, wafted, stood immensely still among the primates, the Egyptian monuments to bestial gods, brushed black histories of dead Africa, stayed awhile in Asia, then sauntered on to newer lands.

"Boys, I know you hear me! The sign reads: SILENCE! So, I'll whisper: one of you still wants what we offer. Eh? *Eh?*"

Jim, thought Will.

Me, thought Jim. No! oh, no! not still! not me!

"Come out." Mr. Dark purred the air through his teeth. "I guarantee rewards! Whoever turns himself in wins it *all!*

Bangity-bang!

My heart! thought Jim.

Is that me? thought Will, *or Jim!!?*

"I hear you." Mr. Dark's lips quivered. "Closer now. Will? Jim? Isn't it Jim who's the *smart* one? Come along, boy . . . !"

No! thought Will.

I don't know anything! thought Jim, wildly.

"Jim, yes . . ." Mr. Dark wheeled in a new direction. "Jim, show me where your friend is." Softly. "We'll shut

him up, give you the ride that would have been his if he'd
used his head. Right, Jim?" A dove voice, cooing. "Closer.
I hear your heart jump!"

Stop! thought Will to his chest.

Stop! Jim clenched his breath. *Stop!!*

"I wonder . . . are you in this alcove . . . ?"

Mr. Dark let the peculiar gravity of a certain group of
stacks tug him forward.

"You *here,* Jim . . . ? Or . . . over behind . . . ?"

He shoved a trolley of books mindlessly off on rubber
rollers to bump through the night. A long way off, it
crashed and spilled its contents to the floor like so many
dead black ravens.

"Smart hide-and-seekers, both," said Mr. Dark. "But
someone's smarter. Did you hear the carousel calliope tonight? Did you know, someone dear to you was down to
the carousel? Will? Willy? William. William Halloway.
Where's your mother tonight?"

Silence.

"She was out riding the night wind, Willy-William.
Around. We put her on. Around. We left her on. Around.
You *hear,* Willy? Around, a year, another year, another,
around, around!"

Dad! thought Will. *Where are you!*

In the far room, Charles Halloway, seated, his heart
pounding, heard and thought, He won't find them, I
won't move unless he does, he can't find them, they won't
listen! they won't believe! he'll go away!

"Your mother, Will," called Mr. Dark, softly. "Around
and around, can you guess *which* direction, Willy?"

Mr. Dark circled his thin ghost hand in the dark air
between the stacks.

"Around, around, and when we let your mother off, boy,
and showed her herself in the Mirror Maze, you should
have heard the *one single sound* she made. She was like a
cat with a hair ball in her so big and sticky there was no
way to gag it out, no way to scream around the hair
coming out her nostrils and ears and eyes, boy, and her
old old old. The last we saw of her, boy Willy, she was
running off away from what she saw in the mirrors. She'll
bang Jim's house door but when his ma sees a thing two

hundred years old slobbering at the keyhole, begging the mercy of gunshot death, boy, Jim's ma will gag the same way, like a hairballed cat sick but can't be sick, and beat her away, send her beggaring the streets, where no one'll believe, Will, such a kettle of bones and spit, no one'll believe this was a rose beauty, your kind relation! So Will, it's up to us to run find, run save her, for we know who she is—right, Will, right, Will, right, right, *right?!*"

The dark man's voice hissed away to silence.

Very faintly now, somewhere in the library, someone was sobbing.

Ah . . .

The Illustrated Man gassed the air pleasantly from his dank lungs.

Yessssssssssss . . .

"Here . . ." he murmured. "What? Filed under B for Boys? A for Adventure? H for Hidden. S for Secret. T for Terrified? Or filed under J for Jim or N for Nightshade, W for William, H for Halloway? Where are my two precious human books, so I may turn their pages, eh?"

He kicked a place for his right foot on the first shelf of a towering stack.

He shoved his right foot in, put his weight there, and swung his left foot free.

"There."

His left foot hit the second shelf, knocked space. He climbed. His right foot kicked a hole on the third shelf, plunged books back, and so up and up he climbed, to fourth shelf, to fifth, to sixth, groping dark library heavens, hands clutching shelfboards, then scrabbling higher to leaf night to find boys, if boys there were, like bookmarks among books.

His right hand, a princely tarantula, garlanded with roses, cracked a book of Bayeaux tapestries aspin down the sightless abyss below. It seemed an age before the tapestries struck, all askew, a ruin of beauty, an avalanche of gold, silver, and sky-blue thread on the floor.

His left hand, reaching the ninth shelf as he panted, grunted, encountered empty space—no books.

"Boys, are you here on Everest?"

Silence. Except for the faint sobbing, nearer now.

"Is it cold here? Colder? Coldest?"

The eyes of the Illustrated Man came abreast of the eleventh shelf.

Like a corpse laid rigid out, face down just three inches away, was Jim Nightshade.

One shelf further up in the catacomb, eyes trembling with tears, lay William Halloway.

"Well," said Mr. Dark.

He reached a hand to pat Will's head.

"Hello," he said.

CHAPTER FORTY-THREE

To Will, the palm of the hand that drifted up was like a moon rising.

Upon it was the fiery blue-inked portrait of himself. Jim, too, saw a hand before his face.

His own picture looked back at him from the palm.

The hand with Will's picture grabbed Will.

The hand with Jim's picture grabbed Jim.

Shrieks and yells.

The Illustrated Man heaved.

Twisting, he fell-jumped to the floor.

The boys, kicking, yelling, fell with him. They landed on their feet, toppled, collapsed, to be held, reared, set right, fistfuls of their shirts in Mr. Dark's fists.

"Jim!" he said. "Will! What were you doing up there, boys? Surely not reading?"

"Dad!"

"Mr. Halloway!"

Will's father stepped from the dark.

The Illustrated Man rearranged the boys tenderly under one arm like kindling, then gazed with genteel curiosity at Charles Halloway and reached for him. Will's father struck one blow before his left hand was seized, held, squeezed. As the boys watched, shouting, they saw Charles Halloway gasp and fall to one knee.

Mr. Dark squeezed that left hand harder and, doing this, slowly, certainly, pressured the boys with his other arm, crushing their ribs so air gushed from their mouths.

Night spiraled in fiery whorls like great thumbprints inside Will's eyes.

Will's father, groaning, sank to both knees, flailing his right arm.

"Damn you!"

"But," said the carnival owner quietly, "I am already."

"Damn you, damn you!"

"Not words, old man," said Mr. Dark. "Not words in books or words you say, but real thoughts, real actions, quick thought, quick action, win the day. So!"

He gave one last mighty clench of his fist.

The boys heard Charles Halloway's finger bones crack. He gave a last cry and fell senseless.

In one motion like a solemn pavane, the Illustrated Man rounded the stacks, the boys, kicking books from shelves, under his arms.

Will, feeling walls, books, floors fly by, foolishly thought, pressed close, Why, why, Mr. Dark smells like . . . calliope steam!

Both boys were dropped suddenly. Before they could move or regain their breath, each was gripped by the hair on their head and roused marionettes-wise to face a window, a street.

"Boys, you read Dickens?" Mr. Dark whispered. "Critics hate his coincidences. But we know, don't we? life's *all* coincidence. Turn death and happenstance flakes off him like fleas from a killed ox. Look!"

Both boys writhed in the iron-maiden clutch of hungry saurians and bristly apes.

Will did not know whether to weep with joy or new despair.

Below, across the avenue, passing from church, going home, was his mother and Jim's mother.

Not on the carousel, not old, crazy, dead, in jail, but freshly out in the good October air. She had been not a hundred yards away in church during all the last five minutes!

Mom! screamed Will, against the hand which, anticipating his cry, clamped tight to his mouth.

"Mom," crooned Mr. Dark, mockingly. "Come save me!"

No, thought Will, save *yourself*, run!

But his mother and Jim's mother simply strolled content, from the warm church through town.

Mom! screamed Will again, and some small muffled bleat of it escaped the sweaty paw.

Will's mother, a thousand miles away over on that sidewalk, paused.

She *couldn't* have heard! thought Will. Yet—

She looked over at the library.

"Good," sighed Mr. Dark. "Excellent, fine."

Here! thought Will. See us, Mom! Run call the police!

"Why doesn't she look at this window?" asked Mr. Dark quietly. "And see us three standing as for a portrait. Look over. Then, come running. We'll let her *in*."

Will strangled a sob. No, no.

His mother's gaze trailed from the front entrance to the first-floor windows.

"Here," said Mr. Dark. "Second floor. A proper coincidence, let's make it proper."

Now Jim's mother was talking. Both women stood together at the curb.

No, thought Will, oh, no.

And the women turned and went away into the Sundaynight town.

Will felt the Illustrated Man slump the tiniest bit.

"Not much of a coincidence, no crisis, no one lost or saved. Pity. Well!"

Dragging the boys' feet, he glided down to open the front door.

Someone waited in the shadows.

A lizard hand scurried cold on Will's chin.

"Halloway," husked the Witch's voice.

A chameleon perched on Jim's nose.

"Nightshade," whisked the dry-broom voice.

Behind her stood the Dwarf and the Skeleton, silent, shifting, apprehensive.

Obedient to the occasion, the boys would have given their best stored yells air, but again, on the instant recognizing their need, the Illustrated Man trapped the sound before it could issue forth, then nodded curtly to the old dust woman.

The Witch toppled forward with her seamed black wax sewn-shut iguana eyelids and her great proboscis with the nostrils caked like tobacco-blackened pipe bowls, her fingers tracing, weaving a silent plinth of symbols on the mind.

The boys stared.

Her fingernails fluttered, darted, feathered cold winter-water air. Her pickled green frog's breath crawled their flesh in pimples as she sang softly, mewing, humming, glistering her babes, her boys, her friends of the slick snail-tracked roof, the straight-flung arrow, the stricken and sky-drowned balloon.

"Darning-needle dragonfly, sew up these mouths so they not speak!"

Touch, sew, touch, sew her thumbnail stabbed, punched, drew, stabbed, punched, drew along their lower, upper lips until they were thread-pouch shut with invisible thread.

"Darning needle-dragonfly, sew up these ears, so they not hear!"

Cold sand funneled Will's ears, burying her voice. Muffled, far away, fading, she chanted on with a rustle, tick, tickle, tap, flourish of caliper hands.

Moss grew in Jim's ears, swiftly sealing him deep.

"Darning needle-dragonfly, sew up these eyes so they not see!"

Her white-hot fingerprints rolled back their stricken eyeballs to throw the lids down with bangs like great tin doors slammed shut.

Will saw a billion flashbulbs explode, then suck to darkness while the unseen darning-needle insect out beyond somewhere pranced and fizzed like insect drawn to sun-warmed honeypot, as closeted voice stitched off their senses forever and a day beyond.

"Darning-needle dragonfly, have done with eye, ear,

lip and tooth, finish hem, sew dark, mound dust, heap with slumber sleep, now tie all knots ever so neat, pump silence in blood like sand in river deep. So. So."

The Witch, somewhere outside the boys, lowered her hands.

The boys stood silent. The Illustrated Man took his embrace from them and stepped back.

The woman from the Dust sniffed at her twin triumphs, ran her hand a last loving time over her statues.

The Dwarf toddled madly about in the boys' shadows, nibbling daintily at their fingernails, softly calling their names.

The Illustrated Man nodded toward the library.

"The janitor's clock. Stop it."

The Witch, mouth wide, savoring doom, wandered off into the marble quarry.

Mr. Dark said: "Left, right. One, two."

The boys walked down the steps, the Dwarf at Jim's side, the Skeleton at Will's.

Serene as death, the Illustrated Man followed.

CHAPTER FORTY-FOUR

Somewhere near, Charles Halloway's hand lay in a white-hot furnace, melted to sheer nerve and pain. He opened his eyes. At the same moment he heard a great breath as the front door swung shut and a woman's voice came singing in the hall:

"Old man, old man, old man, old man . . . ?"

Where his left hand should be was this swelled blood pudding which pulsed with such ecstasies of pain it fed forth his life, his will, his whole attention. He tried to sit up, but the pain hammerblowed him down again.

"Old man . . . ?"

Not old! Fifty-four's not old, he thought wildly.

And here she came on the worn stone floors, her moth-fingers tapping, scanning braille book titles, as her nostrils siphoned the shadows.

Charles Halloway hunched and crawled, hunched and crawled, toward the nearest stack, cramming pain back with his tongue. He must climb out of reach, climb where books might be weapons flung down upon any night-crawling pursuer. . . .

"Old man, hear you breathing. . . ."

She drifted on his tide, let her body be summoned by every sibilant hiss of his pain.

"Old man, feel your *hurt*. . . ."

If he could fling the hand, the pain, out the window! where it might lie beating like a heart, summoning her away, tricked, to go seek this awful fire. Bent in the street, he imagined her brisking her palms at this throb, an abandoned chunk of delirium.

But no, the hand stayed, glowed, poisoned the air, hurrying the strange nun-Gypsy's tread as she gasped her avaricious mouth most ardently.

"Damn you!" he cried. "Get it over with! I'm here!"

So the Witch wheeled swift as a black clothes dummy on rubber rollers and swayed over him.

He did not even look at her. Such weights and pressures of despair and exertion fought for his attention, he could only free his eyes to watch the inside of his lids upon which multiple and everchanging looms of terror jigged and gamboled.

"Very simple." The whisper bent low. "Stop the heart."

Why not, he thought, vaguely.

"Slow," she murmured.

Yes, he thought.

"Slow, very slow."

His heart, once bolting, now fell away to a strange disease, disquiet, then quiet, then ease.

"Much more slow, slow . . ." she suggested.

Tired, yes, you hear that, heart? he wondered.

His heart heard. Like a tight fist it began to relax, a finger at a time.

"Stop all for good, forget all for good," she whispered.

Well, why not?

"Slower . . . slowest."

His heart stumbled.

And then for no reason, save perhaps for a last look around, because he *did* want to get rid of the pain, and sleep was the way to do that . . . Charles Halloway opened his eyes.

He saw the Witch.

He saw her fingers working at the air, his face, his body, the heart within his body, and the soul within the heart. Her swamp breath flooded him while, with immense curiosity, he watched the poisonous drizzle from her lips, counted the folds in her stitch-wrinkled eyes, the Gila monster neck, the mummy-linen ears, the dry-rivulet river-sand brow. Never in his life had he focused so nearly to a person, as if she were a puzzle, which once touched together might show life's greatest secret. The solution was in her, it would all spring clear this moment, no, the next, no, the next, watch her scorpion fingers! hear her chant as she diddled the air, yes, diddled was it, tickling, tickling, "Slow!" she whispered. "Slow!" And his obedient heart pulled rein. Diddle-tickle went her fingers.

Charles Halloway snorted. Faintly, he giggled.

He caught this. Why? Why am I . . . giggling . . . at such a time!?

The Witch pulled back the merest quarter inch as if some strange but hidden electric light socket, touched with wet whorl, gave shock.

Charles Halloway saw but did not see her flinch, sensed but seemed in no way to consider her withdrawal, for almost immediately, seizing the initiative, she flung herself forward, not touching, but mutely gesticulating at his chest as one might try to spell an antique clock pendulum.

"Slow!" she cried.

Senselessly, he permitted an idiot smile to balloon itself up from somewhere to attach itself with careless ease under his nose.

"Slowest!"

Her new fever, her anxiety which changed itself to anger was even more of a toy to him. A part of his attention, secret until now, leaned forward to scan every pore of her Halloween face. Somehow, irresistibly, the prime thing was: nothing mattered. Life in the end seemed a prank of such size you could only stand off at this end of the corridor to note its meaningless length and its quite unnecessary height, a mountain built to such ridiculous immensities you were dwarfed in its shadow and mocking of its pomp. So with death this near he thought numbly but purely upon a billion vanities, arrivals, departures, idiot excursions of boy, boy-man, man and old-man goat. He had gathered and stacked all manner of foibles, devices, playthings of his egotism and now, between all the silly corridors of books, the toys of his life swayed. And none more grotesque than this thing named Witch Gypsy Reader-of-Dust, tickling, that's what! just *tickling* the air! Fool! Didn't she know what she was *doing!*

He opened his mouth.

Of itself, like a child born of an unsuspecting parent, one single raw laugh broke free.

The Witch swooned back.

Charles Halloway did not see. He was far too busy letting the joke rush through his fingers, letting hilarity spring forth of its own volition along his throat, eyes squeezed shut; there it flew, whipping shrapnel in all directions.

"You!" he cried, to no one, everyone, himself, her, them, it, all. "Funny! You!"

"No," the Witch protested.

"Stop tickling!" he gasped.

"Not!" she lunged back, frantically. "Not! Sleep! Slow! Very slow!"

"No, tickling is all it is, for sure!" he roared. "Oh, ha! Ha, stop!"

"Yes, *stop* heart!" she squealed. "*Stop* blood." Her own heart must have shaken like a tambourine; her hands shook. In mid-gesticulation she froze and became aware of the silly fingers.

"Oh, my God!" He wept beautiful glad tears. "Get off my ribs, oh, ha, go on, my heart!"

"Your *heart,* yesssssss!"

"God!" He popped his eyes wide, gulped air, released

more soap and water washing everything clear, incredibly clean. "Toys! The key sticks out your back! Who wound you up!?"

And the largest roar of all, flung at the woman, burnt her hands, seared her face, or so it seemed, for she seized herself as from a blast furnace, wrapped her fried hands in Egyptian rags, gripped her dry dugs, skipped back, gave pause, then started a slow retreat, nudged, pushed, pummeled inch by inch, foot by foot, clattering bookracks, shelves, fumbling for handholds on volumes that thrashed free as she scrambled them down. Her brow knocked dim histories, vain theories, duned-up time, promised but compromised years. Chased, bruised, beaten by his laugh which echoed, rang, swam to fill the marble vaults, she whirled at last, claws razoring the wild air and fled to fall downstairs.

Moments later, she managed to cram herself through the front door, which *slammed!*

Her fall, the door slam, almost broke his frame with laughter.

"Oh God, God, please stop, stop yourself!" he begged of his hilarity.

And thus begged, his humor let be.

In mid-roar, at last, all faded to honest laughter, pleasant chuckling, faint giggling, then softly and with great contentment receiving and giving breath, shaking his happy-weary head, the good ache of action in his throat and ribs, gone from his crumpled hand. He lay against the stacks, head leaned to some dear befriending book, the tears of releaseful mirth salting his cheeks, and suddenly knew her gone.

Why? he wondered. *What did I do?*

With one last bark of mirth, he rose up, slow.

What's happened? Oh, God, let's get it clear! First, the drug store, a half-dozen aspirin to cure this hand for an hour, then, *think*. In the last five minutes you did win something, *didn't* you? What's victory taste like? Think! Try to remember!

And smiling a new smile at the ridiculous dead-animal left hand nested in his right crooked elbow, he hurried down the night corridors, and out into town. . . .

III. DEPARTURES

CHAPTER FORTY-FIVE

The small parade moved, soundless, past the eternally revolving, ending-but-unending candy serpentine of Mr. Crosetti's barber pole, past all the darkening or darkened shops, the emptying streets, for people were home now from the church suppers, or out at the carnival for the last side show or the last high-ladder diver floating like milkweed down the night.

Will's feet, far away below, clubbed the sidewalk. One, two, he thought, someone tells me left, right. Dragonfly whispers: one-two.

Is Jim in the parade?! Will's eyes flicked the briefest to one side. Yes! But who's the other little one? The gone-mad, everything's-interesting-so-touch-it, everything's red-hot, pull-back, Dwarf! Plus the Skeleton. And then behind, who were all those hundreds, no, thousands of people marching along, breathing down his neck?

The Illustrated Man.

Will nodded and whined so high and silently that only dogs, dogs who were no help, dogs who could not speak, might hear.

And sure enough, looking obliquely over, he saw not one, not two, but three dogs who, smelling the occasion, their own parade, now ran ahead, now fell behind, their tails like guidons for the platoon.

Bark! thought Will, like in the movies! Bark, bring the police!

But the dogs just smiled and trotted.

Coincidence, please, thought Will. Just a *small* one!

Mr. Tetley! Yes! Will saw-but-did-not-see Mr. Tetley! Rolling the wooden Indian back into his shop, closing for the night!

"Turn heads," murmured the Illustrated Man.

Jim turned his head. Will turned his head.

Mr. Tetley smiled.

"Smile," murmured Mr. Dark.

The two boys smiled.

"Hello!" said Mr. Tetley.

"Say hello," someone whispered.

"Hello," said Jim.

"Hello," said Will.

The dogs barked.

"A free ride at the carnival," murmured Mr. Dark.

"Free ride," said Will.

"At the carnival!" clacked Jim.

Then, like good machines, they shut up their smiles.

"Have fun!" called Mr. Tetley.

The dogs barked joy.

The parade marched on.

"Fun," said Mr. Dark. "Free rides. When the crowds go home, half an hour from now. We'll ride Jim round. You still *want* that, Jim?"

Hearing but not hearing, locked away in himself, Will thought, Jim, don't listen!

Jim's eyes slid: wet or oily, it was hard to tell.

"You'll travel with us, Jim, and if Mr. Cooger doesn't survive (it's a near thing for him, we haven't saved him yet, we'll try again now) but if he doesn't make it, Jim, how would you like to be partners? I'll grow you to a fine strong age, eh? Twenty-two? twenty-five?! Dark and Nightshade, Nightshade and Dark, sweet lovely names for such as we with such as the side shows to run around the world! What say, Jim?"

Jim said nothing, sewn up in the Witch's dream.

Don't listen! wailed his best friend, who heard nothing but heard it all.

"And Will?" said Mr. Dark. "Let's ride *him* back and back, eh? Make him a babe in arms, a babe for the Dwarf to carry like a clown-child, roundabout in parades, every day for the next fifty years, would you like that, Will? to be a babe forever? not able to talk and tell all the lovely things you know? Yes, I think that's best for Will. A plaything, a little wet friend for the Dwarf!"

Will must have screamed.

But not out loud.

For only the dogs barked, in terror; yiping, off they ran, as if pelted with rocks.

A man came around the corner.

A policeman.

"Who's this?" muttered Mr. Dark.

"Mr. Kolb," said Jim.

"Mr. Kolb!" said Will.

"Darning-needle," whispered Mr. Dark. "Dragonfly."

Pain stabbed Will's ears. Moss stuffed his eyes. Gum glued his teeth. He felt a multitudinous tapping, shuttling, weaving, about his face, all numb again.

"Say hello to Mr. Kolb."

"Hello," said Jim.

". . . Kolb . . ." said the dreaming Will.

"Hello, boys. Gentlemen."

"Turn here," said Mr. Dark.

They turned.

Away toward meadow country, away from warm lights, good town, safe streets, the drumless march. progressed.

CHAPTER FORTY-SIX

Stretched out over a mile of territory the straggling parade now moved as follows:

At the edge of the carnival midway, stumping the grass with their dead feet, Jim and Will paced friends who constantly retold the wondrous uses of darning-needle dragonflies.

Behind, a good half mile, trying to catch up, walking mysteriously wounded, the Gypsy, who whorl-symboled the dust.

And yet farther back came the janitor-father, now slowing himself with remembrances of age, now pacing swiftly young with thoughts of the brief first encounter and victory, carrying his left hand patted to his chest, chewing medicines as he went.

At the midway rim, Mr. Dark looked back as if an inner voice had named the stragglers in his widely separated maneuver. But the voice failed, he was unsure. He nodded briskly, and Dwarf, Skeleton, Jim, Will thrust through the crowd.

Jim felt the river of bright people wash by all around but not touching. Will heard waterfall laughter here, there, and him walking through the downpour. An explosion of fireflies blossomed on the sky; the ferris wheel, exultant as a titanic fireworks, dilated above them.

Then they were at the Mirror Maze and sidling, colliding, bumping, careening through the unfolded ice ponds where stricken spider-stung boys much like themselves appeared, vanished a thousand times over.

That's *me!* thought Jim.

But I can't help me, thought Will, no matter how many of me there are!

And crowd of boys, plus crowd of reflected Mr. Dark's illustrations, for he had taken off his coat and shirt now, crammed and crushed through to the Waxworks at the end of the maze.

"Sit," said Mr. Dark. "Stay."

Among the wax figures of murdered, gunshot, guillotined, garroted men and women the two boys sat like Egyptian cats, unblinked, untwitched, unswallowing.

Some late visitors passed through, laughing. They commented on all the wax figures.

They did not notice the thin line of saliva crept from the corner of one "wax" boy's mouth.

They did not see how bright was the second "wax" boy's stare, which suddenly brimmed and ran clear water down his cheek.

Outside, the Witch limped in through back alleys of rope and peg between the tents.

"Ladies and gentlemen!"

The last crowd of the night, three or four hundred strong, turned as a body.

The Illustrated Man, stripped to the waist, all nightmare viper, sabertooth, libidinous ape, clotted vulture, all salmon-sulphur sky rose up with annunciations:

"The last free event this evening! Come one! Come all!"

The crowd surged toward the main platform outside

the freak tent, where stood Dwarf, Skeleton, and Mr. Dark.

"The Most Amazingly Dangerous, ofttimes Fatal— World Famous BULLET TRICK!"

The crowd gasped with pleasure.

"The rifles, if you please!"

The Thin One cracked wide a racked display of bright artillery.

The Witch, hurrying up, froze when Mr. Dark cried: "And here, our death-defier, the bullet-catcher who will stake her life—Mademoiselle Tarot!"

The Witch shook her head, bleated, but Dark's hand swept down to swing her like a child to the platform, still protesting, which gave Dark pause, but, in front of everyone now, he went on:

"A volunteer, please, to fire the rifle!"

The crowd rumbled softly, daring itself to speak up.

Mr. Dark's mouth barely moved. Under his breath he asked, "Is the clock stopped?"

"Not," she whined, "stopped."

"No?" he almost burst out.

He burnt her with his eyes, then turned to the audience and let his mouth finish the spiel, his fingers rapping over the rifles.

"Volunteers, please!"

"Stop the act," the Witch cried softly, wringing her hands.

"It goes on, damn you, *worse* than double-damn you," he whispered, whistled fiercely.

Secretly, Dark gathered a pinch of flesh on his wrist, the illustration of a black-nun blind woman, which he bit with his fingernails.

The Witch spasmed, seized her breast, groaned, ground her teeth. "Mercy!" she hissed, half aloud.

Silence from the crowd.

Mr. Dark nodded swiftly.

"Since there are no volunteers—" He scraped his illustrated wrist. The Witch shuddered. "We will cancel our last act and—"

"Here! A volunteer!"

The crowd turned.

Mr. Dark recoiled, then asked: "Where?"

"Here."

Far out at the edge of the crowd, a hand lifted, a path opened.

Mr. Dark could see very clearly the man standing there, alone.

Charles Halloway, citizen, father, introspective husband, night-wanderer, and janitor of the town library.

CHAPTER FORTY-SEVEN

The crowd's appreciative clamor faded.

Charles Halloway did not move.

He let the path grow leading down to the platform.

He could not see the expression on the faces of the freaks standing up there. His eyes swept the crowd and found the Mirror Maze, the empty oblivion which beckoned with ten times a thousand million light years of reflections, counterreflections, reversed and double-reversed, plunging deep to nothing, face-falling to nothing, stomach-dropping away to yet more sickening plummets of nothing.

And yet, wasn't there an echo of two boys in the powdered silver at the back of each glass? Did or did he not perceive, with the tremulous tip of eyelash if not the eye, their passage through, their wait beyond, warm wax amongst cold, waiting to be key-wound by terrors, run free in panics?

No, thought Charles Halloway, don't think. Get on with this!

"Coming!" he shouted.

"Go get 'em, Pop!" a man said.

"Yes," said Charles Halloway. "I will."

And he walked down through the crowd.

The Witch spun slowly, magnetized at the night-wandering volunteer's approach. Her eyelids jerked at their sewn black-wax threads behind dark glasses.

Mr. Dark, the illustration-drenched, superinfested civilization of souls, leaned from the platform, gladly whetting his lips. Thoughts spun fiery Catherine wheels in his eyes, quick, quick, what, what, *what!*

And the aging janitor, fixing a smile to his face like a white celluloid set of teeth from a Cracker Jack box, strode on, and the crowd opened as the sea before Moses and closed behind, and him wondering what to do? why was he here? but on the move, steadily, nevertheless.

Charles Halloway's foot touched the first step of the platform.

The Witch trembled secretly.

Mr. Dark felt this secret, glanced sharply. Swiftly he put his hand out to grab for the good right hand of this fifty-four-year-old man.

But the fifty-four-year-old man shook his head, would not give his hand to be held, touched, or helped up. "Thanks, no."

On the platform, Charles Halloway waved to the crowd. The people set off a few firecrackers of applause.

"But—" Mr. Dark was amazed—"your left hand, sir, you can't hold and fire a rifle if you have only the use of one hand!"

Charles Halloway paled.

"I'll do it," he said. "With one hand."

"Hoorah!" cried a boy, below.

"Go it, Charlie!" a man called, out beyond.

Mr. Dark flushed as the crowd laughed and applauded even louder now. He lifted his hands to ward off the wave of refreshing sound, like rain that washed in from the people.

"All right, all right! Let's see if he *can* do it!"

Brutally, the Illustrated Man snapped a rifle from its locks, hurled it through the air.

The crowd gasped.

Charles Halloway ducked. He put up his right hand. The rifle slapped his palm. He grabbed. It did not fall. He had it good.

The audience hooted, said things against Mr. Dark's bad manners which made him turn away for a moment, damning himself, silently.

Will's father lifted the rifle, beaming.

The crowd roared.

And while the wave of applause came in, crashed, and went back down the shore, he looked again to the maze, where the sensed but unseen shadow-shapes of Will and Jim were filed among titanic razor blades of revelation and illusion, then back to the Medusa gaze of Mr. Dark, swiftly reckoned with, and on to the stitched and jittering sightless nun of midnight, sidling back still more. Now she was as far as she could sidle, at the far end of the platform, almost pressed to the whorled red-black rifle bull's-eye target.

"Boy!" shouted Charles Halloway.

Mr. Dark stiffened.

"I need a boy volunteer to help me hold the rifle!" shouted Charles Halloway.

"Someone! Anyone!" he shouted.

A few boys in the crowd shifted around on their toes.

"Boy!" shouted Charles Halloway. "Hold on. My son's out there. He'll volunteer, *won't* you, Will?"

The Witch flung one hand up to feel the shape of this audacity which came off the fifty-four-year-old man like a fever. Mr. Dark was spun round as if hit by a fast-traveling gunshot.

"Will!" called his father.

In the Wax Museum, Will sat motionless.

"Will!" called his father. "Come on, boy!"

The crowd looked left, looked right, looked back.

No answer.

Will sat in the Wax Museum.

Mr. Dark observed all of this with some respect, some degree of admiration, some concern; he seemed to be waiting, just as was Will's father.

"Will, come help your old man!" Mr. Halloway cried, jovially.

Will sat in the Wax Museum.

Mr. Dark smiled.

"Will! Willy! Come here!"

No answer.

Mr. Dark smiled more.

"Willy! Don't you hear your old man?"

Mr. Dark stopped smiling.

For this last was the voice of a gentleman in the crowd, speaking up.

The crowd laughed.

"Will!" called a woman.

"Willy!" called another.

"Yoohoo!" A gentleman in a beard.

"Come on, William!" A boy.

The crowd laughed more, jostled elbows.

Charles Halloway called. *They* called. Charles Halloway cried to the hills. *They* cried to the hills.

"Will! Willy! William!"

A shadow shuttled and wove in the mirrors.

The Witch broke out chandeliers of sweat.

"There!"

The crowd stopped calling.

As did Charles Halloway, choked on the name of his son now, and silent.

For Will stood in the entrance of the Maze, like the wax figure that he almost was.

"Will," called his father, softly.

The sound of this chimed the sweat off the Witch.

Will moved, unseeing, through the crowd.

And handing the rifle down like a cane for the boy to grasp, his father drew him up onto the stand.

"Here's my good left hand!" announced the father.

Will neither saw nor heard the crowd sound forth a solid and offensive applause.

Mr. Dark had not moved, though Charles Halloway could see him, during all this, lighting and setting off cannon crackers in his head; but each, one by one, fizzled and died. Mr. Dark could not guess what they were up to. For that matter, Charles Halloway did not know or guess. It was as if he had written this play for himself, over the years, in the library, nights, torn up the play after memorizing it, and now forgotten what he had set forth to remember. He was relying on secret discoveries of self, moment by moment, playing by ear, no! heart and soul! And . . . *now?!*

The brightness of his teeth seemed to strike the Witch

blinder! Impossible! She flung one hand to her glasses, her sewn eyelids!

"Closer, everyone!" called Will's father.

The crowd gathered in. The platform was an island. The sea was people.

"Watch the bull's-eye targeteer!"

The Witch melted in her rags.

The Illustrated Man looked left, found no pleasure in the Skeleton, who simply looked thinner; found no pleasure looking right to a Dwarf who blandly dwelt in squashed idiot madness.

"The bullet, please!" Will's father said, amiably.

The thousand illustrations on his jerking horseflesh frame did not hear, so why should Mr. Dark?

"If you please," said Charles Halloway. "The bullet? So I may knock that flea off the old Gypsy's wart!"

Will stood motionless.

Mr. Dark hesitated.

Out in the choppy sea, smiles flashed, here, there, a hundred, two hundred, three hundred whitenesses, as if a vast titillation of water had been provoked by a lunar gravity. The tide ebbed.

The Illustrated Man, in slow motion, proffered the bullet. His arm, a long molasses undulation, lazed to offer the bullet to the boy, to see if he would notice; he did not notice.

His father took the missile.

"Mark it with your initials," said Mr. Dark, by rote.

"No, with more!" Charles Halloway raised his son's hand and made him hold the bullet, so he could take a penknife with his one good hand and carve a strange symbol on the lead.

What's happening? Will thought. I know what's happening. I don't know what's happening? What!?

Mr. Dark saw a crescent moon on the bullet, saw nothing wrong with such a moon, rammed it in the rifle, slapped the rifle back at Will's father, who once more caught it deftly.

"Ready, Will?"

The boy's peach face drowsed in the slightest nod.

Charles Halloway flicked a last glance at the maze, thought, Jim, you there still? Get ready!

Mr. Dark turned to go pat, conjure, calm his dust-crone friend, but cracked to a halt at the crack of the rifle being reopened, the bullet ejected by Will's father, to assure the audience it was there. It seemed real enough, yet he had read long ago that this was a substitute bullet, shaped of a very hard steel-colored crayon wax. Shot through the rifle it would dissolve out the barrel as smoke and vapor. At this very moment, having somehow switched bullets, the Illustrated Man was slipping the real marked bullet into the Witch's jerking fingers. She would hide it in her cheek. At the shot, she would pretend to jolt under the imagined impact, then reveal the bullet caught by her yellow rat teeth. Fanfare! Applause!

The Illustrated Man, glancing up, saw Charles Halloway with the opened rifle, the wax bullet. But instead of revealing what he knew, Mr. Halloway simply said, "Let's cut our mark more clearly, eh, boy?" And with his penknife, the boy holding the bullet in his senseless hand, he marked this fresh new wax unmarked bullet with the same mysterious crescent moon, then snapped it back into the rifle.

"Ready?!"

Mr. Dark looked to the Witch.

Who hesitated, then nodded, once, faintly.

"Ready!" announced Charles Halloway.

And all about lay the tents, the breathing crowd, the anxious freaks, a Witch iced with hysteria, Jim hidden to be found, an ancient mummy still seated glowing with blue fire in his electric chair, and a merry-go-round waiting for the show to cease, the crowd to go, and the carnival to have its way with boys and janitor trapped, if possible, and alone.

"Will," said Charles Halloway conversationally, as he lifted the now suddenly heavy rifle. "Your shoulder here is my brace. Take the middle of the rifle, gently, with one hand. Take it, Will." The boy raised a hand. "That's it, son. When I say 'hold,' hold your breath. Hear me?"

The boy's head tremored with the slightest affirmation.

He slept. He dreamed. The dream was nightmare. The nightmare was *this*.

And the next part of this was his father shouting:

"Ladies! Gentlemen!"

The Illustrated Man clenched his fist. Will's picture, lost in it, like a flower, was crushed.

Will twisted.

The rifle fell.

Charles Halloway pretended not to notice.

"Me and Will here will now, together, him being the good left arm I can't use, do the one and only most dangerous, sometimes fatal, Bullet Trick!"

Applause. Laughter.

Quickly the fifty-four-year-old janitor, denying each year, laid the rifle back on the boy's jerking shoulder.

"Hear that, Will? Listen! That's for *us!*"

The boy listened. The boy grew calm.

Mr. Dark tightened his fist.

Will was taken with slight palsy.

"We'll hit 'em bull's-eye on, won't we, boy!" said his father.

More laughter.

And the boy grew very calm indeed, with the rifle on his shoulder, and Mr. Dark squeezed tight on the peach-fuzz face nestled in the flesh of his hand, but the boy was serene in the laughter which still flowed and his father kept the hoop rolling thus:

"Show the lady your teeth, Will!"

Will showed the woman against the target his teeth.

The blood fell away from the Witch's face.

Now Charles Halloway showed her his teeth, too, such as they were.

And winter lived in the Witch.

"Boy," said someone in the audience, "she's great. Acts scared! Look!"

I'm looking, thought Will's father, his left hand useless at his side, his right hand up to the rifle trigger, his face to the sight as his son held the rifle unswervingly pointed at the bull's-eye and the Witch's face superimposed there, and the last moment come, and a wax bullet in the chamber, and what could a wax bullet do? A bullet that dissolved in transit, what use? why were they here, what could they do? silly, silly!

No! thought Will's father. Stop!

He stopped the doubts.

He felt his mouth shape words with no sound.

But, the Witch heard what he said.

Above the dying laughter, before the warm sound was completely gone, he made these words, silently with his lips:

The crescent moon I have marked on the bullet is not a crescent moon.

It is my own smile.

I have put my smile on the bullet in the rifle.

He said it once.

He waited for her to understand.

He said it, silently, again.

And in the moment before the Illustrated Man himself translated the mouthings, quickly, Charles Halloway cried, faintly, "Hold!" Will held his breath. Far back among wax statues, Jim, hid away, dripped saliva from his chin. Strapped in electric chair a dead-alive mummy hummed power in its teeth. Mr. Dark's illustrations writhed with sick sweat as he clenched his fist a final time, but—too late! Serene, Will held breath, held weapon. Serene, his father said, *"Now."*

And fired the rifle.

CHAPTER FORTY-EIGHT

One shot!

The Witch sucked breath.

Jim, in the Wax Museum, sucked breath.

As did Will, asleep.

As did his father.

As did Mr. Dark.

As did all the freaks.

As did the crowd.

The Witch screamed.

Jim, among the wax dummies, blew all the air from his lungs.

Will shrieked himself awake, on the platform.

The Illustrated Man let the air from his mouth in a great angry bray, whipping up his hands to stop all events. But the Witch fell. She fell off the platform. She fell in the dust.

The smoking rifle in his one good hand, Charles Halloway let his breath go slow, feeling every bit of it move from him. He still stared along the rifle sights at the target where the woman had been.

At the platform rim, Mr. Dark looked down at the screaming crowd and what they were screaming about.

"She's fainted—"

"No, she slipped!"

"She's . . . shot!"

At last Charles Halloway came to stand by the Illustrated Man, looking down. There were many things in his face: surprise, dismay, and some small strange relief and satisfaction.

The woman was lifted and put on the platform. Her mouth was frozen open, almost with a look of recognition.

He knew she was dead. In a moment, the crowd would know. He watched the Illustrated Man's hand move down to touch, trace, feel for life. Then Mr. Dark lifted both her hands, like a doll, in some marionette strategy, to give her motion. But the body refused.

So he gave one of the Witch's arms to the Dwarf, the other to the Skeleton, and they shook and moved them in a ghastly semblance of reawakening as the crowd backed.

". . . dead . . ."

"But . . . there's no wound."

"Shock, you think?"

Shock, thought Charles Halloway, my God, did *that* kill her? Or the other bullet? When I fired the shot, did she suck the *other* bullet down her throat? Did she . . . choke on my smile! Oh, Christ!

"It's all right! Show's over! Just fainted!" said Mr.

Dark. "All an act! All part of the show," he said, not looking at the woman, not looking at the crowd, but looking at Will, who stood blinking around, out of one nightmare and fresh into the next as his father stood with him and Mr. Dark cried: "Everyone home! Show's over! Lights! Lights!"

The carnival lights flickered.

The crowd, herded before the failing illumination, turned like a great carousel, and as the lamps dimmed, hustled toward the few remaining pools of light as if to warm themselves there before braving the wind. One by one, one by one, the lights indeed were going off.

"Lights!" said Mr. Dark.

"Jump!" said Will's father.

Will jumped. Will ran with his father who still carried the weapon that had fired the smile that had killed the Gypsy and put her to dust.

"Is Jim in there?"

They were at the maze. Behind them, on the platform, Mr. Dark bellowed: "Lights! Go home! All over! Done!"

"*Is* Jim in there?" wondered Will. "Yes. Yes, he is!"

Inside the Wax Museum, Jim still had not moved, had not blinked.

"Jim!" The voice came through the maze.

Jim moved. Jim blinked. A rear exit door stood wide. Jim blundered toward it.

"I'm coming for you, Jim!"

"No, Dad!"

Will caught at his father, who stood at the first turn of the mirrors with the pain come back to his hand, racing up along the nerves to strike a fireball near his heart. "Dad, don't go in!" Will grabbed his good arm.

Behind them, the platform was empty, Mr. Dark was running . . . where? Somewhere as the night shut in, the lights went off, went off, went off, the night sucked around, gathering, whistling, simpering, and the crowd, like a shake of leaves from one huge tree, blew off the midway, and Will's father stood facing the glass tides, the waves, the gauntlet of horror he knew waited for him to swim through, stride through to fight the desiccation, the annihilation of one's self that waited there. He had

seen enough to know. Eyes shut, you'd be lost. Eyes open,
you'd know such utter despair, such gravities of anguish
would weight you, you might never drag past the twelfth
turn. But Charles Halloway took Will's hands away.
"Jim's there. Jim, wait! I'm coming in!"

And Charles Halloway took the next step into the
maze.

Ahead flowed sluices of silver light, deep slabs of
shadow, polished, wiped, rinsed with images of themselves
and others whose souls, passing, scoured the glass with
their agony, curried the cold ice with their narcissism,
or sweated the angles and flats with their fear.

"Jim!"

He ran. Will ran. They stopped.

For the lights in here were going blind, one by one,
going dim, changing color, now blue, now a color like
lilac summer lightning which flared in haloes, then a
flickerlight like a thousand ancient windblown candles.

And between himself and Jim in need of rescue, stood
an army of one million sick-mouthed, frost-haired, white-
tine-bearded men.

Them! all of them! he thought. That's *me!*

Dad! thought Will, at his back, don't be afraid. It's
only you. All only my father!

But he did not like their look. They were so old, so
very old, and got much older the farther away they
marched, wildly gesticulating, as Dad threw up his hands
to fend off the revelation, this wild image repeated to insanity.

Dad! he thought, it's you!

But, it was more.

And all the lights went out.

And both, squeezed still, in muffle-gasping silence,
stood afraid.

CHAPTER FORTY-NINE

A hand dug like a mole in the dark.

Will's hand.

It emptied his pockets, it delved, it rejected, it dug again. For while it was dark he knew those million old men might march, hustle, rush, leap, smash Dad with what they *were!* In this shut-up night, with just four seconds to think of them, they might do *anything* to Dad! If Will didn't hurry, these legions from Time Future, all the alarms of coming life, so mean, raw, and true you couldn't deny that's how Dad'd look tomorrow, next day, the day after the day after that, that cattle run of possible years might sweep Dad under!

So, quick!

Who has more pockets than a magician?

A boy.

Whose pockets contain *more* than a magician's?

A boy's.

Will seized forth kitchen matches!

"Oh God, Dad, here!"

He struck the match.

The stampede was close!

They had come running. Now, fixed by light, they widened their eyes, as did Dad, amazed their mouths at their own ancient quakes and masquerades. Halt! the match had cried. And platoons left, squads right, had stilt-muscled themselves to fitful rest, to baleful glare, itching for the match to whiff out. Then, given lease to run next time, they'd hit this old, very old, much older, terribly old man, suffocate him with Fates in one instant.

"No!" said Charles Halloway.

No. A million dead lips moved.

Will thrust the match forward. In the mirrors, a wizened multiplication of boy-apes did likewise, posing a single rosebud of blue-yellow flame.

"No!"

Every glass threw javelins of light which invisibly pierced, sank deep, found heart, soul, lungs, to frost the veins, cut nerves, send Will to ruin, paralyze and then kick-football heart. Hamstrung, the old old man foundered to his knees, as did his suppliant images, his congregation of terrified selves one week, one month, two years, twenty, fifty, seventy, ninety years from now! every second, minute, and long-after-midnight hour of his possible survival into insanity, there all sank grayer, more yellow as the mirrors ricocheted him through, bled him lifeless, mouthed him dry, then threatened to whiff him to skeletal dusts and litter his moth ashes to the floor.

"No!"

Charles Halloway struck the match from his son's hand.

"Dad, don't!"

For in the new dark, the restive herd of old men shambled forward, hearts hammering.

"Dad, we gotta *see!*"

He struck his second and final match.

And in the flare saw Dad sunk down, eyes clenched, fists tight, and all those other men who would have to shunt, crawl, scramble on knees once this last light was gone. Will grabbed his father's shoulder and shook him.

"Oh, Dad, Dad, I don't care how old you are, ever! I don't care what, I don't care anything! Oh, Dad," he cried, weeping. "I love you!"

At which Charles Halloway opened his eyes and saw himself and the others like himself and his son behind holding him, the flame trembling, the tears trembling on his face, and suddenly, as before, the image of the Witch, the memory of the library, defeat for one, victory for another, swam before him, mixed with sound of rifle shot, flight of marked bullet, surge of fleeing crowd.

For only a moment longer he looked at all of himselves, at Will. A small sound escaped his mouth. A little larger sound escaped his mouth.

And then, at last, he gave the maze, the mirrors, and all Time ahead, Beyond, Around, Above, Behind, Beneath or squandered inside himself, the only answer possible.

He opened his mouth very wide, and let the loudest sound of all free.

The Witch, if she were alive, would have known that sound, and died again.

CHAPTER FIFTY

Jim Nightshade, out the back door of the maze, lost on the carnival grounds, running, stopped.

The Illustrated Man, somewhere among the black tents, running, stopped.

The Dwarf froze.

The Skeleton turned.

All had heard.

Not the sound that Charles Halloway made, no.

But the terrific sounds that followed.

One mirror alone, and then a second mirror, followed by a pause, and then a third mirror, and a fourth and another after that and another after that and still another and another after that, in domino fashion, they formed swift spiderwebs over their fierce stares and then with faint tinkles and sharp cracks, fell.

One minute there was this incredible Jacob's ladder of glass, folding, refolding and folding away yet again images pressed in a book of light. The next, all shattered to meteor precipitation.

The Illustrated Man, halted, listening, felt his own eyes, crystal, almost spiderweb and splinter with the sounds.

It was as if Charles Halloway, once more a choirboy in a strange sub-sub-demon church had sung the most beautiful high note of amiable humor ever in his life which first shook moth-silver from the mirror backs, then shook images from glass faces, then shook glass itself to ruin. A dozen, a hundred, a thousand mirrors, and with them the ancient images of Charles Halloway, sank earthward in delicious moonfalls of snow and sleety water.

All because of the sound he had let come from his lungs through his throat out his mouth.

All because he accepted everything at last, accepted the carnival, the hills beyond, the people in the hills, Jim, Will, and above all himself and all of life, and, accepting, threw back his head for the second time tonight and showed his acceptance with sound.

And lo! like Jericho and the trump, with musical thunders the glass gave up its ghosts, Charles Halloway cried out, released. He took his hands from his face. Fresh starlight and dying carnival glow rushed in to set him free. The reflected dead men were gone, buried under the cymbaled slide, the splash and surfing of glass at his feet.

"Lights . . . lights!"

A far voice cried away more warmth.

The Illustrated Man, unfrozen, vanished among the tents.

The crowd was now gone.

"Dad, what'd you *do?*"

But the match burned Will's fingers, he dropped it, but now there was dim light enough to see Dad shuffle the trash, stir the mess of mirrored glass, heading back through the empty places where the maze had been and was no more.

"Jim?"

A door stood open. Pale carnival illumination, fading, poured through to show them wax figures of murderers and murderees.

Jim did not sit among them.

"Jim!"

They stared at the open door through which Jim had run to be lost in the swarms of night between black canvases.

The last electric light bulb went out.

"We'll *never* find him now," said Will.

"Yes," said his father, standing in the dark. "We'll find him."

Where? Will thought, and stopped.

Far down the midway, the carousel steamed, the calliope tortured itself with musics.

There, thought Will. If Jim's anywhere, it's there, to the music, old funny Jim, the free-ride ticket hid in his pocket still, I bet! Oh, damn Jim, damn him, damn him! he cried, and then thought, no! don't *you*, he's damned already, or near it! So how do we find him in the dark, no matches, no lights, just the two of us, all of them, and us alone in their territory?

"How—" said Will, aloud.

But his father said "There," very softly. With gratitude.

And Will stepped to the door, which was lighter now. The moon! Thank God.

It was rising from the hills.

"The police . . . ?"

"No time. It's the next few minutes or nothing. Three people we got to worry about—"

"The freaks!"

"Three people, Will. Number one, Jim, number two, Mr. Cooger frying in his Electric Chair. Number three, Mr. Dark and his skinful of souls. Save one, kick the other two to hell and gone. Then I think the freaks go, too. You ready, Will?"

Will eyed the door, the tents, the dark, the sky with new light paling it.

"God bless the moon."

Hands tight together, they stepped out the door.

As if to greet them, the wind flung up and down all the tent canvases in a great prehistoric thunder-kite display of leprous wings.

CHAPTER FIFTY-ONE

They ran in urine smell of shadow, they ran in clean ice smell of moon.

The calliope steam-throb whispered, tatted, trilled.

The music! thought Will, is it running backward or forward?

"Which way?" Dad whispered.

"Through here!" Will pointed.

A hundred yards off, beyond a foothill of tents, there was a flare of blue light, sparks jumped up and fell away, then dark again.

Mr. Electrico! thought Will. They're trying to move him, sure! Get him to the merry-go-round, kill or cure! And if they cure him, then, oh gosh, then, it's angry him and angry Illustrated Man against just Dad and me! And Jim? Well, where was Jim? This way one day, that way the next, and . . . tonight? Whose side would he wind up on? Ours! Old friend Jim! Ours, of course! But Will trembled. Did friends last forever, then? For eternity, could they be counted to a warm, round, and handsome sum?

Will glanced left.

The Dwarf stood half enfolded by tent flaps, waiting, motionless.

"Dad, look," cried Will, softly. "And there—the Skeleton."

Further over, the tall man, the man all marble bone and Egyptian papyrus stood like a dead tree.

"The freaks—why don't they stop us?"

"Scared."

"Of *us*?!"

Will's father crouched and squinted out from around an empty cage.

"They're walking wounded, anyway. They saw what happened to the Witch. That's the only answer. Look at them."

And there they stood, like uprights, like tent poles spotted all through the meadow grounds, hiding in shadow, waiting. For what? Will swallowed, hard. Maybe not hiding at all, but spread out for the running fight to come. At the right time, Mr. Dark would yell and—they'd just circle in. But the time wasn't right. Mr. Dark was busy. When he'd done what must be done, then he'd give that yell. So? So, thought Will, we got to see he never yells at all.

Will's feet slithered in the grass.

Will's father moved ahead.

The freaks watched with moon-glass eyes as they passed.

The calliope changed. It whistled sadly, sweetly, around a curve of tents, around a riverflow of darkness.

It's going ahead! thought Will. Yes! It *was* going backward. But now it stopped and started again, and this time forward! What's Mr. Dark *up* to?

"Jim!" Will burst out.

"Sh!" Dad shook him.

But the name had tumbled from his mouth only because he heard the calliope summing the golden years ahead, felt Jim isolate somewhere, pulled by warm gravities, swung by sunrise notes, wondering what it could be like to stand sixteen, seventeen, eighteen years tall, and then, oh then, nineteen and, most incredible!—twenty! The great wind of time blew in the brass pipes, a fine, a jolly, a summer tune, promising everything and even Will, hearing, began to run toward the music that grew up like a peach tree full of sun-ripe fruit—

No! he thought.

And instead made his feet step to his own fear, jump to his own tune, a hum cramped back by throat, held fast by lungs, which shook the bones of his head and drowned the calliope away.

"There," said Dad softly.

And between the tents, ahead, in transit, they saw a grotesque parade. Like a dark sultan in a palanquin, a half-familiar figure rode a chair borne on the shoulders of assorted sizes and shapes of darkness.

At Dad's cry, the parade jolted, then broke into a run!

"Mr. Electrico!" said Will.

They're taking him to the carousel!

The parade vanished.

A tent lay between them.

"Around here!" Will jumped, pulling his father.

The calliope played sweet. To pull Jim, to draw Jim. And when the parade arrived with Electrico?

Back the music would spin, back the carousel run, to shard away his skin, to freshen forth his years!

Will stumbled, fell. Dad picked him up.

And then . . .

There arose a human barking, yapping, baying, whining, as if *all* had fallen. In a long-drawn moan, a gasp, a shuddering sigh, an entire crowd of people with crippled throats made chorus together.

"Jim! They've got Jim!"

"No . . ." murmured Charles Halloway, strangely. "Maybe Jim . . . or us . . . got *them*."

They stepped around the last tent.

Wind blew dust in their faces.

Will clapped his hand up, squinched his nose. The dust was antique spice, burnt maple leaves, a prickling blue that teemed and sifted to earth. Swarming its own shadows, the dust filtered over the tents.

Charles Halloway sneezed. Figures jumped and scurried away from an upended, half-tilted object abandoned half-way between one tent and the carousel.

The object was the electric chair, capsized, with straps dangling from wooden arms and legs, and a metal headcap hanging from its top.

"But," said Will. "Where's Mr. Electrico!? I mean . . . Mr. Cooger!?"

"*That* must have been him."

"*What* must have been him?"

But the answer was there, sifting down the midway in the whorling wind devils . . . the burnt spice, the autumn incense that had floured them when they turned this corner.

Kill or cure, Charles Halloway thought. He imagined them rushed in the last few seconds, toting the ancient dustsack boneheap over starched grasses in his disconnected chair, perhaps only one in a running series of attempts to foster, encourage, preserve life in what was really nothing but a mortuary junkpile, rust-flakes and dying coals that no wind could blow alight again. Yet they must try. How many times in the last twenty-four hours had they run out on such excursions, only, in panic, to cease activity because the merest jolt, the slightest breath, threatened to shake old ancient Cooger down to mealmush and chaff? Better to leave him propped in electric-warm chair, a continual exhibit, an ever-going-on performance for gaping audiences, and try again, but espe-

cially try now, when, lights out, and crowds herded off in
the dark, all threatened by one smile on a bullet, there
was need of Cooger as he once was, tall, flame-headed,
and riven with earthquake violence. But somewhere,
twenty seconds, ten seconds ago, the last glue crumbled,
the last bolt of life fell free, and the mummy-doll, the
Erector-set grotesque disencumbered itself in smoke puffs
and November leaflets, a broadcast of mortality along the
wind. Mr. Cooger, threshed in a final harvest, was now a
billion parchment flecks, tumbled sea-scrolls capered in
meadows. A mere dust explosion in a silo of ancient
grain: gone.

"Oh, no, no, no, no, no," someone murmured.

Charles Halloway touched Will's arm.

Will stopped saying "Oh, no, no, no." He, too, in the
last few moments, had thought the same as his father, of
the toted corpse, the strewn bone-meal, the mineral-en-
riched hills of grass. . . .

Now there was only the empty chair and the last parti-
cles of mica, the radiant motes of peculiar dirt crusting
the straps. And the freaks, who had been toting the
baroque dump, now fled to shadows.

We made them run, thought Will, but something made
them drop it!

No, not something. Someone.

Will flexed his eyes.

The carousel, deserted, empty, traveled on its way
through its own special time, forward.

But between the fallen chair and the carousel, standing
alone, was that a freak? No . . .

"Jim!"

Dad knocked his elbow and Will shut up.

Jim, he thought.

And where, now, was Mr. Dark?

Somewhere. For he had started the carousel, hadn't
he? Yes! To draw them, to draw Jim, and—what else?
Right now there was no time, for—

Jim turned from the spilled chair, turned and walked
slowly toward the free, free ride.

He was going where he had always known he must go.
Like a weather vane in wild seasons he had tremored this

way, wandered that, hesitated upon bright horizons and
warm directions, only at last now to tilt and, half sleep-
walking, tremble about in the bright brass pull and summer march of music. He could not look away.

Another step, and then another, toward the merry-go-
round, there went Jim.

"Go get him, Will," said his father.

Will went.

Jim raised his right hand.

The brass poles flashed by into the future, pulling the
flesh like syrup, stretching the bones like taffy, the sun-
metal color burning Jim's cheeks, flinting his eyes.

Jim reached. The brass poles flick-knocked his fingernails, tinkling their own small tune.

"Jim!"

The brass poles chopped by in a yellow sunrise at
night.

The music leaped in a clear fountain, high.

Eeeeeeeeeeeeeee.

Jim opened his mouth with the same cry:

"Eeeeeeeeeeeeeee!"

"Jim!" cried Will, running.

Jim's palm slapped one brass pole. The pole whipped
on.

He slapped another brass pole. This time, his palm
glued itself tight.

Wrist followed fingers, arm followed wrist, shoulder
and body followed arm. Jim, sleepwalked, was torn from
his roots in the earth.

"Jim!"

Will reached, felt Jim's foot flick from his grasp.

Jim swung round the wailing night in a great dark
summer circle, Will racing after.

"Jim, get off! Jim, don't leave me *here!*"

Flung by centrifuge, Jim grasped the pole with one
hand, spun, and, as if by some lone lost and final instinct,
gestured his other hand free to trail on the wind, the one
part of him, the small white separate part that still remembered their friendship.

"Jim, *jump!!*"

Will snatched for that hand, missed, stumbled, almost

fell. The first race was lost. Jim must circle once, alone. Will stood waiting the next charge of horses, the fling-about of boy not-so-much boy—

"Jim! Jim!"

Jim awoke! Circled half round, his face showed now July, now December. He seized the pole, bleating out his despair. He wanted, he did not want. He wished, he rejected, he ardently wished again, in flight, in heat-spell river of wind and blaze of metal, in jog of July and August horses whose hoofs thudded the air like thrown fruit, his eyes blazed. Tongue clamped in teeth, he hissed his frustration.

"Jim! Jump! Dad, stop the machine!"

Charles Halloway turned to see where the control box stood, fifty feet off.

"Jim!" Will's side was stabbed with pain. "I need you! Come back!"

And, far over away on the far side of the carousel, traveling, fast-traveling, Jim fought with his own hands, the pole, the empty wind-whipped journey, the growing night, the wheeling stars. He let go the pole. He grabbed it. And still his right hand trailed down and out, begging Will's last full ounce of strength.

"Jim!"

Jim came around. There, below, in the black-night station from which this train pulled away forever in a flurry of ticket-punch confetti, he saw Will—Willy—William Halloway, young pal, young friend who would seem younger still at the end of this journey, and not just young but unknown! vaguely remembered from some other time in some other year . . . but now that boy, that friend, that younger friend, ran along by the train, reached up, asking passage? or demanding he get off? which?!

"Jim! Remember *me?*"

Will lunged his final lunge. Fingers touched fingers, palm touched palm.

Jim's face, white cold, stared down.

Will trot-paced the circling machine.

Where was Dad? Why didn't he shut it *off?*

Jim's hand was a warm hand, a familiar, a good hand. It closed on his. He gripped it yelling.

"Jim, please!"

But still they spun on the journey, Jim borne, Will dragged in a jog-crazy-trot.

"Please!"

Will jerked. Jim jerked. Trapped by Jim, Will's hand was shot with July heat. It went, like a kept animal, held and fondled by Jim, along, around, into older times. So his hand, far-traveling, would be alien to himself, knowing things by night that he himself, abed, might only guess. Fourteen-year boy, fifteen-year hand! Jim had it, yes! cramped it tight, would not let go! And Jim's face, was it older, from the journey round? Was he fifteen now, going on sixteen!?

Will pulled. Jim pulled opposite.

Will fell on the machine.

Both rode the night.

All of Will rode with friend Jim now.

"Jim! Dad!"

How easy it might be to just stand, ride, go round with Jim, if he couldn't pull Jim off, just leave him on and, dear pals, travel! The juices of his body swam, blinding his sight, they drummed his ears, shot electric jolts through his loins. . . .

Jim shouted. Will shouted.

They traveled half a year in slithering orchard-warm dark before Will seized Jim's arm tight and dared to leap from so much promise, so many fine tall-growing years, flail out, off, down, pull Jim with. But Jim could not let go the pole, could not give up the ride.

"Will!"

Jim, half between machine and friend, one hand on each, screamed.

It was like a great tearing of cloth or flesh.

Jim's eyes went blind as a statue's.

The carousel whirled.

Jim screamed, fell, spun crazily, on the air.

Will tried to break his fall, but Jim struck earth rolling. He lay, silent.

Charles Halloway hit the carousel control switch.

Empty, the machine slowed. Its horses paced themselves down from their trot toward some far midsummer night.

Together, Charles Halloway and his son knelt by Jim to touch his wrist, to put ear to his chest. Jim's eyes, skinned white, were fixed on the stars.

"Oh, God," cried Will. "Is he dead?"

CHAPTER FIFTY-TWO

"Dead . . . ?"

Will's father moved his hand over that cold face, the cold chest.

"I don't feel . . ."

A long way off, someone cried for help.

They looked up.

A boy came running down the midway, bumping into ticket booths, falling over tent ropes, looking back over his shoulder.

"Help! He's after me!" the boy cried. "The terrible man! The terrible man! I want to go home!"

The boy flung himself forward, and grabbed at Will's father.

"Oh, help, I'm lost, I don't like it. Take me home. That man with the tattoos!"

"Mr. Dark!" gasped Will.

"Yes!" gibbered the boy. "He's down that way! Oh, stop him!"

"Will—" his father rose—"take care of Jim. Artificial respiration. All right, boy."

The boy trotted off. "This way!"

Following, Charles Halloway watched the distraught boy who led him; observed his head, his frame, the way his pelvis hung from his spine.

"Boy," he said, by the shadowed merry-go-round, twenty feet around from where Will bent to Jim. "What's your name?"

"No time!" cried the boy. "Jed. Quick, quick!"

Charles Halloway stopped.

"Jed," he said. The boy no longer moved, but turned, chafing his elbows. "How old are you, Jed?"

"Nine!" said the boy. "My gosh, this is no time! We—"

"This is a fine time, Jed," said Charles Halloway. "Only nine? So young. I was *never* that young."

"Holy cow!" shouted the boy, angrily.

"Or unholy something," said the man, and reached out. The boy backed away. "You're only afraid of one man, Jed. Me."

"You?" The boy still backed off. "Cut it out! Why, why?"

"Because, sometimes good has weapons and evil none. Sometimes tricks fail. Sometimes people can't be picked off, led to deadfalls. No divide-and-conquer tonight, Jed. Where were you taking me, Jed? To some lion's cage you got fixed and ready? To some side show, like the mirrors? To someone like the Witch? What, what, Jed, what? Let's just roll up your right shirt sleeve, shall we, Jed?"

The great moonstone eyes flashed at Charles Halloway.

The boy leaped back, but not before the man had leaped with him, seized his arm, grabbed the back of his shirt and instead of simply rolling up the sleeve as first suggested, tore the entire shirt off the boy's body.

"Why, yes, Jed," said Charles Halloway, almost quietly. "Just as I thought."

"You, you, you, you!"

"Yes, Jed, me. But especially you, look at you."

And look he did.

For there, on the back of the small boy's hand, on the fingers, and up along the wrist scrambled blue serpents, blue-venomed snake eyes, blue scorpions scuttling about blue shark maws which gaped eternally hungry to feed upon all the freaks crammed and stung-sewn cheek by jowl, skin to skin, flesh to flesh all up and down the chest, the tiny torso, and tucked in the secret gathering places on this small small very small body, this cold and now shocked and trembling body.

"Why, Jed, that's fine artwork, that is."

"You!" The boy struck.

"Yes, still me." Charles Halloway took the blow in the face and clamped a vise on the boy.

"No!"

"Oh, yes," said Charles Halloway, using just his good right hand, his ruined left hand hanging limp. "Yes, Jed, jump, squirm, go ahead. It was a fine idea. Get me off alone, fix me, then go back and get Will. And when the police come, why, you're just a boy nine or ten and the carnival, oh, no, it's not yours, doesn't belong to you. Stay here, Jed. Why you trying to get out from under my arm? The police look and the owners of the show have vanished, isn't that it, Jed? A fine escape."

"You can't hurt me!" the boy shrieked.

"Funny," said Charles Halloway. "I think I can."

He pressed the boy, almost lovingly, close, very close.

"Murder!" wailed the boy. "Murder."

"I'm not going to murder you, Jed, Mr. Dark, whoever, whatever you are. You're going to murder yourself because you can't stand being near people like me, not this close, *close,* not this *long.*"

"Evil!" groaned the boy, writhing. "You're evil!"

"Evil?" Will's father laughed, which made the boy, wasp-stung and brambled by the sound, jerk all the more violently. "Evil?" The man's hands were flypaper fastened to the small bones. "Strange hearing that from you, Jed. So it must seem. Good to evil seems evil. So I will do only good to you, Jed, I will simply hold you and watch you poison yourself. I will do good to you, Jed, Mr. Dark, Mr. Proprietor, boy, until you tell what's wrong with Jim. Wake him up. Let him free. Give him life!"

"Can't . . . can't. . . ." The boy's voice fell down a well inside his body, fading away, away . . . "can't. . . ."

"You mean you won't?"

". . . can't . . ."

"All right, boy, all right, then here and here and this and this . . ."

They looked like father and son long apart, passionately met, embraced, yet more embraced, as the man lifted his wounded hand to gently touch the stricken face as the crowd, the teem, of illustrations shivered and flew now this way and that in microscopic forays quickly abandoned. The boy's eyes swiveled wildly, fixed upon the man's mouth. He saw there the strange and somehow lovely smile once flung as beatification to the Witch.

He gathered the boy somewhat closer and thought, Evil has only the power that we give it. I give you nothing. I take back. Starve. Starve. Starve.

The two matchstick lights in the boy's affrighted eyes blew out.

The boy, and his stricken and bruised conclave of monsters, his felt but half-seen crowd, fell to earth.

There should have been a roar like a mountain slid to ruin.

But there was only a rustle, like a Japanese paper lantern dropped in the dust.

CHAPTER FIFTY-THREE

Charles Halloway stood for a long while, breathing deep, lungs aching, looking down at the body. The shadows swooned and fluttered in all the canvas alleys where odd assorted sizes of freaks and people, fleshed in their own terrors and sins, held to poles, moaning in disbelief. Somewhere, the Skeleton moved out in the light. Somewhere else, the Dwarf *almost* knew who he was, and scuttled forth like a crab from a cave to blink and blink again at Will bent working over Jim, at Will's father bent to exhaustion over the still form of the silent boy, while the merry-go-round, at last, slow, slow, came to a stop, rocking like a ferryboat in the watery-blowing grass.

The carnival was a great dark hearth lit with gathered coals, as shadows came to stare and fire their gaze with the tableau by the carousel.

There in the moonlight lay the illustrated boy named Dark.

There lay dragons slaughtered, towers ruined, monsters from dim ages toppled into rusted coinage, pterodactyls smashed like biplanes from old and always mean-

ingless wars, crustacea the color of emeralds abandoned
on a white sand shore where the tide of life was going
out, all, all the illustrations changing now, shifting, shriveling as the small flesh cooled. There the obscene wink of the
navel eye gasped in on itself, there the nipple-iris of a
trumpeting mastodon went blind and raved at its blind-
ness; each and every picture remembered from the tall
Mr. Dark now rendered down to miniature canvas
pronged and forked over a boy's tennis-racket bones.

More freaks, with faces the color of beds where so
many had lost the battle of souls, emerged from the
shadows to glide in a great and ever more curious carousel motion about Charles Halloway and his dropped
burden.

Will paused in his desperate push and relaxation, push
and relaxation, trying to shape Jim back to life, unafraid
of the watchers in the dark, no time for that! Even if
there were time, these freaks, he sensed, were breathing
the night as if they had not been fed on such rare fine
air in years!

And as Charles Halloway watched, and the fox-fire,
lobster-moist, phlegm-trapped eyes watched from distances, the boy-who-had-been-Mr.-Dark grew yet colder,
as death cut the timbers of nightmares, and the calligra-
phies, the smoky lightnings of sketch that coiled and
crouched and soared like terrible banners of a lost war,
began to vanish one by one from the strewn small body.

A score of freaks glanced fearfully round as if the
moon had suddenly filled itself full and they could see;
they chafed their wrists as if chains had fallen from them,
chafed their necks as if weights had crumbled from their
bowed shoulders. Stumbled forth after long entombments,
they blinked swiftly, disbelieving the packet of their misery sprawled near the spent carousel. If they dared they
might have bent to tremble their hands over that suddenly
death-sweet mouth, the marbling brow. As it was they
watched, benumbed, as their portrait pictures, the vital
stuffs of their mortal greed, rancor, and poisonous guilt,
the emerald abstracts of their self-blinded eyes, self-
wounded mouths, self-trapped bodies melted one by one
from this insignificant mound of snow. There melted the

Skeleton! there the sidewise-scuttling crayfish Dwarf!
Now the Lava Sipper took leave of autumn flesh, followed by the black Executioner from London Dock,
there soared off and gone went the Human Montgolfier,
the Balloon Man, Avoirdupois the Magnificent! deflated to
purest air, there! there fled mobs and bands, as death
washed the drawing board clean!

Now there lay just a plain dead boy, unbruised by pictures, staring up at the stars with Mr. Dark's empty eyes.

"Ahhhh . . ."

In a chorus of release, the strange people in the shadows sighed.

Perhaps the calliope gave a last ringmaster's bark.
Perhaps thunder turned, sleeping, in the clouds. Suddenly
all wheeled about. The freaks stampeded. North, south,
east, west, free of tent, master, dark law, free above all
of each other, they ran like albino pigs, tuskless boars,
and stricken sloths before storms.

It must have been, it seemed, each yanked a rope,
loosed a tent-peg, running.

For now the sky was shaken with a fatal respiration,
the breathing down, the insunk rattle and pule of col-
lapsing darkness as the tents gave way.

With hiss of viper, swirl of cobra, the ropes insanely
raveled, slithered, snapped, cut grass with frictioned
whips.

The networks of the vast Main Freak Tent convulsed,
parted bones, small from medium, and medium from
brontosaur magnificent. All swayed with impending fall.

The menagerie tent shut up like a dark Spanish fan.

Other small tents, caped figures in the meadow, fell
down at the wind's command.

Then at last, the Freak Tent, the great melancholy
mothering reptile bird, after a moment of indecision,
sucked in a Niagara of blizzard air, broke loose three
hundred hempen snakes, crack-rattled its black sidepoles
so they fell like teeth from a cyclopean jaw, slammed the
air with acres of moldered wing as if trying to kite away
but, earth-tethered, must succumb to plain and most simple gravity, must be crushed by its own locked bulk.

Now this greatest tent staled out hot raw breaths of

earth, confetti that was ancient when the canals of Venice were not yet staked, and wafts of pink cotton candy like tired feather boas. In rushing downfalls, the tent shed skin; grieved, soughed as flesh fell away until at last the tall museum timbers at the spine of the discarded monster dropped with three cannon roars.

The calliope simmered, moronic with wind.

The train stood, an abandoned toy, in a field.

The freak oil paintings clapped hands high on the last standing pennant poles, then plummeted to earth.

The Skeleton, the only strange one left, bent to pick up the body of the porcelain boy-who-was-Mr.-Dark. He moved away into the fields.

Will, in a swift moment, saw the thin man and his burden go over a hill among all the footprints of the vanished carnival race.

Will's face shadowed this way, then that, pulled by the swift concussions, the tumults, the deaths, the fleeing away of souls. Cooger, Dark, Skeleton, Dwarf-who-was-Lightning-Rod-Salesman, don't run, come back! Miss Foley, where are you? Mr. Crosetti! it's over! Be still! Quiet! It's all right. Come back, come back!

But the wind was blowing their footprints out of the grass and they might run forever now trying to outflee themselves.

So Will turned back astride Jim and pushed the chest and let go, pushed and let go, then, trembling, touched his dear friend's cheek.

"Jim . . . ?"

But Jim was cold as spaded earth.

CHAPTER FIFTY-FOUR

Beneath the cold was a fugitive warmness, in the white skin lay some small color, but when Will felt Jim's wrist there was nothing and when he put his ear to the chest there was nothing.

"He's *dead!*"

Charles Halloway came to his son and his son's friend and knelt down to touch the quiet throat, the unstirred rib cage.

"No." Puzzled. "Not quite . . ."

"Dead!"

The tears burst from Will's eyes. But then, as swiftly, he felt himself knocked, struck, shaken.

"Stop that!" cried his father. "You want to save him?!"

"It's too late, oh, Dad!"

"Shut up! Listen!"

But Will wept.

And again his father hauled off and hit him. Once on the left cheek. Once on the right cheek, hard.

All the tears in him were knocked flying; there were no more.

"Will!" His father savagely jabbed a finger at him and at Jim. "Damn it, Willy, all this, all these, Mr. Dark and his sort, they *like* crying, my God, they *love* tears! Jesus God, the more you bawl, the more they drink the salt off your chin. Wail and they suck your breath like cats. Get up! Get off your knees, damn it! Jump around! Whoop and holler! You hear! Shout, Will, sing, but most of all laugh, you got that, laugh!"

"I can't!"

"You must! It's all we got. I *know!* In the library! The Witch ran, my God, *how* she ran! I shot her dead with it. A single smile, Willy, the night people can't stand it. The sun's there. They hate the sun. We *can't* take them seriously, Will!"

"But—"

"But hell! You saw the mirrors! And the mirrors shoved me half in, half out the grave. Showed me all wrinkles and rot! Blackmailed me! Blackmailed Miss Foley so she joined the grand march Nowhere, joined the fools who wanted everything! Idiot thing to want: everything! Poor damned fools. So wound up with nothing like the dumb dog who dropped his bone to go after the reflection of the bone in the pond. Will, you saw: *every* mirror fell. Like ice in a thaw. With no rock or rifle, no knife, just my teeth, tongue and lungs, I gunshot those mirrors with pure contempt! Knocked down ten million scared fools and let the *real* man get to his feet! Now, on *your* feet, Will!"

"But Jim—" Will faltered.

"Half in, half out. Jim's been that, always. Sore-tempted. Now he went too far and maybe he's lost. But he fought to save himself, right? Put his hand out to you, to fall free of the machine? So we finish that fight *for* him. Move!"

Will sailed up, giddily, yanked.

"Run!"

Will sniffed again. Dad slapped his face. Tears flew like meteors.

"Hop! Jump! Yell!"

He banged Will ahead, shuffled with him, shoved his hand in his pockets, tearing them inside out until he pulled forth a bright object.

The harmonica.

Dad blew a chord.

Will stopped, staring down at Jim.

Dad clouted him on the ear.

"Run! Don't look!"

Will ran a step.

Dad blew another chord, yanked Will's elbow, flung each of his arms.

"Sing!"

"What?"

"God, boy, anything!"

The harmonica tried a bad "Swanee River."

"Dad." Will shuffled, shaking his head, immensely tired. "Silly . . . !"

"Sure! We *want* that! Silly damn fool man! Silly harmonica! Bad off-key tune!"

Dad whooped. He circled like a dancing crane. He was not *in* the silliness yet. He *wanted* to crack through. He had to *break* the moment!

"Will: louder, funnier, as the man said! Oh, hell, don't let them drink your tears and want more! Will! Don't let them take your crying, turn it upside down and use it for their own smile! I'll be damned if death wears *my* sadness for glad rags. Don't feed them one damn thing, Willy, loosen your bones! Breathe! Blow!"

He seized Will's hair, shook him.

"Nothing . . . funny . . ."

"*Sure* there is! Me! You! Jim! All of us! The whole shooting works! Look!"

And Charles Halloway pulled faces, popped his eyes, mashed his nose, winked, cavorted like chimpanzee-ape, waltzed with the wind, tap-danced the dust, threw back his head to bay at the moon, dragging Will with him.

"Death's funny, God damn it! Bend, two, three, Will. Soft-shoe. Way down upon the Swanee River—what's *next*, Will? . . . Far far away! Will, your God-awful voice! Damn girl soprano. Sparrow in a tin can. Jump, boy!"

Will went up, came down, cheeks hotter, a wincing like lemons in his throat. He felt balloons grow in his chest.

Dad sucked the silver harmonica.

"That's where the old folks—" Will spoke.

"Stay!" bellowed his father.

Shuffle, tap, bounce, jog.

Where was Jim! Jim was forgotten.

Dad jabbed his ribs, tickling.

"De Camptown ladies sing this song!"

"Doo-dah!" yelled Will. "Doo-dah!" he sang it now, with a tune. The balloon grew. His throat tickled.

"Camptown race track, five miles long!"

"Oh, doo-dah day!"

Man and boy did a minuet.

And in midstep *it* happened.

Will felt the balloon grow huge within him.

He smiled.

"What?" Dad was surprised by those teeth.

Will snorted. Will giggled.

"What *say*?" asked Dad.

The force of the exploding warm balloon alone shoved Will's teeth apart, kicked his head back.

"Dad! Dad!"

He bounded. He grabbed his Dad's hand. He raced crazily, hollering, quacking like a duck, clucking like a chicken. His palms hit his throbbing knees. Dust flew off his soles.

"Oh, Susanna!"

"Oh, don't you cry—"

"—for me!"

"For I come from—"

"Alabama with my—"

"Banjo on my—"

Together. "Knee!"

The harmonica knocked teeth, wheezing, Dad hocked forth great chords of squeeze-eyed hilarity, turning in a circle, jumping up to kick his heels.

"Ha!" They collided, half-collapsed, knocked elbows, cracked heads, which blew the air out faster. "Ha! Oh God, ha! Oh God, Will, ha! Weak! Ha!"

In the middle of wild laughter—

A sneeze!

They spun. They stared.

Who lay there on the moonlit earth?

Jim? Jim Nightshade?

Had *he* stirred? *Was* his mouth wider, his eyelids quivering? *Were* his cheeks pinker?

Don't look! Dad swung Will handily round in a further reel. They do-si-do'ed, hands extended, the harmonica seeping and guzzling raw tunes from a father who storked his legs and turkeyed his arms. They hopped Jim one way, hopped back, as if he were but a lump-stone on the grass.

"Someone's in the kitchen with Dinah! Someone's in the kitchen—"

"—I know-oh-oh-*oh!*"

Jim's tongue slid out on his lips.

No one saw this. Or if they saw, ignored it, fearing it might pass.

Jim did the final things himself. His eyes opened. He watched the dancing fools. He could not believe. He had been off on a journey of years. Now, returned, no one said "Hi!" All jigged Sambo-style. Tears might have jumped to his eyes. But before they could start, Jim's mouth curved. He gave up a ghost of laughter. For, after all, there indeed was silly Will and his silly old janitor dad racing like gorillas knuckle-dusting the meadows, their faces a puzzlement. They toppled above him, clapped hands, wiggled ears, bent to wash him all over with their now bright full-river flowing laughter that could not be stopped if the sky fell or the earth rent open, to blend their good mirth with his, to fuse-light and set him off in a detonation which could not stop exploding from lady-fingers to four-inchers to doomsday cannon crackers of delight!

And looking down, jolt-dancing his bones loose and delicious, Will thought: Jim don't remember he was dead, so we won't tell, not now—some day, sure, but not . . . Doo-dah! Doo-dah!

They didn't even say "Hello, Jim" or "Join the dance," they just put out hands as if he had fallen from their swung pandemonium commotion and needed a boost back into the swarm. They yanked Jim. Jim flew. Jim came down dancing.

And Will knew, hand in hand, hot palm to palm, they had truly yelled, sung, gladly shouted the live blood back. They had slung Jim like the newborn, knocked his lungs, slapped his back, shocked joyous breath to where it made room.

Then Dad bent and Will leaped over him and Will bent and Dad jumped him and they both waited, crouched in a line, wheezing songs, deliciously tired, while Jim swallowed spit, and ran full tilt. He got half over Dad when they all fell, rolled in the grass, all hoot-owl and donkey, all brass and cymbal as it must have been the first year of Creation, and Joy not yet thrown from the Garden.

Until at last they drew up their feet, socked each other's shoulders, embraced knees tight, rocking, and looking with swift bright happiness at each other, growing wine-drunkenly quiet.

And when they were done smiling at each other's faces as at burning torches, they looked away across the field.

And the black tent poles lay in elephant boneyards with the dead tents blowing away like the petals of a great black rose.

The only three people in a sleeping world, a rare trio of tomcats, they basked in the moon.

"What happened?" asked Jim, at last.

"What *didn't!*" cried Dad.

And they laughed again, when suddenly Will grabbed Jim, held him tight and wept.

"Hey," Jim said, over and over, quietly. "Hey . . . hey . . ."

"Oh, Jim, Jim," Will said. "We'll be pals forever."

"Sure, hey sure." Jim was very quiet now.

"It's all right," said Dad. "Have a small cry. We're out of the woods. Then we'll laugh some more, going home."

Will let Jim go.

They got to their feet and stood looking at each other. Will examined his father, with fierce pride.

"Oh, Dad, Dad, you *did* it, you did it!"

"No, we did it together."

"But without you it'd all be over. Oh, Dad, I never knew you. I sure know you now."

"Do you, Will?"

"Darn right!"

Each, to the other, shimmered in bright halos of wet light.

"Why then, hello. Reply, son, and curtsey."

Dad held out his hand. Will shook it. Both laughed and wiped their eyes, then looked quickly at the footprints scattered in the dew over the hills.

"Dad, will they ever come back?"

"No. And yes." Dad tucked away his harmonica. "No, not them. But yes, other people like them. Not in a carnival. God knows what shape they'll come in next. But sunrise, noon, or at the latest, sunset tomorrow they'll show. They're on the road."

"Oh, no," said Will.

"Oh, yes," said Dad. "We got to watch out the rest of our lives. The fight's just begun."

They moved around the carousel slowly.

"What will they look like? How will we know them?"

"Why," said Dad, quietly, "maybe they're already here."

Both boys looked around swiftly.

But there was only the meadow, the machine, and themselves.

Will looked at Jim, at his father, and then down at his own body and hands. He glanced up at Dad.

Dad nodded, once, gravely, and then nodded at the carousel, and stepped up on it, and touched a brass pole.

Will stepped up beside him. Jim stepped up beside Will.

Jim stroked a horse's mane. Will patted a horse's shoulders.

The great machine softly tilted in the tides of night.

Just three times around, ahead, thought Will. Hey.

Just four times around, ahead, thought Jim. Boy.

Just ten times around, back, thought Charles Halloway. Lord.

Each read the thoughts in the other's eyes.

How easy, thought Will.

Just this once, thought Jim.

But then, thought Charles Halloway, once you start, you'd always come back. One more ride and one more ride. And, after awhile, you'd offer rides to friends, and more friends until finally . . .

The thought hit them all in the same quiet moment.

. . . finally you wind up owner of the carousel, keeper of the freaks . . . proprietor for some small part of eternity of the traveling dark carnival shows. . . .

Maybe, said their eyes, *they're already here.*

Charles Halloway stepped back into the machinery of the merry-go-round, found a wrench, and knocked the flywheels and cogs to pieces. Then he took the boys out and he hit the control box one or two times until it broke and scattered fitful lightnings.

"Maybe this isn't necessary," said Charles Halloway. "Maybe it wouldn't run anyway, without the freaks to give it power. But—" He hit the box a last time and threw down the wrench.

"It's late. Must be midnight straight up."

Obediently, the City Hall clock, the Baptist church clock, the Methodist, the Episcopalian, the Catholic church, all the clocks, struck twelve. The wind was seeded with Time.

"Last one to the railroad semaphore at Green Crossing is an old lady!"

The boys fired themselves off like pistols.

The father hesitated only a moment. He felt the vague pain in his chest. If I run, he thought, what will happen? Is Death important? No. Everything that happens before Death is what counts. And we've done fine tonight. Even Death can't spoil it. So, there went the boys . . . and why not . . . *follow?*

He did just that.

And Lord! it was fine printing their life in the dew on the cool fields that new dark suddenly-like-Christmas morning. The boys ran as tandem ponies, knowing that someday one would touch base first, and the other second or not at all, but now this first minute of the new morning was not the minute or the day or morning of ultimate loss. Now was not the time to study faces to see if one was older and the other too much younger. Today was just another day in October in a year suddenly better than anyone supposed it could ever be just a short hour ago, with the moon and the stars moving in a grand rotation toward inevitable dawn, and them loping, and the last of this night's weeping done, and Will laughing and singing and Jim giving answer line by line, as they breasted the waves of dry stubble toward a town where they might live another few years across from each other.

And behind them jogged a middle-aged man with his own now solemn, now amiable, thoughts.

Perhaps the boys slowed. They never knew. Perhaps Charles Halloway quickened his pace. He could not say.

But, running even with the boys, the middle-aged man reached out.

Will slapped, Jim slapped, Dad slapped the semaphore signal base at the same instant.

Exultant, they banged a trio of shouts down the wind.

Then, as the moon watched, the three of them together left the wilderness behind and walked into the town.